PATHOPHYSIOLOGY - ALTERED PHYSIOLOGICAL STATES

Edited by **David C. Gaze**

Pathophysiology - Altered Physiological States
http://dx.doi.org/10.5772/65994
Edited by David C. Gaze

Contributors

Zesergio Melo, Juan A. Ruiz-Pacheco, Raquel Echavarria, Claudia A. Mendoza-Cerpa, Hideo Orimo, Gratiela G. Pircalabioru, Mariana Carmen Chifiriuc, Marcela Popa, Ariana Picu, Laura Petcu, Jesús Pérez-Ortega, José Bargas, Bassim Alsadi, Csilla Tothova, Oskar Nagy, Johannes Baumann, E. Muthu Kumaran, Tetyana Beregova, Dmytro Nozdrenko, Nataly Medvedeva, Sergii Berehovyi, Natali Nikitina, Tetyana Falalyeyeva, Liudmyla Ostapchenko, Helder Miguel Fernandes, Patricia Tatiana Soler, Jefferson Da Silva Novaes, Cristina Michiko Harada Ferreira, Taize Machado Augusto, Gustavo Simoes, Nilva Cervigne, Paula Sakuramoto, Caroline Santos

First published in London, United Kingdom, 2018 by IntechOpen
IntechOpen is the global imprint of INTECHOPEN LIMITED, registered in England and Wales, registration number: 11086078, The Shard, 25th floor, 32 London Bridge Street
London, SE19SG – United Kingdom
Printed in Croatia

British Library Cataloguing-in-Publication Data
A catalogue record for this book is available from the British Library

Additional hard copies can be obtained from orders@intechopen.com

Pathophysiology - Altered Physiological States , Edited by David C. Gaze
p. cm.
Print ISBN 978-1-78923-180-9
Online ISBN 978-1-78923-181-6

Meet the editor

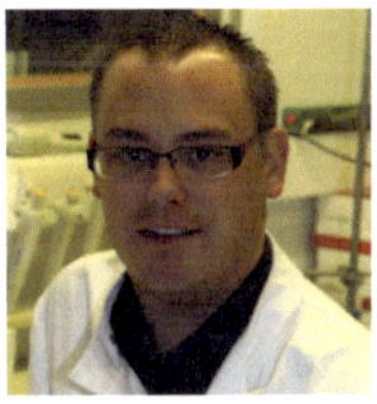

Dr. David Gaze studied biochemistry at undergraduate and master's level in West Yorkshire followed by a PhD degree in Clinical Biochemistry in London, United Kingdom. He is currently a lecturer in Clinical Biochemistry at the University of Westminster and honorary cardiac research scientist within the Department of Chemical Pathology, Clinical Blood Sciences at St George's Hospital and Medical School, London.

He has authored and co-authored in excess of 150 peer-reviewed papers and 200 abstracts, as well as presented at over 50 internationally invited conferences. He has contributed five book chapters to cardiovascular-related textbooks as well, and is writing a textbook on cardiac troponin. He is a peer reviewer for 25 medical journals. He is the commissioning editor for review articles for the *Annals of Clinical Biochemistry and Laboratory Medicine* and is the co-editor-in-chief of *Practical Laboratory Medicine.*

His academic research interests are in the development and clinical utility of cardiac biomarkers for the detection of cardiovascular disease with a special interest in the cardiorenal population.

He is a member of the Royal Society of Medicine of London and the Association for Clinical Biochemistry, of which he chairs the Clinical Sciences Review Committee for the Annals of Clinical Biochemistry. He is also a member of the American Association of Clinical Chemistry, Institute of Biomedical Sciences, Institute of Biology, European Society of Pathology, and the Pathological Society of Great Britain and Ireland and an associate member of the Royal Institution of London.

Gaze and colleagues have won a number of awards including two distinguished Abstract awards from the National Academy of Clinical Biochemistry as well as Diploma for Oral Presentation regarding D-dimer, natriuretic peptide and cardiac troponin in dialysis patients presented at the 17th IFCC-FESCC European Congress of Clinical Chemistry and Laboratory Medicine and the 60th National congress of the Netherlands Society of Clinical Chemistry and Laboratory Medicine in Amsterdam in 2007.

Contents

Preface

The term *"pathophysiology"* comes from the Ancient Greek πάθος (*pathos*) and φυσιολογία (*phusiologia*). Pathophysiology is the convergence of pathology (the discipline of observed changes in a diseased state) with physiology (the mechanisms of systems operation). It represents the functional changes that occur because of injury or disease.

This volume provides state-of-the-art up-to-date literature reviews on pathophysiological processes in a number of disease states. The book is organised methodically in a head-to-toe systems approach, comprising five sections:

a. Neuropathophysiology

This section includes chapters concerning the central nervous system. Chapter 1 explores the psychiatric associations in patients with body dysmorphic disorder (BDD), which is increasing in prevalence globally. The authors discuss the psychopathology and associated pathologies in BDD. Chapter 2 examines the nasal cycle rhythm alterations, in which asymmetrical airflow forms one nasal passage to the other. This cycle is regulated by the hypothalamus by coordinating the autonomic and sympathetic nerves in the nasal mucosa. Observed changes in nasal airflow duration, pattern and rhythm correspond to various disease states. Chapter 3 is a translational biology chapter detailing the changes in striatal network connectivity in Parkinson's disease via a dyskinetic rodent model. The striatum of the basal ganglia receives the major dopaminergic innervation. Using network analysis, the authors have quantified the pathological changes on a functional histological scale associated with Parkinson's disease.

b. Endocrine pathophysiology

In Chapter 4, the authors explore the transport protein transthyretin (prealbumin), which binds thyroid hormones and retinol. Transthyretin can be measured in the blood as an indicator of protein calorie malnutrition and as a prognosticator in critically ill patients. The authors discuss various clinical applications of this disease state biomarker. In Chapter 5, the authors investigate the intricate relationship between diabetes, dietary state and gut microbiota. Diabetes is a global health concern. Only now are we learning of the role of gut microbiota composition and its role in health and disease. The authors summarise recent advances in the microbiome-diet-diabetes interactions with a view to establishing novel therapeutic approaches in patients with diabetes.

c. Endocrine Structural pathophysiology

The structural pathophysiology section starts with Chapter 6 in which the clinical sequelae of hypophosphatasia are discussed. This inherited bone disease results from a deficiency of bone alkaline phosphatase. Some 300 mutations in the *ALPL* gene that encodes alkaline phosphatase result in differential clinical manifestations. Chapter 7 investigates the dynamic properties of skeletal muscle contraction in a rat model with diabetes. The investigators studied the tibia muscle activation in rats with induced diabetes (streptozotocin) compared to a control group of nondiabetic rats. The findings reported help to understand the pathology of diabetic polyneuropathy.

d. Renal pathophysiology

The penultimate section investigates renal pathophysiology. The immunopathology of kidney transplantation is discussed in Chapter 8. Allograft rejection rates in transplantation surgery remain high and occur because of cellular and humoral responses to specific antigens. These are discussed as potential adaptive responses by therapeutic intervention to reduce allograft rejection. Chapter 9 examines renal calcification in the pathogenesis of calcium nephrolithiasis, detailing stone composition and the role of calcium oxalate.

e. Genitourinary pathophysiology

In the final section on "Genitourinary Pathophysiology", an overview of prostate pathophysiology is given in Chapter 10, detailing the epidemiology of prostate cancer, clinical diagnosis and the role of biomarkers such as prostate-specific antigen (PSA) with emphasis on treatment modalities for patients with prostate cancer. The final chapter investigates the pathophysiology and reproductive health implications of polycystic ovary syndrome, which is clinically heterogeneous reflecting many potential aetiologies. The chapter reviews the endocrine involvement and links to obesity, insulin resistance and diabetes, demonstrating the complexity of the syndrome beyond that of a purely reproductive disorder.

This short volume on pathophysiology is intended for general medical and biomedical students at both undergraduate and postgraduate levels. In addition, it is a useful short update of recent advances in research and translational biology to those working in academia or as healthcare scientists.

David C. Gaze
University of Westminster
London, United Kingdom

Section 1

Neuropathophysiology

Chapter 1

Body Dysmorphic Disorder: Characteristics, Psychopathology, Clinical Associations, and Influencing Factors

Patricia Tatiana Soler,
Cristina Michiko Harada Ferreira,
Jefferson da Silva Novaes and
Helder Miguel Fernandes

Additional information is available at the end of the chapter

http://dx.doi.org/10.5772/intechopen.76446

Abstract

Body dysmorphic disorder (BDD) is defined by a recurring and persistent concern characterized by psychic suffering caused by a possible physical imperfection in appearance. It is a severe psychiatric condition, duly confirmed by neuroanatomical findings, very peculiar repetitive behaviors, and specific personalities. The prevalence of BDD is increasing around the world and differs between countries, because of cultural differences and different health-care systems. This increase is worrying because BDD is a pathology that presents comorbidity like severe depression, suicidal ideation, and functional and social impairment. However, BDD is an unrecognized and often not diagnosed in our society. Many patients are ashamed of their complaints and do not usually seek psychiatric help with ease, and unfortunately, they seek help in cosmetic and surgical treatments to improve their appearance, and these professionals are not yet prepared to assist in the diagnosis of this disorder. Therefore, this chapter presents not only the psychopathology of BDD but also its associations with other pathologies and their main factors of influence. Finally, we present a clinical experience with a detailed description of a clinical case. The aim is to contribute to the diagnosis and treatment of this pathology and also to future research that may benefit society and these patients.

Keywords: body dysmorphic disorder, appearance disorders, social anxiety disorder, obsessive–compulsive disorder, behavior

1. Introduction

In the context of a society where beauty is directly related to success and simultaneously hard to achieve, this is the background for the manifestation of the most of the appearance disorders. Among them, we observe the body dysmorphic disorder (BDD), classified as the most fragilizing and afflictive pathology related to body image [1–3].

The body dysmorphic disorder (BDD), previously denominated as dysmorphophobia, consists in a severe psychiatric condition, with high incidence and frequently incapacitating. It is characterized by psychic suffering caused by a possible physical imperfection in appearance, always focused in a specific body part, as a common example, nose, hair, freckles, or breast size. Any part can or body characteristic can be the focus, including the presence of body hair excess or the body shape as a whole [4–6].

Although BDD is an unrecognized and often not diagnosed in our society, it causes significant clinical suffering to the patient, social, and professional prejudice and affects others spheres of the individual life. Nowadays, new characteristics have been added to the disorder as repetitive behavior and mental acts related to self-image preoccupation. To acquire a better knowledge and help in BDD diagnosis should be a priority, not only for psychological and psychiatric professionals but also for aesthetical, cosmetic, and physical educators, because these patients may search for the solution with appearance-enhancing treatments, an action that can worsen the psychological symptoms caused by the disorder [7, 8].

2. Definitions and characteristics

BDD is defined by a recurring and persistent concern about a specific trait or a group of characteristics, noticed in the self-image. The etiology is associated to a perfectionist pre-morbid personality, teasing in school, or a traumatic event. Recent research suggests that more than three-quarters of individuals with BDD reported a perception of childhood maltreatment [2]. The patient relates that these traits are ugly, unattractive, abnormal, or even crippled. The self-noticed flaws are not necessarily bad or abnormal to other individuals. These appearence concerns range from seem unattractive or inappropriate, to horrible, repulsive or often described as monstrous. Patients can focus in specific details or several parts. It is very frequent that the skin is the focus of the disorder, for example, acne, scars, wrinkles, pale skin, or body hair, characteristics of hair, hair loss, and unwanted facial hair, nose (size and shape). However, any part can be the focus of this disorder. Some even present concern about the perception of asymmetry of body parts. The perceptions are intrusive, unwanted, and take time (about 3–8 h a day); it is usually hard to avoid or control [9–11].

The BDD can be classified according to the level of insight. In the good or reasonable insight, the individual can recognize that the beliefs of BDD may not be true. In the case of poor insight, the individual believes that it is most likely true. In the absence of an insight or a delusional state, the individual is completely convinced that his/her beliefs are true. The degree of compromise affects the treatment of the patient [9, 12].

BDD can also be divided into delusional and not delusional. The delusional type is more severe because the individual presents visual hallucinations, in which he/she perceives his/her defect as monstrous, whereas in the non-delusional mode, the subject only overevaluates a little imperfection, which was already there. It is believed that 36–60% of the cases of BDD are delusional [13]. However, both BDD delusional and non-delusional usually have good treatment response to the same type of therapeutic. Nevertheless, it is important to establish the differential diagnostics in order to determine the severity of the disease, the comorbidities, and the risk factors [13, 14].

Some variations were found in brain structure and function. Research suggests that BDD patients may have some alteration in the white substance of the brain, leading to a functional impairment due to disorganization in the tract which connects the vision with emotional issues and memory [13, 15].

BDD, which was primarily called dysmorphophobia, is a severe psychiatric disorder usual and disabling. It is marked by deep psychological sorrow, directly proportional to the imaginary or delusional physical defect. This "defect" is always focused in a given area of the body, such as, nose, hair, freckles, or breasts. Any part of the body can be "chosen"; it can include the presence of unwanted body hair or the body weight or the body shape [4–6].

Even though BDD being still an underrecognized and underdiagnosed pathology in our society, it causes too much pain, social, and professional impairment to the patients. It affects another important area of their lives too: most of them have deep emotional issues and cannot keep a marriage or a long-term relationship because of BDD. Recently, some repetitive behaviors and mental acts related to appearance concerns were added to the list of symptoms too [8, 9].

Most of these patients look for appearance-enhancing treatments, trying to get rid of their sorrow and frustration, but it usually exacerbates the psychological symptoms and leads to more dissatisfaction [7, 8]. Therefore, it is paramount that not only psychologists and psychiatrists know more about BDD, but also, professionals of esthetics area, cosmetology and gyms, which include alternative specialty doctors, physiotherapists and personal trainers. They could identify potential patients and referral to specialized treatment.

3. Neuroanatomic findings

In the past, BDD used to be part of somatoform disorder spectrum [16], which now is known as somatic symptoms disorders [9]. This spectrum is featured by the presence of physical symptoms, which suggests a medical general condition underlying the behavior symptoms, because there is no detectable neurobiological imbalance or other psychiatry disorders to justify the symptoms. It is important to emphasize that this classification has changed much and do not include BDD anymore [9].

Nowadays, BDD has been included in the range of obsessive compulsive disorders (OCDs), because the neuroanatomic findings presented new evidences about BDD, pointing biological features to its etiopathogeny. One study detected that orbitofrontal cortex and anterior cingulate cortex volumes of BDD patients were significantly smaller than healthy individuals. It means that their brain has more white substance than the control group. Besides, there is a tendency of an increase of thalamic volume in BDD patients compared with that in the control group [17, 18].

Neuroanatomic evidence in the limbic system was also found, more specifically in the amygdalas, between BDD, anxiety, and self-evaluating visual process. Self-image is captured by ventral visual system, which is later interpreted by the brain's amygdalas. That structure is involved in emotional control in a higher level, like companionship, love, affection, mood swings, fear, rage, and hostility. They are involved in some anxiety manifestations too. Interestingly, only the right amygdala volume has shown a significant correlation with BDD symptom severity, which suggests a different lateral involvement of these brain regions [19].

One study conducted by researchers at the University of California, Los Angeles, shows that people with BDD may process visual information differently than people without the disorder. Researchers showed 25 people, half with BDD and half without the disorder, three different images of faces in high, regular, and low resolutions. Magnetic resonance image (MRI) results showed that participants with BDD used the left side of the brain (the analytical side) to process all three images. The other participants used the brains' left hemisphere for only the high-resolution images. This could mean that the minds of people with BDD strive to acutely process visual details, even when there is nothing to process. This might be why they can see flaws in themselves, even when those flaws might not exist [20].

Another biological factor under consideration is that people with BDD seem to have a chemical imbalance of the neurotransmitter serotonin, because they often respond well to the selective serotonin reuptake inhibitor (SSRI) class of antidepressants. While doctors know that the differences in brain and neurotransmitter functions exist, they do not know whether BDD causes the differences or if the differences cause BDD. For this reason, it is so important to know and to analyze the other factors involved in BDD [21].

4. Behavior and personality of the BDD patient

Currently, there are many studies comparing BDD patients' behavior with personality. These are very important clinical evidences of the disorder. As said before, BDD patients usually have perfectionist personality, as a natural trait or a pathological feature; between them, it is possible to observe a very large range of anankastic (obsessive) behaviors, according to each affected individual. Nevertheless, when the BDD is already detected, the patient is very often anguished, afflicted, and tormented; they have social, emotional, and labor impairment. They have maladapted thoughts about their appearance: "if I'm not good looking, I can't be happy." That kind of thought leads to negative self-evaluation, which provokes specific behavior known as repetitive acts. Some studies sustain that 90% of people with BDD engage in compulsive behaviors [10, 22].

Among the repetitive acts of compulsive behavior of BDD patients, there are check, camouflage, dressing-up excessively, and self-mutilation. In check behavior, patients spend most of their time checking their own image in front of the mirror; it is known as "mirror checking" or "mirror gazing." Around 80% of people with BDD usually have mirror gaze behavior. There are reports of patients who can spend 11 h per day looking themselves at the mirror [23]. It can be explained as a cycle, and it begins when a person views an external or an internal representation of their appearance. External events include looking at a mirror. Internal events include somatic sensations or intrusive thoughts. Such events activate a distorted mental image or a "felt" impression of the self. People with BDD selectively focus on this image, which leads to a magnification of perceived imperfections. It showed that people with BDD endorse assumptions such as "if my appearance is inadequate, life is not worth living." Negative assumptions result in rumination, decreased mood, and safety behaviors such as mirror gazing, which uphold the distorted mental image, increase doubts, and reinforce the cycle [24]. The mirror checking is perceived as being uncontrollable, addictive, and trapping. On a "bad day," motivations for mirror gazing are punitive and tortuous as patients usually report. Some patients describe what they see in the mirror by comparing themselves to inanimate creatures like monsters [10].

In the camouflage, patients waste too much time trying to hide the defect [3, 25, 26]. It includes the habit of buying compulsively objects like make-up items, scarfs, and so on [19, 27]. In the dressing-up excessively, patients spend most of the day beautifying themselves and trying to look better. They imagine that people are constantly observing and evaluating them; this feeling creates a great emotional pain and functional impairment [28].

The self-mutilation behavior is considered the most severe and harmful of the symptoms. A typical self-mutilation injury is called neurotic excoriations (or pathological skin picking), which is defined for the irresistible impulse of causing or worsening skin damage, by scratching, biting, clawing with nails, fingers, or objects. The self-mutilation can be used to provoke the amputation of the "ugly" part of the body [29, 30]. The lesions are polymorphic. Newer lesions are angulated excoriated crusted erosions, while older lesions have depigmented scarred center and hyperpigmented periphery. Lesion numbers vary from few to hundred and are in all stages of development. Prurigo nodularis is an extreme variant of this entity. Distribution of the lesions reflects their self-inflicted nature with lesions concentrated over the most accessible sites. Neurotic excoriation is differentiated from dermatitis artefacta by its conscious and compulsive nature. However, a patient should be evaluated for all cutaneous and systemic causes of pruritus before making this diagnosis [31].

Acne excoriee is a variant of neurotic excoriation where patients have either only facial or predominant facial involvement. Few patients develop lesions after picking acne lesions while majority did not have acne at any time. It is most common in females with an average age of 30 years. Another very common habit is "tricolomania," which is characterized by the act of, recurrently, pulling the own hair or body hair, for pleasure, satisfaction, or tension relief. The most usual areas are scalp, eyelashes, and eyebrow. This behavior pattern is relevant only if it is frequent enough to cause injuries or irreversible hair loss or diary. Normally, it is followed by the attempt of hiding the injuries. There is a female preponderance, and the average age of onset of this syndrome varies between 30 and 50 years [29, 31].

There is an important trait of BDD, established by essays, which is the capability of these individuals of observing "irregularities and defects" in their own appearance. Any minimal asymmetry can be the starter for the development or worsening of the disease. Only patients with BDD may have such a powerful intensified selective attention able to find or imagine defects on their own face. Moreover, it also happens with another person's body's area, for example, the defect they imagine on him/her and they also observe too much in the others [33]. Indeed, the symmetry obsession is considered one of the most obvious traits of the BDD, and very often, it is found in OCD patients, who suffer from a chronic and disabling disorder characterized by uncontrollable, persistent, and repetitive obsessions and compulsions. Around 25% of BDD patients present this symptom, and it has a direct impact in the low quality of life of these individuals [27].

BDD is also characterized by mental acts, in which the patient wastes most of his/her time thinking about his/her appearance or concerned about it; in addition to it, the person cannot stop comparing his/her appearance with the others [8]. Unwanted mental intrusions might be a transdiagnostic variable across different disorders such as OCD, BDD, eating disorders, and hypochondriasis, and they might contribute to explaining the phenomenological similarities among them. Unwanted mental intrusions in BDD have been defined as discrete, untimely, and unexpected conscious cognitive products that can be experienced as thoughts, images, sensations, or impulses. They interfere with the normal flow of thoughts, tend to be recurrent, and promote subjective resistance efforts, although they are highly uncontrollable [33].

Still regarding personality, individuals with BDD have been postulated to have schizoid, narcissistic, and obsessional personality traits and to be sensitive, introverted, perfectionist, and insecure. However, data on personality traits and disorders in BDD are limited. In one research involving patients diagnosed with BDD, 57% had one or more personality disorders, with avoidant personality disorder (43%) being most common, followed by dependent (15%), obsessive–compulsive (14%), and paranoid (14%) personality disorders [34, 35]. In another assessment in patients seeking cosmetic surgery and diagnosed with BDD, it was also found that the presence of a psychopathological reaction to imagined defects in appearance in subjects pursuing a surgical correction is associated with the severity of schizotypal and paranoid personality disorders [36].

In another trial, more recent, three groups of personality were verified in patients diagnosed with BDD. The first group includes pessimistic, shy, insecure subjects; people with fragile and immature personality and poor self-esteem; individuals concerned about the way they look and those who spend more time thinking about it. The second group includes subjects that are more confident, with a stronger personality and a greater self-esteem. A third, less differentiated group, includes subjects who are more impulsive and spend an intermediate amount of time thinking about the way they look [37].

An antisocial personality can also be attributed to BDD. Clinical observations suggest that both BDD and social anxiety disorder (SAD) are characterized by a fear of negative evaluation in social situations, as well as avoidance of social interactions, although in BDD, social fear and avoidance are largely related to the perceived bodily "defects." Individuals with BDD also have a tendency to misinterpret neutral interpersonal cues as more negative and threatening when compared to healthy controls. Moreover, the high SAD comorbid rates in BDD (37–40%) suggest that BDD and SAD may be related disorders [38, 39].

5. Prevalence, comorbidities, influencing factors, and association with other disorders

The prevalence of BDD is increasing around the world. Prevalence in the general population may differ between countries, because of cultural differences and different health-care systems. Studies have found a BDD prevalence of 1.9 in German women [40]; 2.5% in American women [41]; 2.0% in American women in another time frame [42]; 4.4% in German women in another time frame [43]; 2.1% in Swedish women [8]. In mixed populations (both genders), the prevalence of BDD was 1.7% in English population and 2.4% in French population [44]; 0.7% in Italian population [45], and around 28% in the population of American college students [48]. In the worldwide population, the prevalence of BDD is around 1–2% [3, 14, 46]; it can reach 3% of global population [25]. In the dermatological patient population, the prevalence is predominantly higher, with 8.8% of Turkish dermatology patients [47]; 14% of US dermatology patients [8]; 6.7% of Brazilian dermatology patients [48]; 4.2% of Turkish dermatology patients in another time frame [49]; 4.9% of Swedish dermatology patients [8]; and from 2.9 to 24.9% in patients of multiple nationalities [3].

BDD affects each individual in a different way; so, its prevalence can be modified according to not only the population regarding its finding, but also regarding the original physical trait that the person assumed as a "defect." The prevalence of BDD in patients who underwent plastic surgery procedures is around 6–20%. In patients undergoing rhinoplasty, it raises to 20.7% [50]. An essay was conducted with patients seeking for plastic surgery, and 7.7% showed BDD. Most of these patients (85.7%) were diagnosed before surgery, and the remaining (14.3%) in the post-surgery period, after they have reported dissatisfaction with the surgical results [51].

According to different researches, the prevalence of BDD in plastic surgery is around 7–15% [29]; another study points to a prevalence of 16–24% [50], and there is another that points to about 53% [52]. In Iran, a research was conducted with patients who were seeking plastic surgery. It was noticed that 41% of them had shown mental disorder, of which 24.5% were diagnosed as BDD patients. Most of the subjects of the survey were seeking for rhinoplasty and 80% of them were women [53]. The rhinoplasty surgery, in special, is a common practice in BDD patients' community, and the diagnoses of severe cases of BBD before surgery are very frequently connected to the high level of dissatisfaction with the results after surgery [54, 55].

Among BDD patients, 76% have already considered plastic surgery as a "treatment" for their "defects," of which most of them, 64–66%, have previously undergone some plastic surgery [53]. Although the dissatisfaction level with the results is high, the idea of perfection is based on delusional thoughts about one's esthetics complaints, which are not reachable by cosmetic treatments or surgeries [50]. For this reason, a more comprehensive psychiatric evaluation is indicated for the patients who look for an esthetic procedure, because in the case of BDD patient, the psychological intervention is more indicated than a surgical procedure [53, 56].

Regarding the prevalence of BDD between genders, different studies have shown that although seeking for surgical esthetic treatments is more frequent in feminine population (86.4%) than in masculine population (13.6%), BDD is more prevalent in masculine gender. Among men of the sample, 33.3% presented BDD, while only 14% of women presented the disorder [36]. Therefore, although men are the minority in the researches regarding esthetics treatments, they have presented always equal or larger prevalence of BDD than women. In a German study involving 133 college students, in which 71.4% were women, there were no differences of prevalence between genders; with 5.1% of women and 5.7% of men diagnosed with BDD [57]. In another population of patients with BDD clinically diagnosed, 89% of the sample was female [58]. There is another study, in which case 64.2% of the sample is composed of women [38]. In all these reports, the prevalence of BDD was larger among men.

Comparing prevalence between genders, considering patients of general dermatological clinics, women are the most frequent costumers (69.7%), against 30.3% of men. Considering individuals who look for treatment in dermatological clinic specialized in acne, the prevalence between genders do not change compared to the first case (general dermatologic clinic). Women were 66.7% of the patients and men were 33.3%. However, in the dermatological clinics with aesthetic purposes, an increase of women clients (85.2%) and a decrease of men clients (14.8%) can be noticed [25]. In general, the prevalence of BDD is larger in esthetics dermatological clinics (14%); compared to general dermatological clinics (6.7%) and in the control group (2%), the prevalence of BDD was almost equal to the general population [48].

Comparing the prevalence of BDD and considering the level of schooling of the subjects, it has been reported in most of the samples that the BDD patients usually were attending middle school (63.3%), followed by patients who were attending primary school (36.4%). In this sample, none of the patient with BDD was attending university education [36]. In another study where patients were clinically diagnosed with BDD, 72.4% of the sample [38] and 77% of another sample [58] had university education complete or incomplete.

Regarding the prevalence of BDD and marital status of the patients, BDD patients usually have emotional impairment, remaining single (56.3%) [59]. Some studies have shown a 72.7% rate that has never been married [60]. This scenery does not seem to be modified through the years, considering that in a precedent study, the rate of BDD patients that were never married was 60.4%, the married were 25.4%, the divorced were 13.4%, and the widowers were 0.7% [38]. The age of the onset of the symptoms seems to be related to the marital status. When it shows up before 18 years old, the prevalence of singles in the sample seems to be higher (77.9%) than if it begins after 18 years old, when the prevalence of singles is a little lower (64.5%) [58].

The same happens to the work capability of the BDD patients: when the disorder starts earlier in life, the social and labor impairment usually is worse. BDD patients in which the disease started before 18 years old had more issues regarding work (65.8%) than patients in which the disorder started after this age (58.1%) [58].

Among BDD patients in treatment, 57.5% were unemployed, only 38.5% were working full time, 22.5% were working half time, and 3% were removed from work due to Medical Certificate of Health related to BDD [38].

More recently, another study showed that among OCD patients, less than half were in a full-time employment, and 27.2% was receiving work incapacity benefit [60]. Almost 39% of patients reported removal from work and 79.7% indicated some level of labor functional impairment because of the pathology. It is been noticed that patients who were removed from work because of the psychopathology of BDD presented more severe form of the disease and tended more to chronicity as well. The worse cases were usually composed by males with a lower scholarship, more severe depressive symptoms, higher rates of comorbidities, worse quality of life, worse social skills, higher rates of suicides, and higher propensity to psychiatric internment. One study concluded that being removed from work can worsen the outcome of the treatment for the patient, because it would intensify the tendency to self-isolation and depression [60]. It has to be considered, however, on the other hand, that some of these cases may be condemned to evolve badly since the onset of the disorder, due to possibly neuroanatomic lesions or malfunctions (already described earlier). The characteristics as lower scholarship, worse social skills, poverty, and worse quality of life may be associated to brain damage. We also know that male gender is more vulnerable to express this type of symptomatology. Therefore, it is possible that the same patients have to be removed from work with special care, because the removal is necessary at some point of the treatment, but the prolonged removal without care will lead to psychological worsening [60].

Hispanics or "non whites" were considered the minority of patients (19.1%) with BDD comparing the prevalence of the disease among the different ethnic groups [59], or even less than that (9.1%) in another study [60]. The Caucasian was 87.9% of BDD population under treatment in another study [38].

Concerning the way of living, 44.8% of the BDD individuals live with a spouse, 28.4% with their parents, 25.4% alone, and 1.5% need home supervision because they have special needs or comorbidities that imply in additional risks [38].

Although BDD is more often present in athletes than in regular people, the intensity of psychological problems usually is more severe in non-athletes. Therefore, the current practice of physical activity is very good for mental health. In both samples, the rate of satisfaction with body self-image presented equally low [61].

Regarding differences between genders in BDD, there are more points of similarities than differences, although much disparity can be found. Initially, the areas elected as central "loci" of BDD were different between genders, for example, men were obsessed about genitals, muscle mass amount, and hair loss. Women, on the other hand, were obsessively concerned about skin, breasts, buttocks, thighs, legs, hips, toes, and body hair, among many other parts of the body. Women were also more predisposed to behave repetitively (compulsion), using resources like camouflage of the presumed defects and constant image check; they tend more to the neurotic excoriation and to eating disorder, as well [62].

BDD individuals usually have lower scores of self-evaluation regarding appearance and high levels of dissatisfaction to their own body compared with normal population, in both genders [4, 63]. It means that the disorder directly affects the self-body image of the patients and it is frequently associated with other disorder in which the individuals refer the fear of being negatively evaluated by other people, which is the same as what occur in the social phobia disorder (SAD). In fact, SAD is considered an outstanding feature of BDD [32, 60], even though there are remarkable differences between this theoretical constructs.

Some pathologies can be associated to BDD. A research involving BDD population sample found that the majority of the patients (71%) have not shown concerns related to body weight, but they have bigger concerns related to body parts, such as skin, hair, nose, belly, and teeth. Most of these patients were female, white, single, and have incomplete superior education. All subjects of the sample demonstrate some concern regarding another very specific area of the body, besides depressive symptoms [64].

Early surveys have been investigated SAD in BDD and concluded that these patients can have high scores of SAD, regarding appearance concerns [39, 65]. BDD rates were higher in patients with SAD compared to control population [66]. Patients with BDD had higher scores at Social Phobia Inventory (SPIN), even not having SAD diagnosed as comorbidity. It was also detected that the typical social aversion of the SAD has contributed to the functional impairment of the patients with BDD [39].

Some features in common of both pathologies have been pointed, such as anxiety and denial. One study also compared sociodemographic and clinical aspects of BDD and SAD, observing that SAD is more common in younger people with lower educational level than BDD [18]. In addition, BDD patients seem to be less propensed to marry and presented more often historic of psychiatric internment than patients with SAD [18]. Another assessment claims that individuals diagnosed with BDD are often single, avoid dating, and report high levels of social isolation [67]. With regard to comorbidities, BDD and SAD have different probabilities. Patients with BDD tend more to evolve with eating disorder or OCD, whereas patients with SAD are more likely to develop anxiety disorders [18].

Based on the above, it is important to emphasize that there are ways to distinguish BDD from SAD. One way is to consider that in BDD, there are repetitive behaviors, already mentioned, such as checking and neurotic excoriation. Besides, in BDD, the main concern of the person is focused on his/her physical appearance and his/her imaginary "defects"; whereas in the SAD, the patient is worried about the judgment that the other can do about his/her behavior and about his/her social exposure. Besides, the comorbidities in BDD are much more in number and gravity than in SAD: eating disorders (bulimia, anorexia, and vigorexia), severe depression, self-mutilation, and suicide [18, 62].

Usually, BDD begins in childhood or puberty. It starts always gradually and its development is related with low quality of life; however, there is no evidence of any difference of quality of life or functional loss between patients in which the disorder started early or later in life [68]. Although, depending of the history of life of the individual, the outcome of the disorder can be suicidal or other comorbidity even more severe than BDD [58, 72], the majority of BDD patients have suicidal ideas (80%), and a considerable percentage of them have already presented suicidal attempts (24%) [60, 69]. Among American population, it has been noticed that suicide rates are 45 times larger in BDD patients when related to the rest of the population. It means there is a higher mortality rate in BDD than compared with what is observed in pathologies like "anorexia nervosa," severe depression, and bipolar disorder [29, 70]. Suicidal rates are most frequently observed in patients with dermatological complaints [71].

Comparing the existence of comorbidities in BDD with OCD, the rates were 27.5% and 10.4%. Both conditions presented SAD and severe depression (major depression) as the main comorbidities [72]. The association of BDD cases with psychiatric internment is estimated in 14% of the cases, while the suicide attempts are present in 22–27.5% of the cases [14, 70, 73]. Based on these possible comorbidities linked to BDD, there are studies showing that among patients with BDD, 76.4% present mood disorder, 1.8% present psychotic disorder, 70.9% present anxiety disorder, 16.4% present some type of drug abuse or addiction, 10.9% present eating disorders, 3.6% present somatoform disorder, 66.7% present some type of personality disorder, and only 1.5% do not present any kind of comorbidity [60].

Therefore, BDD at most of the time presents an important association with another psychiatric morbidity, and it can evolve to more severe conditions, like anorexia, vigorexia, bulimia, major depression, and a very high risk of suicide, besides leading to a low capability and quality of life [64, 74]. BDD is linked to other psychiatric symptoms: 80% of the cases are connected with depressive symptoms, 12% has SAD, 48.9% are linked with drug abuse, and 32.5% of the patients diagnosed with BDD have eating disorders as well [50].

There are some diseases more acknowledged and shared by media, characterized as eating disorder, but, actually, they are all derived from a primary BDD and ultimately evolve with very own traits which make easier to diagnose and to treat them. Anorexia, bulimia, and vigorexia are examples of such case [75–77]. In anorexia, BDD gets evident regarding body weight, in which case the patient's self-image is distorted and the person imagines herself/himself with lots more weight than actually has. Trying to compensate it, the patient seeks compulsively to lose these "imaginary" extra pounds by refusing to eat, exercising too much, taking pills (laxatives and diuretics), and/or self-inflicted vomiting episodes. In bulimia, BDD shows up just like anorexia, but there are previous episodes of binge eating followed by extreme regret, which leads the patient to the already described compulsive behavior to try to lose weight immediately. In vigorexia, BDD is related to body size and strength. Patient's self-image is small and weak, which makes the person eat and exercise compulsively, trying to get the maximum of possible muscle mass that one can reach, frequently using steroids to get bigger enough. There is a condition called plasticomania too, in which BDD is evident in one or multiple areas of the body, and the patient do not hesitate to undergo several plastic surgeries, trying to solve the frustration [76, 78, 79].

Although several researches have been concluded, BDD is still an underdiagnosed disease. Too many professionals that should be involved in this disorder recognition ignore the condition and its severity. In studies with patients diagnosed with depression, there are elevated rates of

BDD, but most of these patients have their BDD not noticed as the primary pathology, which, usually, lead to a failure of treatment [59]. Some patients may resist referral to psychiatrists and psychologists, because they continue to believe that their problems are physical and not psychological. It is often fruitless to try to convince these patients that their beliefs are irrational [8]. Appearance-enhancing treatments should not be implemented, because these may even exacerbate the psychological symptoms [76]. Concluding, the difficulty in recognizing and diagnosing BDD has been appointed as the main factor of morbidity and mortality of this pathology [29].

6. The diagnosis and treatment by a clinical perspective

This topic presents a personal perspective of a clinical psychiatrist who has practiced in several mental health settings and who aims to present one illustrative case.

During almost 20 years of clinical practice of psychiatry, I have observed several patients with what was once called "epileptical personality," possibly involving temporal lobe disorders. They do not necessarily have seizures or absence of crises. Some of them have what it is called Geshwin's syndrome. They usually have migraine, with photophobia and misophonia (these last two symptoms may occur not necessarily during migraine crisis). They often have reports of somnambulism (i.e., sleepwalking), night terror, nocturnal enuresis while infants or during puberty (or even in adults), and/or history of feverish crisis while in infants.

An important number of them have some relatives (grandparents, parents, cousins, siblings) with classical epilepsia, involving seizures or partial epilepsy complex, which suggests that they may have inherited a low threshold to resist a convulsion. However, they usually also have an acquired factor: premature birth delivery with complications, head trauma in the first year of life, encephalitis, and so on.

A large number of these patients evolve, usually, after puberty with changes in behavior. Some of them develop episodes of rage and mood swing. In girls, it is notorious after the menarche and gets worse during the menstrual period, showing that hormones play a very important role in these phenomena.

In males, the symptoms can be more constant because there is no hormones see-saw involved, but the onset of behavioral disturbance is related to puberty too. In addition, it can be related to violence or hostility more frequently, reminding of the explosive intermittent disorder's described features.

With this in mind, the aim of presenting this previous information is to report a few cases of BDD patients I have seen all over these years too. They are 12 patients, and in all of them, I could find traits of epileptical personality; some of them had alterations in the electroencephalogram (EEG) test, frequently on the right temporal lobe or in both. A reduced number of cases had alterations in the frontal lobe too.

I am going to report a case of a young man who was 19 years old at the time of his first appointment. He was taken to my private practice by his parents, because he had no conscious of his sickness. At the day before the appointment, he had punched his father's face. It never happened before. The patient was really regretted and scared with his own behavior. His parents were really worried and shocked because, on top of all, he had just given up on Law School and was obsessed by his own image on the mirror, spending 6–9 h a day in gym working out and more than 3 or 4 h in front of the mirror, checking each part of his body. However, he wasn't happy with himself, like in the case of Narcissus myth; he was in real pain, frustrated, and the parents could hear him whispering "I'm weak, I'm thin." No matter how strong his body was, he could not notice it. He was very concerned about his hair too.

His mother said she noticed 6 months before that he was becoming a little agitated and hostile. She tried to talk to him. But he was evasive and avoidant, then she looked through his medicines and found out he was taking steroids for muscles and finasteride for hair loss. I asked about his neonatal history; his mother answered she had a little trouble during labor delivery and he was born with a reduced Apgar score, but nothing that compromised his development; he had some episodes of feverish crisis until 5 years old. But lately, in the past 4 or 5 months, he started to have night terror episodes, which he never had before. However, his younger brother used to have it at the age of 3–4 years. In addition to the night terror, he started to have intense migraine episodes during the day, with photophobia and misophonia.

The parents said he was "normal" until 6–8 months before; described him as "just a little over concerned about physical shape, but like other youngster." They confirm that he was introvert and shy during his childhood and became a little more confident after 16 years old when he started to work out. He said to me, after getting better with medication, that he used to be teased at school for being shorter than the other boys.

I deduced that this patient had some temporal lobe level of instability which leads him to feel very intense about his emotional pains. The use of steroids and finasteride may have impaired some of his brain functions, reducing his convulsive threshold. The result was more aggressivity, mood swing, and the severe BDD symptoms escalating from an original simple unhappiness with his body features.

He mentioned social anxiety since he was a boy. Therefore, he decided to work out to get stronger. At certain point, influenced by a friend, he started to take steroids and finasteride.

He started to get better after quitting the hormones and finasteride. The social anxiety and the BDD were controlled after a week taking oxcarbazepine 600 mg/day and citalopram 10 mg/day. After 6 months of treatment, he stopped medication and continued psychotherapy. I have not heard from him since 4 years ago.

7. Conclusions

In summary, this chapter has addressed the main characteristics and related psychopathology of the body dysmorphic disorder, as well as some clinical associations and influencing factors. Moreover, this chapter has also presented one illustrative case of the diagnosis and treatment of body dysmorphic disorder symptoms by an experienced clinical psychiatrist.

We hope that this chapter contributes to the diagnosis, prevention, treatment, and management of body dysmorphic disorder in different health-care settings, by providing a more comprehensive and integrated understanding of this underdiagnosed mental disorder.

Author details

Patricia Tatiana Soler[1]*, Cristina Michiko Harada Ferreira[2], Jefferson da Silva Novaes[3] and Helder Miguel Fernandes[4,5]

*Address all correspondence to: patfisioterapia@hotmail.com

1 Unigran Capital University, Campo Grande, Brazil

2 Psychiatry Residence Training Program of Santa Casa, Campo Grande, Brazil

3 Federal University of Rio de Janeiro, Rio de Janeiro, Brazil

4 Research Centre in Sports Sciences, Health Sciences and Human Development, CIDESD, Portugal

5 Research in Education and Community Intervention, RECI, Portugal

References

[1] Buhlman U, Teachman BA, Naumann E, Fehlinger T, Rief W. The meaning of beauty: Implicit and explicit self-esteem and attractiveness beliefs in body dysmorphic disorder. Journal of Anxiety Disorders. 2009;**23**:694-702. DOI: 10.1016/j.janxdis.2009.02.008

[2] Silver J, Reavey P. "He's a good-looking chap aint he?": Narrative and visualisations. Social Science & Medicine. 2010;**70**:1641-1647. DOI: 10.1016/j.socscimed.2009.11.042

[3] Veríssimo F, Andrade P, Correia L, Rocha I. Perturbação Dismórfica Corporal – um desafio em Dermatologia. Revista da SPDV. 2012;**70**(1):35-44

[4] Buhlmann U, Winter A, Kathmann N. Emotion recognition in body dysmorphic disorder: Application of the reading the mind in the eyes task. Body Image. 2013;**10**:247-250. DOI: 10.1016/j.bodyim.2012.12.001

[5] Onden-Lim M, Grisham JR. The relationship between body dysmorphic concerns and the effects of image suppression: Implications for models of body dysmorphic disorder. Journal of Obsessive-Compulsive and Related Disorders. 2012;**1**:189-195. DOI: 10.1016/j.jocrd.2012.05.001

[6] Reese HE, McNally RJ, Wihelm S. Probabilistic reasoning in patients whith body dysmorphic disorder. Behavior Theraphy and Experimental Psychiatry. 2012;**42**:270-276. DOI: 10.1016/j.jbtep.2010.11.005

[7] Crerand CE, Phillips KA, Menard W, Fay C. Nonpsychiatric medical treatment of body dysmorphic disorder. Psychosomatics. 2005;**46**:549-555. DOI: 10.1176/appi.psy.46.6.549

[8] Brohede S. Body dysmorphic disorder: capturing a prevalent but a under-recognized disorder. [dissertation]. Linköping: Linköping University; 2017. DOI: 10.3384/diss.diva-133368ISBN

[9] American Psychatric Association. Diagnostic and Statistical Manual of Mental Disorders V. 5th ed. Arlington VA: Author; 2013

[10] Silver J, Farrants J. 'I Once Stared at Myself in the Mirror for Eleven Hours.' Exploring mirror gazing in participants with body dysmorphic disorder. Journal of Health Psychology. 2016;**21**(11):2647-2657. DOI: 10.1177/1359105315581516

[11] Bewley A. The neglected psychological aspects of skin disease. British Medical Journal. 2017;**358**:j3208. DOI: 10.1136/bmj.j3208

[12] Bonfim GW, Nascimento IPC, Borges NB. Body dysmorphic disorder: Literature review. Contextos Clínicos. 2016;**9**(2):240-252. DOI: 10.4013/ctc.2016.92.09

[13] Smith AK. Delusions of body image in the prodrome. Schizophrenia Research. 2013;**146**:366-367. DOI: 10.1016/j.schres.2013.01.033

[14] Bohon C, Hembacher E, Moller H, Moody TD, Feusner JD. Nonlinear relationships between anxiety and visual processing of own. Psychiatry Research: Neuroimaging. 2012;**204**:132-139. DOI: 10.1016/j.pscychresns.2012.09.003

[15] Feusner JD, Arienzo D, Li W, Zhan L, GadElkarim J, Thompson PM, Leow AD. White matter microstructure in body dysmorphic disorder and its clinical correlates. Psychiatry Research: Neuroimaging. 2013;**211**:132-140. DOI: 10.1016/j.pscychresns.2012.11.001

[16] American Psychiatric Association. Diagnostic and Statistical Manual Mental Disorders. 1st ed. Washington: Author; 1952

[17] Atmaca M, Bingol I, Aydin A, Yildirim H, Okur I, Yildirim MA, et al. Brain morphology of patients with body dysmorphic disorder. Journal of Affective Disorders. 2010;**123**:258-263. DOI: 10.1016/j.jad.2009.08.012

[18] Kelly MM, Zhang J, Phillips KA. The prevalence of body dysmorphic disorder and its clinical correlates in a VA primary care behavioral health clinic. Psychiatry Research. 2013;**228**:162-165. DOI: 10.1016/j.psychres.2012.08.009

[19] Feusner JD, Townsend J, Bystritsky A, McKinley M, Moller H, Bookheimer S. Regional brain volumes and symptom severity in body dysmorphic disorder. Psychiatry Research: Neuroimaging. 2009;**172**:161-167. DOI: 10.1016/j.pscychresns.2008.12.003

[20] Feusner JD, Townsend J, Bystritsky A, Bookheimer S. Visual information processing of faces in body dysmorphic disorder. Archives of General Psychiatry. 2007;**64**:1417-1426. DOI: 10.1001/archpsyc.64.12.1417

[21] Toothman J. howstuffsworks: Biological Causes of Body Dysmorphic Disorder [Internet]. Updated: 2017. Available from: http://science.howstuffworks.com/life/inside-the-mind/human-brain/body-dysmorphic-disorder2.htm [Accessed: July 15, 2017]

[22] Buhlmann U, Teachman BA, Kathmann N. Evaluating implicit attractiveness beliefs in body dysmorphic disorder using the Go/No-go association task. Journal of Behavior Therapy and Experimental Psychiatry. 2011;**42**:192-197. DOI: 10.1016/j.jbtep.2010.10.003

[23] Veale D, Riley S. Mirror, mirror on the wall, who is the ugliest of them all? The psychopathology of mirror gazing in body dysmorphic disorder. Behaviour Research and Therapy. 2001;**39**:1381-1393

[24] Veale D, Bewley A. Body dysmorphic disorder. British Medical Journal. 2015;**350**:h2278. DOI: 10.1136/bmj.h2278

[25] Bowe WP, Leyden JJ, Crerand CE, Sarwer DB, Margolis DJ. Body dysmorphic disorder symptoms among patients with acnes vulgaris. Journal of American Academy of Dermatology. 2007;**57**(2):222-230. DOI: 10.1016/j.jaad.2007.03.030

[26] Windheim K, Veale D, Anson M. Mirror gazing in body dysmorphic disorder and healthy controls: Effects of duration of gazing. Behaviour Research and Therapy. 2011;**49**:555-564. DOI: 10.1016/j.brat.2011.05.003

[27] Hart AS, Phillips KA. Symmetry concerns as a symptom of body dysmorphic disorder. Journal of Obsessive-Compulsive and Related Disorders. 2013;**2**:292-298. DOI: 10.1016/j.jocrd.2013.04.004

[28] Phillips KA, Pinto A, Hart AS, Coles ME, Eisen JL, Menard W, Rasmussen SA. A comparison of insight in body dysmorphic disorder and obsessive-compulsive disorder. Journal of Psychiatric Research. 2012;**46**:1293-1299. DOI: 10.1016/j.jpsychires.2012.05.016

[29] Brito MJA, Nahas FX, Ortega NRS, Cordás TA, Dini GM, Neto MS, Ferreira LM. Support system for decision making in the identification of risk for body dysmorphic disorder: A fuzzy model. International Journal of Medical Informatic. 2013;**89**(9):844-853. DOI: 10.1016/j.ijmedinf.2013.04.007

[30] Chan JK, Jones SM, Heywood AJ. Body dysmorphia, self-mutilation and the reconstructive surgeon. Journal of Plastic, Reconstructive & Aesthetic Surgery. 2011;**64**:4-10. DOI: 10.1016/j.bjps.2010.03.029

[31] Yadav S, Narang T, Kumaram MS. Psychodermatology: A comprehensive review. Indian Journal of Dermatology, Venerology and Leprology. 2013;**79**(2):176-192. DOI: 10.4103/0378-6323.107632

[32] Grocholewskia A, Kliemb S, Heinrichsa N. Selective attention to imagined facial ugliness is specific to body dysmorphic. Body Image. 2012;**9**:261-269. DOI: 10.1016/j.bodyim.2012.01.002

[33] Pascual-Vera B, Sanchís MR, Fuster AB. Are unwanted mental intrusions a transdiagnostic variable? Psicothema. 2017;**29**(2):166-171. DOI: 10.7334/psicothema2016.199

[34] Phillips KA, McElroy SL. Personality disorders and traits in patients with body dysmorphic disorder. Comprehensive Psychiatry. 2000;**41**(4):229-236. DOI: 10.1053/comp.2000.7429

[35] Buhlmann U, Etcoff NL, Wilhelm S. Facial attractiveness ratings and perfectionism in body dysmorphic disorder and obsessive-compulsive disorder. Journal of Anxiety Disorders. 2008;**22**:540-547. DOI: 10.1016/j.janxdis.2007.05.004

[36] Bellino S, Zizza M, Paradiso E, Rivarossa A, Fulcheri M, Bogetto F. Dysmorphic concern symptoms and personality disorders: A clinical investigation in patients seeking cosmetic surgery. Psychiatry Research. 2006;**144**:73-78. DOI: 10.1016/j.psychres.2005.06.010

[37] Pecorari G, Gramaglia C, Garzaro M, Abbate-Daga G, Cavallo GP, Giordano C, Fassino S. Self-esteem and personality in subjects with and without body dysmorphic disorder traits undergoing cosmetic rhinoplasty: Preliminary data. Journal of Plastic, Reconstructive & Aesthetic Surgery. 2010;**63**:493-498. DOI: 10.1016/j.bjps.2008.11.070

[38] Phillips KA, Menard W, Fay C, Weisberg R. Demographic characteristics, phenomenology, comorbidity, and family history in 200 individuals with body dysmorphic disorder. Psychosomatics. 2005b;**46**(4):317-325

[39] Kelly MM, Dalrymple K, Zimmerman M, Phillips KA. A comparison study of body dysmorphic disorder versus social phobia. Journal of Psychiatry Research. 2013;**205**:109-116. DOI: 10.1016/j.psychres.2012.08.009

[40] Rief W, Buhlmann U, Wilhelm S, Borkenhagen A, Brahler E. The prevalence of body dysmorphic disorder: A population-based survey. Psychological Medicine. 2006;**36**:877-885. DOI: 10.1017/S0033291706007264

[41] Mufaddel A, Osman OT, Almugaddam F, Jafferany M. A rewiew of body dysmorphic disorder and its presentation in different clinical settings. The Primary Care Companion for CNS Disorders. 2013;**15**. pii: PCC.12r01464

[42] Buhlmann U, Glaesmer H, Mewes R, Fama JM, Wilhelm S, Bröhler, Rief W. Updates on the prevalence of body dysmorphic disorder: A population-based survey. Psychiatry Research. 2010;**178**:171-175. DOI: 10.1016/j.psychres.2009.05.002

[43] Schiebe K, Kollei I, De Zwaan M, Martin A. Classidication of body dysmorphic disorder – What is the advantage of the new DSM-5 criteria? Journal of Psychosomatic Research. 2015;**78**:223-227. DOI: 10.1016/j.jpsychores.2015.01.002

[44] Tignol J, Martin-Guehl C, Aouizerzate B. Body dysmorphic disorder. Revue systématique. 2012;**41**:22-35. DOI: 10.1016/j.lpm.2011.05.021

[45] Faravelli C, Salvatori S, Galassi F, Aiazzi L, Drei C, Cabras P. Epidemiology of somatoform disorders: A community survey in Florence. Social Psychiatry and Psychiatric Epidemiology. 1997;**32**(1):24-29. DOI: 10.1007/BF00800664

[46] Fitts SN, Gibson P, Redding CA, Deiter PJ. Body dysmorphic disorder: Implications for its validity as a DSM-III-R clinical syndrome. Psychological Reports. 1989;**64**:655-658

[47] Uzun O, Basoglu C, Akar A, Cansever A, Ozsahin A, Cetin M, Ebrinc S. Body dysmorphic disorder in patients with acne. Comprehensive Psychiatry. 2003;**44**:415-419. DOI: 10.1016/S0010-440X(03)00102-0

[48] Conrado LA, Hounie AG, Diniz JB, Fossaluza V, Torres AR, Miguel EC, et al. Body dysmorphic disorder among dermatologic patients: Prevalence and clinical features. Journal of American Academy of Dermatology. 2010;**63**(2):235-243. DOI: 10.1016/j.jaad.2009.09.017

[49] Dogruk Kacar S, Ozuguz P, Bagcioglu E, Coskun KS, Uzel Tas H, Polat S, et al. The frequency of body dysmorphic disorder in dermatology and cosmetic dermatology clinics: A study from Turkey. Clinical and Experimental Dermatology. 2014;**39**:433-438. DOI: 10.1111/ced.12304

[50] Alavi M, Kalafi Y, Dehbozorgi GR, Javadpour A. Body dysmorphic disorder and other psychiatric morbidity in aesthetic rhinoplasty candidates. Journal of Plastic, Reconstructive & Aesthetic Surgery. 2011;**64**:738-741. DOI: 10.1016/j.bjps.2010.09.019

[51] Lai C, Lee S, Yeh Y, Chen C. Body Dysmorphic disorder in patients with cosmetic surgery. Kaohsiung Journal of Medical Sciences. 2010;**26**(9):478-482. DOI: 10.1016/S1607-551X(10)70075-9

[52] Vindigni V, Pavan C, Semenzin M, Granà S, Gambaro F, Marini M, Bassetto F, Mazzoleni F. The importance of recognizing body dysmorphic disorder in cosmetic surgery patients: Do our patients need a preoperative psychiatric evaluation? European Journal of Plastic Surgery. 2002;**25**(6):305-308. DOI: 10.1007/s00238-002-0410-8

[53] Callaghan GM, Lopez A, Wong L, Northcross J, Anderson KR. Predicting consideration of cosmetic surgery in a college population: A continuum of body image disturbance and the importance of coping strategies. Body Image. 2011;**8**:267-274. DOI: 10.1016/j.bodyim.2011.04.002

[54] Picavet VA, Hellings PW. Reply: Preoperative symptoms of body dysmorphic disorder determine postoperative satisfaction and quality of life in aesthetic rhinoplasty. Plastic and Reconstructive Surgery. 2014;**133**(1):62e. DOI: 10.1097/01.prs.0000437262.08822.8a

[55] Masieiro LM. Cultural changes: A reflection about the evolution of plastic surgery. Revista Antropología del Cuerpo, Salamanca. 2015;**0**:62-77

[56] Ellison N, Werner TG, Dodhia R, Serfaty MA, Clarke A. Development of a cosmetic procedure screening questionnaire (COPS) for body dysmorphic disorder. Correspondence and Communications. 2011:530-532. DOI: 10.1016/j.bjps.2011.09.007

[57] Bohnea A, Wilhelma S, Keuthena NJ, Florinb I, Baera L, Jenike MA. Prevalence of body dysmorphic disorder in a German college student sample. Psychiatry Research. 2002;**109**:101-104. DOI: 10.1016/S0165-1781(01)00363-8

[58] Bjornssona AS, Didie ER, Grant JE, Menard W, Stalkere E, Phillips KA. Age at onset and clinical correlates in body dysmorphic disorder. Comprehensive Psychiatry. 2013;**54**(7):893-903. DOI: 10.1016/j.comppsych.2013.03.019

[59] Conroy MC, Menard W, Fleming-Ives K, Modha P, Cerullo H, Phillips KA. Prevalence and clinical characteristics of body dismorphic disorder in a adult inpatient. General Hospital Psychiatry. 2008;**30**:67-72. DOI: 10.1016/j.genhosppsych.2007.09.004

[60] Didie ER, Menard W, Stern AP, Phillips KA. Occupational functioning and impairment in adults with body dysmorphic disorder. Comprehensive Psychiatry. 2008;**49**:561-569. DOI: 10.1016/j.comppsych.2008.04.003

[61] Ghasemi A, Ardakani ZP, Momeni M, Falahati M, Azimzade E. The investigation of the relationship between body dysmorphic disorder and psychological problems and comprise it among female athletes and non athletes students. Procedia Social and Behavioral Sciences. 2010;**5**:1799-1803. DOI: 10.1016/j.sbspro.2010.07.367

[62] Phillips KA, Wilhelm S, Koran LM, Didie ER, Fallon BA, Feusner J, et al. Body dysmorphic disorder: Some key issues for DSM-V. Depression and Anxiety. 2010;**27**(6):573-591. DOI: 10.1002/da.20709

[63] Anson M, Veale D, de Silva P. Social-evaluative versus self-evaluative appearance concerns in body dysmorphic disorder. Behaviour Research and Therapy. 2012;**50**:753-760. DOI: 10.1016/j.brat.2012.09.003

[64] Kittler JE, Menard J, Phillips KA. Weight concerns in individuals with body dysmorphic disorder. Eating Behaviors. 2007;**8**:115-120. DOI: 10.1016/j.eatbeh.2006.02.006

[65] Coles ME, Phillips KA, Menard W, Pagano ME, Fay C, Weisberg RB, et al. Body dysmorphic disorder and social phobia: Ccross-sectional and prospective data. Depression and Anxiety. 2006;**23**(1):26-33

[66] Connor KM, Davidson JR, Churchill LE, Sherwood A, Weisler RH, Foa E. Psychometric properties of the social phobia inventory (SPIN): New self-rating scale. British Journal of Psychiatry. 2000;**176**(4):379-386

[67] Didie ER, Tortolani CC, Pope CG, Menard W, Fay C, Phillips KA. Childhood abuse and neglect in body dysmorphic disorder. Child Abuse & Neglect. 2006;**30**:1105-1115. DOI: 10.1016/j.chiabu.2006.03.007

[68] Borda T, Neziroglu F, Santos N, Donnelly K, Rivera RP. Status of body dysmorphic disorder in Argentina. Journal of Anxiety Disorders. 2011;**25**:507-512. DOI: 10.1016/j.janxdis.2010.12.004

[69] Phillips KA, Didie ER, Menard W. Clinical features and correlates of major depressive disorder in individuals with body dysmorphic disorder. Journal of Affective Disorders. 2007;**97**:129-135. DOI: 10.1016/j.jad.2006.06.006

[70] Phillips KA, Menard W, Fay C. Gender similarities and differences in 200 individuals with body dysmorphic disorder. Comprehensive Psychiatry. 2006;**47**:77-87. DOI: 10.1016/j.comppsych.2005.07.002

[71] Picardi A, Lega I, Tarolla E. Suicide risk in skin disorders. Clinics in Dermatology. 2013;**31**:47-56. DOI: 10.1016/j.clindermatol.2011.11.006

[72] Frias A, Palma C, Farriols N, Gonzàlez L. Comorbidity between obsessive-compulsive disorder and body dysmorphic disorder: Prevalence, explanatory theories, and clinical characterization. Neuropsychiatric Disease and Treatment. 2015;**11**:2233-2244. DOI: 10.2147/NDT.S67636

[73] Koran LM, Abujaoude E, Large MD, Serpe RT. The prevalence of body dysmorphic disorder in the United States adult population. CNS Spectrums. 2008;**13**(4):316-322. DOI: 10.1017/S1092852900016436

[74] Madsen SK, Bohon C, Feusner JD. Visual processing in anorexia nervosa and body dysmorphic disorder: Similarities, differences, and future research directions. Journal of Psychiatry Research. 2013;**47**(10):1483-1491. DOI: 10.1016/j.jpsychires.2013.06.003

[75] Farah MHS, Mate CH. Uma discussão sobre as práticas de anorexia e bulimia como estéticas de existência. Educação e Pesquisa. 2015;**41**(4):883-898. DOI: 10.1590/s1517-97022015021539

[76] Soler PT, Fernandes HM, Damasceno VO, Novaes JS. Vigorexy and levels of exercise dependence in gym goers and body builders. Revista Brasileira de Medicina do Esporte. 2013;**19**(5):343-348. DOI: 10.1590/S1517-86922013000500009

[77] Vargas CS, Moraes CB, Mozzaquatro NF, Kirsten VR. Prevalência de dismorfia muscular em mulheres frequentadoras de academia Revista Brasileira de Nutrição Esportiva, São Paulo. 7. 37. p.28-34. 2013 Jan/Feb. ISSN 1981-9927

[78] Goetz ER, Camargo BV. Attitude scale health and beauty: Construction and validation. Fractal Revista de Psicologia, DOI. 2014;**26**(1):199-222. DOI: 10.1590/S1984-02922014000100015

[79] Goetz ER, Camargo BV, Bertoldo RB, Justo AM. Social representation of the body in press media. Psicologia & Sociedade. 2008;**20**(2):226-236

Chapter 2

Alteration in Nasal Cycle Rhythm as an Index of the Diseased Condition

Elangovan Muthu Kumaran

Additional information is available at the end of the chapter

http://dx.doi.org/10.5772/intechopen.70599

Abstract

Breathing is the vital function based on the conductance of air through a system of branching tubes that taper off and eventually connect to the alveoli. Nose act as an interface between atmospheric air and lower respiratory system, constitute the moist respiratory epithelium, which performs various vital physiological functions like filtering the inspired air, warming, and humidifying. Several anatomical and physiological factors are responsible for the passage of airflow in two nostrils, which are asymmetric in nature. The inequality airflow passage in both the nostrils exists for a specific duration. This phenomenon of altering asymmetrical airflow from one nasal passage to the other is called 'nasal cycle'. For every regular interval of time period, the swap of predominant nasal airflow between two nostrils determines the nasal patency. This cycle is controlled by the central regulator located at hypothalamus by coordinating the autonomic nervous system that comprises sympathetic and parasympathetic nerves that clog the nasal mucosa. The nostril decongest when the sympathetic nerves in one nostril become active. In this biorhythm, if the sympathetic nerves of one nostril drop, immediately the parasympathetic nerves take over, so that the other nostril congests. It is unclear why these cycles exist but the total nasal airway resistance is almost unchanged. There are a range of activities and reflexes, which can affect the nasal airway. This biorhythm is categorized under ultradian cycle since the mean duration of nasal cycle is about two and a half hours. In this study, it observed changes in nasal airflow duration, pattern, and rhythm that correspond to various disease states in human.

Keywords: nasal cycle, biorhythm, sympathetic and parasympathetic nerves, ultradian cycle

1. Introduction

Variety of temporal variations is observed in organism, organs, tissues, even in cellular level. Most of these variations are periodicity synchronous with nature rhythms. These periodic variations in human bio-signals are referred as biorhythms. Biorhythms cover broad spectrum ranges from fraction of seconds to even several years. The cycle exists less than a day (~24 hours) is referred as ultradian cycle (e.g., neuron activity, heart rate, respiration rate, rapid eye moment during sleep), equal to a day as circadian cycle (e.g., sleep-wake cycle) and greater than a day as infradian cycle (e.g., menstruation cycle).

The airflow pattern during breathing in both the nostrils will not be same in most of the time. Only one nostril will be dominant for the particular time period, later the dominance shift to other nostril, and this cycle continuous from one nostril to other. This swapping of airflow from one nostril to another for a short duration is called nasal cycle Nasal cycle last for about 25 minutes–4 hours, it varies from person to person; even for the same person, the time periods varies from cycle to cycle. Since the duration of nasal cycle is less than 24 hours, it is classified under ultradian cycle. This chapter completely deals with the analysis of nasal airflow pattern from both the nostrils at healthy and different diseased states.

2. Understanding of nasal cycle

The nasal cycle is an alternating one, with the total resistance in the nose remaining constant. The nasal cycle's value becomes evident when one considers that the function of the nose is to warm, humidify, and filter nasally inspired air. These humidifying and filtering functions are dependent on the presence of moist respiratory epithelium. The presence of two nasal fossae or chambers that function in an alternating pattern prevents excessive drying, crusting, and infection, which are the likely results of a static passage that is open to constant airflow, especially in desert regions. This cycle was believed to be an ultradian rhythm seen in people with normal health.

The swap of predominant nasal airflow between two nostrils determines the nasal patency, "why" we breathe from any one nostril at any point of time, there is no conclusive scientific evidence to answer. The "how" is explained by the presence of sympathetic and parasympathetic nerves that clog the nasal mucosa. When the sympathetic nerves in one nostril become active that nostril decongests. In this biorhythm, if the sympathetic nerves of the one nostril drop, immediately the parasympathetic nerves take over, so that the other nostril congests. This cycle, which is controlled by the autonomic nervous system as described above, had a mean duration of two and a half hours. The periodic congestion and decongestion of cavernous tissue of the nasal mucosa is the cause for nasal cycle [1]. Nasal cycle rhythm pattern is considered to be controlled by the central regulator located in the hypothalamus resulted in the bilateral vasoconstriction of the nasal mucosa [2].

Breathing through alternate nostrils showed effects on brain hemisphere symmetry on EEG topography [3]. There is a significant difference of airflow between left-nostril and right-nostril breathing. Effect of this cycle and manipulation through forced nostril breathing on one side on the endogenous ultradian rhythms of the autonomic and central nervous system [4]. In addition changes in the amount of blood flowing through the cavernous tissues of the nasal conchae was, the way in which the nasal cycle was described [5]. The normal nasal cycle rhythm is disturbed in diseased case, the nasal cycle dominance have been investigated with autism in children [6]. The effect of unilateral nostril breathing is associated with EEG amplitude in contralateral hemisphere [7, 8]; it is reported that left uninostril breathing is associated with enhanced spatial abilities and right uninostril breathing is associated with enhanced verbal abilities [9, 10].

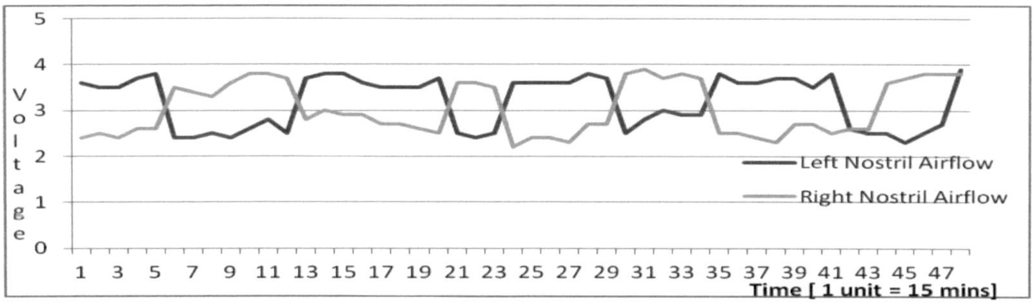

Figure 1. Nasal cycle rhythm between two nostrils for the period of 12 hours.

The exact relationship between uninostril breathing and cerebral hemispheric activity is not known. But, some of the previous studies explain the effect of hyperventilation by the nose on EEG activity in the cortex proposes that it is produced by a neural reflex mechanism in the superior nasal meatus [11].

In this study, the most interesting factor of characteristics of airflow in both the nostrils was analyzed extensively. Airflow in one nostril will be greater and other will be lesser, the nostril with greater quantity of airflow is called as dominant nostril. This dominance will exists only for limited duration (approx. 25 minutes–4 hours), later the dominant airflow found to be exists in the other nostril. This swapping of dominant airflow between one nostril to another is called as nasal cycle as illustrated in **Figure 1**. Graph indicating alteration of left and right dominant airflow measured at every 15 minutes for the period of 12 hours.

Previous study on nasal cycle elaborates the cause for this oscillatory function in different view that nasal cycle is regulated by the autonomic nervous system, such that unilateral sympathetic dominance in one nostril causes vasoconstriction and decongestion, while simultaneously parasympathetic dominance in the other nostril causes vasodilatation and congestion [6].

It is proposed that the periodic congestion and decongestion of nasal venous sinusoids may provide a pump mechanism for the generation of plasma exudate, which is an important component of respiratory defense [12]. Nasal cycle also reported to be regulated by the alternating lateralization of plasma catecholamine's [12].

The nasal cycle is not only observed in human nose, it is also found in rabbit and rat [13], the domestic pig [14], the cat [15], and the dog [16] and seems to be a common phenomenon in all mammals and other animals.

3. Effect of unilateral nostril breathing in various physiological and psychological changes

It is well understood that there exists a strong relation between nasal cycle with physiological and behavioral changes. There is a slight, but significant correlation between the dominant nostril and the relative cognitive performance in free breathing subjects is observed [9]. The vasomotor and secretory activity of the nasal mucosa in healthy volunteers are observed and reported that the nasal secretions over the mucous membrane had a definite relation to the congestion of the turbinal structures [17]. The modification in actual nasal cycle rhythms in terms of change in period length, increase or decrease in strength of the rhythm, or desynchronization, and uncoupling of rhythms are observed in depressed patients [18].

Nasal resistive reflexes, which are anatomically mediated may change the nasal resistance [19]. Studies on nasal cycle prove its importance on clinical aspect that breathing through the right nostril increases blood glucose level significantly whereas through left nostrils decreases [20]. Also, breathing through right nostril increases metabolism whereas breathing through the left nostril decreases sympathetic activity to the sweat glands [21].

Alternative nasal airflow activates alternative hemispheres of the brain, right dominant airflow activates left hemisphere of brain and vice versa, since the right hemisphere of brain is responsible for creative thinking whereas the left hemisphere of brain is responsible for logical thinking. During EEG measurements, rapid eye movement (REM) and non-rapid eye movement (NREM) was noticed and correlated with left and right hemisphere brain activity [22]. It is suggested one can selectively activate a hemisphere depending on which functions are mostly needed at a certain point in time [4, 23].

Nasal cycle has a strong correlation with psychological changes in wake state as well as in sleeping state both for normal and abnormal subjects [24, 25]. Even though many researchers found the origin of the system responsible for this nasal rhythm oscillation [26], the factor which controls this rhythm is still ambiguity [27]. In nineteenth century, German scientist Kayser sparked interest in the nostril cycle [4] studied the nostril cycle and the effects of forced unilateral nostril breathing (FUNB). In this experiment, subjects are instructed to block one nostril and breathe through the other nostril for a period of 1–30 minutes; during the period both physiological and psychological parameters are measured.

The participants' nostrils are categorized to the independent decongested nostril, that is, the nostril with dominant airflow. Nostril dominance is measured by the collection of quantitative data during FUNB to measure nostril dominance, and the corresponding effects on the brain and the heart was recorded. Long-term studies of the nostril cycle have been very limited. One month study was conducted by Funk and Clarke [28], but observed only weak patterns in nostril dominance and failed to identify possible factors responsible for the variability.

To explore the possible effects of the nasal cycle on the brain, it is important to understand the alterations in cognitive processes that are responsible for each cerebral hemisphere. Generally, it is well known that the left hemisphere is responsible for language processing whereas the right hemisphere is for visual processing. Certain research indicates the individual differences in the degree to which one cerebral hemisphere rather than the other in processing the various information [29]. This is referred to as hemispheric dominance.

The qualities assigned to each nostril are assumed to correspond with brain hemispheric dominance. Physiologically, electro-cortical activity in one hemisphere (measured by greater EEG power) relates to contra lateral nostril dominance [7]. This relationship has been intensively analyzed by forced unilateral nostril breathing (FUNB). For example, participants perform better in cognitive tasks that require rational and logical thinking, where tasks associated with the left hemisphere, the right nostril dominance is found. During the left nostril dominance, they perform better in spatial tasks, associated with the right hemisphere [23].

It is noticed that the nostril cycle also has an influence on neurotransmitters and hormones. For example, FUNB has an effect on involuntary blink rates, which are directly related to dopaminergic activity. Blink rates have been significantly increased during left FUNB, which indicates the association between right hemispheric preference and a possible lateralization of dopamine. Studies have also shown that there is a strong relationship between dominant nostril airflow with plasma catecholamines, such as norepinephrine, epinephrine, and dopamine. The ratio of plasma catecholamines from samples taken in each arm correlates with nostril dominance [12].

Furthermore, the effects of nostril cycle are also apparent in the endocrine system. The levels of pituitary hormones (adrenocorticoids, luteinizing hormones) as well as catecholamines varied according to the nasal cycle [30]. The alteration in nasal cycle correlated with autonomic nervous system results with indicating alternating lateralization of catecholamines in one of the two arms [12].

The nasal cycle also supports three general conclusions with respect to brain activity are: (1) nasal cycle dominance correlates with changes in hemispheric EEG differences; (2) in free breathing subjects, relative performance on spatial and verbal tasks is related to nostril dominance; and (3) at least theoretically, unilateral forced nostril breathing (UFBN) may differentially affect the ipsilateral and contralateral cerebral hemispheres, thereby changing relative EEG activity and influencing relative spatial and verbal performance [31].

In addition to the effects of the nostril cycle in psychological effects, research has also explored in many physiological effects, with an emphasis in autonomic activity, especially in human heart. It is evident that heart rate and mean arterial pressure in dogs varies in a cycle that lasts approximately 1.5 hours [32, 33]. From this, researchers have concluded that the internal variations of the heart drive by the sympathetic nervous system [30]. FUNB studies have shown that the nostril cycle affects intraocular blood pressure: right nostril breathing reduces it and left nostril breathing increases. Similarly, nostril dominance has been shown to affect blood glucose level: right FUNB increased blood glucose levels, while left FUNB decreased the levels. Homeostasis of glucose levels is regulated by the autonomic nervous system [20].

During the night sleep, there is synchronization of nasal and sleep cycles in some of the REM phases of sleep, the length of periods of the nasal cycle is one or more length of sleep cycle [34]. From the above literatures, it is clear evident that analyzing the characteristic of nasal cycle becomes most important since there is a strong association between the physiological and psychological changes in human with nasal cycle.

4. Analyzing characteristic of nasal airflow in healthy subjects

From the experiments conducted by recording nasal air flow from two nostrils, there exists predominant airflow in only one nostril that justifies the existence of nasal cycle. Twenty healthy subjects (mean age 21 years) were examined for every 15 minutes for a stretch of 8 hours per day. The same procedure was repeated for 8 days. It is observed that the nasal cycle exists for 90% of the population. **Figure 2** shows the airflow from both the nostrils indicating predominant airflow in left nostril recorded from a healthy subject.

The work was carried out with Hotwire Anemometer method to measure the small temperature difference between inhale and exhale. The output is measured separately and simultaneously from both right and left nostril and can be stored for analysis of breath characteristics. The nasal cycle was recorded and analyzed using data acquisition system model PowerLab 8/35 with LabChart Software from AD Instruments, Australia.

It is estimated from 20 healthy subjects that an average duration of nasal cycle is about 2.45 hours. Rhythm duration varies from person to person in the range of 20 minutes–4.26 hours. Much precaution was taken to measure airflow without disturbing the normal airflow during breathing. Even in the healthy subjects for the same subject, the nasal cycle duration varies from time to time based on physiological and psychological changes. The people with respiratory problem were excluded from the study.

The existence of predominant airflow under normal and different state of forced breathing is illustrated in **Figures 3–7**.

- Normal breathing
- Deep breathing
- Holding breath at exhale condition
- Holding breath at inhale condition
- Holding breath both at exhale and inhale condition

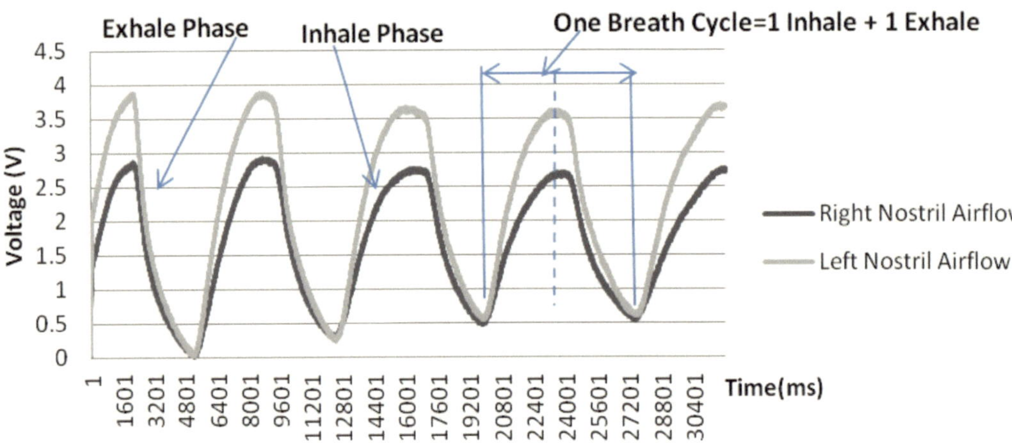

Figure 2. Indicating nasal cycle with predominant airflow in left nostril in a healthy subject.

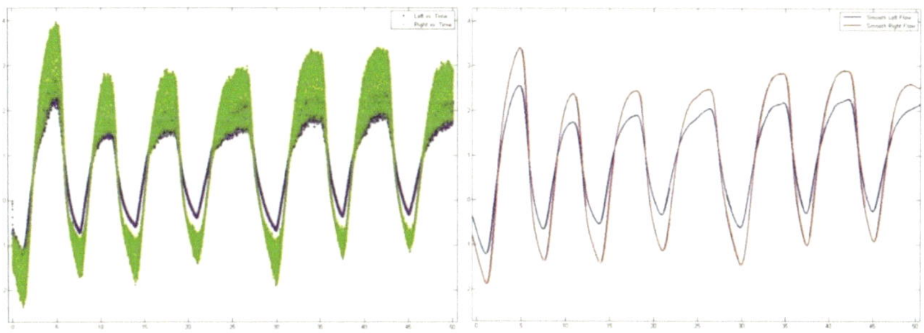

a) b)

Figure 3. Indicating predominant airflow in right nostril (red line—filtered signal) versus left nostril (blue line—filtered signal) during normal breathing in filtered signal. (a) Raw signal and (b) filtered signal.

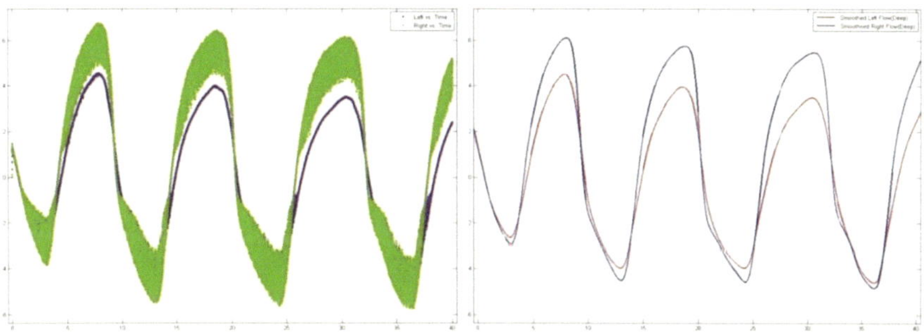

a) b)

Figure 4. Indicating predominant airflow in right nostril (red line—filtered signal) versus left nostril (blue line—filtered signal) during forced deep breath in filtered signal. (a) Raw signal and (b) filtered signal.

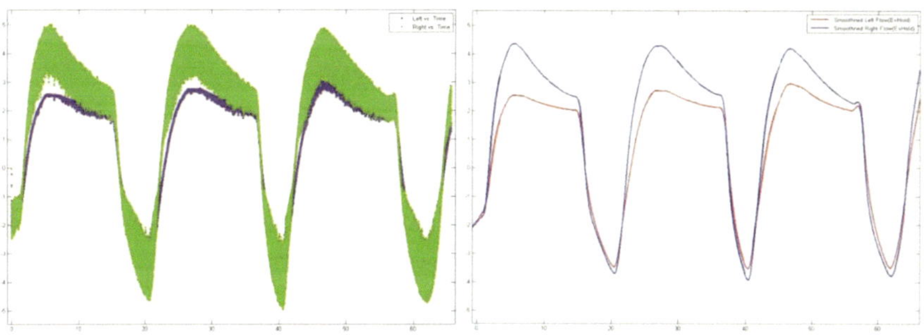

a) b)

Figure 5. Indicating predominant airflow in right nostril (red line—filtered signal) versus left nostril (blue line—filtered signal) during forced holding of breath after inhale in filtered signal. (a) Raw signal and (b) filtered signal.

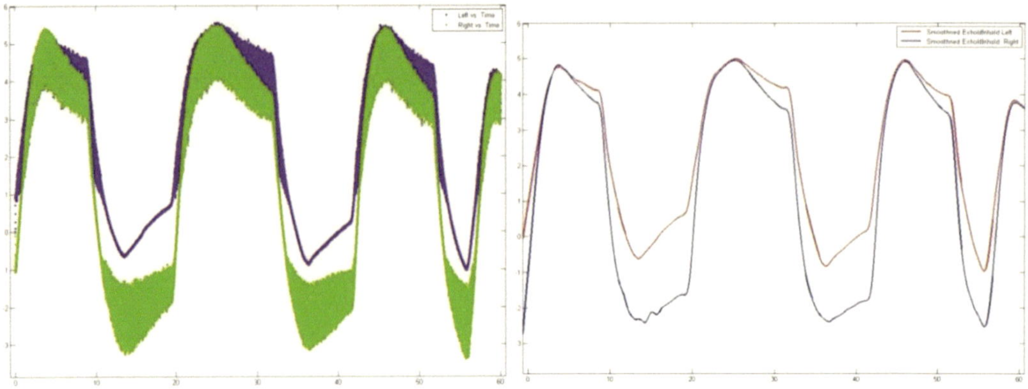

a) b)

Figure 6. Indicating predominant airflow in right nostril (red line—filtered signal) versus left nostril (blue line—filtered signal) during forced holding of breath after exhale in filtered signal. (a) Raw signal and (b) filtered signal.

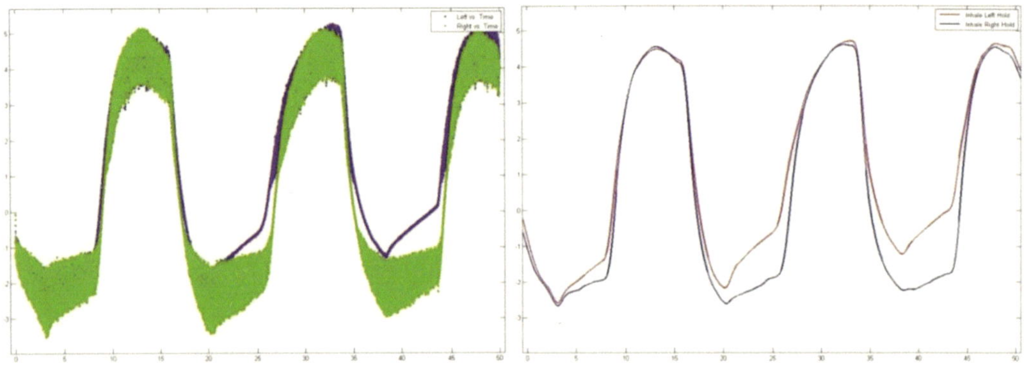

a) b)

Figure 7. Forced exhale hold and inhale hold indicating predominant airflow in right nostril (blue line—filtered signal) in both the cases in filtered signal. (a) Raw signal and (b) filtered signal.

5. Analyzing characteristic of nasal airflow in diseased subjects

The experimental investigation was carried out at Government Siddha Medical College Palayamkottai, Tamil Nadu, India. Totally 260 diseased patients participated in this study from both in-patient and out-patient sections. After receiving a waiver of informed consent form from the Institutional Human Ethical Committee, a retrospective study from various patients is undertaken under the supervision of physician. The nasal airflow for the duration of about 3 minutes is recorded at every 20 minutes to the stretch of 8 hours. Then, the average period of nasal cycle rhythm is calculated. In normal case, the nasal cycle exists for the period of 2–2.5 hours (average) ranges between 20 minutes and 3.6 hours. Whereas in diseased case, the cycle duration greater than 4.5 hours or existence of predominant airflow in particular nostril is very high when compared to the other nostril. The huge multivariate samples are collected with different disease from 260 samples. Out of 260, 154 subjects were classified under first group that belongs to subjects possessing a predominant nasal airflow in right nostril and remaining 106 subjects belong to second group possessing predominant nasal airflow in left nostril.

It is determined that about 87% in group 1 exist a predominant airflow in right nostril and the subjects were suffering from anyone of the following diseases like peptic ulcer, eye diseases, hyper chloride, esopatic, gastritis, diarrhea, insomnia, liver disorder, gastro intestinal disorder, and cardiac diseases. Similarly 92% of group 2 possesses predominant airflow in left nostril and the subjects were suffering from anyone of the following diseases like loss of appetite, tuberculosis, allergy, respiratory disorders like wheezing, and bronchitis asthma.

6. Conclusion

Recently the field of chronobiology attracted many researchers all over the world toward Circaseptan cycle (seven-day weekly cycle). It is commonly noticed in most of the plants, insects, and animals other than humans possessing weekly cycles. Apart from being the key coordinating rhythm for many rhythmic activity in body, seven-day cycle has been found in blood pressure fluctuations, variation in blood acid content, heartbeat, red blood cells, urine chemistry and volume, oral temperature, the ratio between two important neurotransmitters, female breast temperature, norepinephrine and epinephrine, and the rise and fall of several body chemicals such as cortisol, the stress coping hormone.

The research in biological rhythms attracted many scientists especially in the field of chronotherapy, the application of biological rhythm to therapeutic procedures may be achieved by synchronizing drug concentration in drug delivery system with rhythms in disease activity that will improve the healing nature [35]. Furthermore research on this nasal cycle may pave a way for a new diagnostic and therapeutic technique in the medical field. A data base can be maintained for various diseases based on airflow pattern, which can be utilized by the researchers to train the neural network-based disease classification.

Author details

Elangovan Muthu Kumaran

Address all correspondence to: reachemk@gmail.com

Dr. B.R. Ambedkar Institute of Technology, Port Blair, Andaman and Nicobar Islands, India

References

[1] Eccles RB. A role for the nasal cycle in respiratory defence. The European Respiratory Journal. 1996;9(2):371-376

[2] Eccles R, Lee RL. The influence of the hypothalamus on the sympathetic innervation of the nasal vasculture of the cat. Acta Otolaryngolica. 1981;**91**:127-134

[3] Stancák AJ, Kuna M. EEG changes during forced alternate nostril breathing. International Journal of Psychophysiology. 1994;**18**(1):75-79

[4] Shannahoff-Khalsa DS. Selective unilateral autonomic activation: Implications for psychiatry, CNS spectrums. The International Journal of Neuropsychiatric Medicine. 2007; **12**(8):625-634

[5] Flanagan P, Eccles R. Spontaneous changes of unilateral nasal airflow in man: A reexamination of the nasal cycle. Acta Otolaryngolica. 1997;**117**:590-595

[6] Dane S, Balci N. Handedness, eyedness and nasal cycle in children with autism. International Journal of Developmental Neuroscience. 2007;**25**:223-226

[7] Werntz DA, Bickford RG, Shannahoff-Khalsa D. Alternating cerebral hemispheric activity and the lateralization of autonomic nervous function. Human Neurobiology. 1983;**2**:39-43

[8] Werntz DA, Bickford RG, Shannahoff-Khalsa D. Selective hemispheric stimulation by unilateral forced nostril breathing. Human Neurobiology. 1987;**6**(3):165-171

[9] Klein R, Pilon D, Prosser S, Shannahoff-Khalsa D. Nasal airflow asymmetries and human performance. Biological Psychology. 1986;**23**:127-137

[10] Jella SA, Shannahoff-Khalsa DS. The effects of unilateral forced nostril breathing on cognitive performance. The International Journal of Neuroscience. 1993;**73**:61-68

[11] Kristof M, Sevit Z, Manas K. Activating effect of nasal airflow on epileptic electrographic abnormalities in the human EEG. Evidence for the Reflect Origin of the Phenomenon PhysiologiaBohemoslovaca. 1981;**30**:73-77

[12] Kennedy B, Ziegler MG, Shannahoff-Khalsa DS. Alternating lateralization of plasma catecholamines and nasal patency in humans. Life Sciences. 1986;**38**:1203-1214

[13] Bojsen Moller F, Fahrenkrug J. Nasal swell bodies and cyclic changes in the air passages of the rat and rabbit nose. Anatolia. 1971;**110**:25-37

[14] Eccles R. The domestic pig as an experimental animal for studies on the nasal cycle. Acta Otolaryngolica (Stockh). 1978;**85**:431-436

[15] Bamford OS, Eccles R. The central reciprocal control of nasal vasomotor oscillations. Pflügers Archiv. 1982;**394**:139-143

[16] Webber RL, Jeffcoat MK, Harman JT, Ruttimann UE. Demonstration of the nasal cycle in the beagle dog. Journal of Computer Assisted Tomography. 1987;**11**:869-871

[17] Bezshapochny SB, Gasiuk IA, Loburets VV, Vakhnina AB. The mechanisms of local protection of the mucous membrane of the nasal cavity and paranasal sinuses. Vestnikotorinolaringologii. 2013;**4**:44-47

[18] Healy D. Rhythms and blues neurochemical, neuro-pharmacological and neuropsychological implications of hypothesis of circadian rhythm dysfunction in affective disorders. Psychopharmacology. 1987;**93**:271-285

[19] Cole P. Nasal and oral airflow resistors. Archives of Otolaryngology - Head and Neck Surgery. 1992;**118**:790-793

[20] Backon J. Changes in blood glucose levels induced by different forced nostril breathing: A technique which affects brain hemisphericity and automatic activity. Medical Science Research. 1988;**16**:1197-1199

[21] Raghuraj P, Telles S. Immediate effect of specific nostril manipulating yoga breathing practices on autonomic and respiratory variables. Applied Psychophysiology and Biofeedback. 2008;**33**(2):65-75

[22] Atanasov AT, Dimov PD. Nasal and sleep cycle – Possible synchronization during night sleep. Medical Hypotheses. 2003;**61**:275-277

[23] Shannahoff-Khalsa D, Boyle MR, Buebel ME. The effects of unilateral forced nostril breathing on cognition. International Journal of Neuroscience. 1991;**57**:239-249

[24] Barcaro U, Denoth F, Murri L, Navona C, Stefanini A. Changes in the interhemispheric correlation during sleep in normal subjects. Electroencephalography and Clinical Neurophysiology. 1986;**63**:112-118

[25] Berg S, Haight JSJ, Yap V, Hoffstein V, Cole P. Comparison of direct and indirect measurements of respiratory airflow: Implications for hypopneas. American Sleep Disorders Association and Sleep Research Society. 1997;**20**:60-64

[26] Edmunds L. Cellular and Molecular Bases of Biological Clocks. Springer-Verlag; 1988. p. 305-311

[27] NASA, 1981, Effects of circadian rhythm phase alteration on physiological and psychological variables: Implications to pilot performance, NASA-TM-81277. NASA 01-03-1981. Retrieved 25-05-2011

[28] Funk F, Clarke J. The nasal cycle observations over prolonged periods of time. Research Bulletin of the Himalayan International Institute. 1980;**1**(Winter):4

[29] Torrance TF. Reality and evangelical theology. Scottish Journal of Theology. 1982;**36**(03): 388-390

[30] Shannahoff-Khalsa DS, Yates FE. Ultradian sleep rhythms of lateral EEG, autonomic, and cardiovascular activity are coupled in humans. International Journal of Neuroscience. 2000;**101**(1-4):21-43

[31] Block RA, Arnott DP, Quigley B, Lynch WC. Unilateral nostril breathing influences lateralized cognitive performance. Brain and Cognition. 1989;**9**:181-190

[32] Zehr JP, McReynolds LA. The use of degenerate oligonucleotides for amplification of the nifH gene from the marine cyanobacterium *Trichodesmium thiebautii*. Applied and Environmental Microbiology. 1989;**55**:2522-2526

[33] Shimada S, Marsh DJ. Oscillations in mean arterial pressure in conscious dogs. Circulation Research. 1979;**44**:692-700

[34] Touitou, Haus E. Biological Rhythms in Clinical and Laboratory Medicine. Heidelberg: Springer-Verlag; 1992

[35] Rohan S. Chronotherapeutical approach: Circadian rhythm in human and its role in occurrence and severity of disease. International Journal of Pharmaceutical Technology and Research. 2012;**4**(2):765-777

Chapter 3

Changes in the Striatal Network Connectivity in Parkinsonian and Dyskinetic Rodent Models

Jesús Pérez-Ortega and José Bargas

Additional information is available at the end of the chapter

http://dx.doi.org/10.5772/intechopen.70601

Abstract

In Parkinson's disease, there is a loss of dopaminergic innervation in the basal ganglia. The lack of dopamine produces substantial changes in neural plasticity and generates pathological activity patterns between basal ganglia nuclei. The treatment to relieve Parkinsonism is the administration of levodopa. However, the treatment produces dyskinesia. The question to answer is how the interactions between neurons change in the brain microcircuits under these pathological conditions. Calcium imaging is a way to record the activity of dozens of neurons simultaneously with single-cell resolution in brain slices from rodents. We studied these interactions in the striatum, since it is the nucleus of the basal ganglia that receives the major dopaminergic innervation. We used network analysis, where each active neuron is taken as a node and its coactivity with other neurons is taken as its functional connections. The network obtained represents the functional connectome of the striatal microcircuit, which can be characterized with a small set of parameters taken from graph theory. We then quantify the pathological changes at the functional histological scale and the differences between normal and pathological conditions.

Keywords: Parkinson's disease, L-DOPA induced dyskinesia, striatal microcircuit, functional connectome, network properties

1. Introduction

Idiopathic Parkinson's disease (PD) was first described by James Parkinson in 1817 and it is the second most common neurodegenerative disease after Alzheimer's disease. PD prevalence is lower in African, Asian, and Arabic countries than in North America, Europe, and South America [1, 2]. In the USA, the incidence of PD by ethnicity is highest among Hispanic people, followed by non-Hispanic white people, Asian people and black people [1, 2]. Gender is another risk factor with a male to female incidence ratio around 3:2 [1, 2]. However, age is the greatest risk factor to develop PD: the incidence is low before the age of 50 years but increases quickly peaking around 80 years [1, 2]. In addition, there are several environmental risk factors for PD: pesticide exposure, head injury, rural living, etc.; but also there are some factors that help to decrease the risk: tobacco smoking, coffee drinking, alcohol consumption, etc. [1, 2].

The main characteristics of PD are the motor symptoms: resting tremor, rigidity, postural instability, bradykinesia, among others [3]. The motor symptoms of PD are the result of dopaminergic denervation of the basal ganglia (BG). This loss of dopamine is due to the death of dopaminergic neurons in the *substantia nigra pars compacta* (SNc). Dopamine is essential for the proper functioning of the BG [4]. The causes of PD are still unknown. Some neurotoxic animal models have been developed to mimic and study its pathophysiology. In rodents, the most used is the hemiparkinsonian model: the unilateral lesion of the SNc with the 6-hidroxidopamine toxin (6-OHDA). It is commonly evaluated by turning behavior induced by dopaminergic agonists [5–7]. In this chapter, recent results to study pathophysiology at the microcircuit level will be disclosed together with their theoretical framework [8, 9]. The best treatment to relieve some signs and symptoms of PD is the administration of dopaminergic agonists, mainly L-DOPA. However, the long-term administration of L-DOPA produces other movement disorders: L-DOPA-induced dyskinesias (LIDs). There are three well-characterized types of LID [10]. (1) Peak dose dyskinesia, which is the most common, occurs in 80% of patients at peak of dopamine concentrations derived from L-DOPA ("on" time). (2) Diphasic dyskinesia, that occurs at the rising and falling of L-DOPA's clinical useful concentrations. (3) Early morning dystonia, that occurs when dopamine levels are very low, commonly after patients spent nighttime without L-DOPA.

LID is characterized by abnormal and involuntary movements which seem to appear randomly. It is often extremely disabling. 50% of the patients present it between 4 and 5 years after starting treatment and 75% after 10 years of treatment [11, 12]. To study this kind of dyskinesia, the 6-OHDA rodent model is treated with high doses of L-DOPA during several days and it is evaluated by counting abnormal involuntary movements (AIMs): locomotive, limb, axial, and orolingual [13]. Here, this model was used to study the dyskinetic pathophysiology at the microcircuit level [9]. We propose the study of the BG at the microcircuit level in order to better understand the detailed pathophysiology of these movement disorders.

2. Striatal microcircuit

The BG contains subcortical nuclei involved in motor coding: selection, generation, learning, and control of movements [14]. The nuclei of the BG are the striatum, the external and internal segments of the *globus pallidus* (GPe & GPi), the subthalamic nucleus (STN), and the *substantia nigra pars compacta* (SNc), and *substantia nigra pars reticulata* (SNr). The main input of the BG is the striatum, which receives glutamatergic afferents from the cortex and the thalamus, and dopaminergic terminals from the SNc [15]. The striatal microcircuit contains different neural classes. A general classification separates the spiny projection neurons (SPNs) from the interneurons. The SPNs are the 95% of the striatal neural population and they have collateral synapses between them at distances less than 100 μm [16–18]. The SPNs are divided in two populations: direct pathway SPNs (dSPNs) that connect monosynaptically to the BG output nuclei, GPi and SNr, and the indirect pathway SPNs (iSPNs) that send synaptic terminals to the GPe. Normally, SPNs have little spontaneous activity until they are activated by an excitatory drive, defined as afferents, neurotransmitter agonists, or modulators that induce the microcircuit to produce alternant neural activity [19]. When SPNs are activated, they show particular temporal patterns with oscillations between two distinct states: one with a hyperpolarized membrane potential or downstate at around −80mV, and the second with membrane potential depolarizations that last hundreds of milliseconds or seconds, the upstate, at around −50 mV [20]. It is during the upstate that SPNs fire action potentials, better respond to synaptic inputs and concert their firing with other SPNs conforming active neuronal ensembles.

On the other hand, the interneurons conform the remaining 5% of the population [15]. One class of interneuron expresses choline acetyltransferase (ChAT) with axons extending more than 1 mm. Other classes of interneurons are GABAergic and they are divided in numerous types: the fast spiking interneurons, which express parvalbumin (PV) and/or serotonin receptors (5-HT3); the low threshold spike interneurons (LTS), which could be further subdivided and may express or coexpress neuropeptide Y (NPY), somatostatin (SOM), nitric oxide synthase (NOS), or else, serotonin receptors (5-HT3), or calretinin, there are also neurogliaform interneurons (NGF), and other types still being studied [21–23]. The axonal arborizations of most interneurons may reach up to 1 mm. The exact combination of connections between these neuronal classes is still under study using electrophysiological recordings and optogenetics. There may be several valid combinations depending on function or context and further research is necessary to find out each of them.

The traditional model of the two pathways [24–25] propose that in control conditions there is an equilibrium between the activity of the direct pathway (dSPNs), which promotes movement, and the indirect pathway (iSPNs) which inhibits movement. Therefore, the balanced activation of both pathways produce coordinated movements. It is posited that in PD there is an imbalanced activity between these pathways: the activity of iSPNs becoming more important producing greater inhibition of movements. In contrast, during LID there is more activity in the direct pathway producing more involuntary movements. Unfortunately, these explanations are not supported by some experiments in monkeys, where these differences in activity were not observed [4]. Therefore, instead of staying at cellular level descriptions, in this work, we describe the interactions or functional connections between neuronal ensembles of the striatal microcircuit at the functional histological level in living brain tissue. This approach may help to identify what changes characterize control and pathological microcircuits to then ask, in future experiments, what cellular elements produce them.

3. Striatal cell assemblies

In the history of neuroscience, ideas about how neural activity is organized, one of them stands out: the cell assembly hypothesis. This hypothesis was formally proposed in its modern form by Hebb in 1949 [26] and defines a cell assembly as a group of interconnected neurons dedicated to code motor processes or to store and maintain neural representations. This hypothesis is based on long-term synaptic plasticity and has been modified to include both long-term potentiation and depression (LTP and LTD). It postulates that the changes in synaptic weights due to synaptic plasticity produce preferential connections and circuits for the flow of activity within and between neuronal ensembles, making up neural circuits. Experiments in small areas of tissue have shown these ensembles, which exhibit recurrence and alternation in their activity. The flow of activity generates spatiotemporal sequences and reverberations that correlate with behavior [27–34].

In cerebral slices, the activity of some neural circuits may be facilitated by an excitatory drive [19]. In striatal slices of rodents, microcircuits are almost silent, therefore to induce their activation one may use an excitatory drive such as N-methyl-D-aspartate (NMDA) [35]. However, circuits may also be activated by an adequate electrical stimulus in the cortex or the thalamus without the use of any chemical transmitter (unpublished). Recording the activity of dozens of neurons in the striatum using calcium imaging, the alternation and recurrence of so-called "network states," conformed by coactive sets of neurons or neurons that have correlated firing between them as expected for cell assemblies or ensembles [36], have been observed. It has also been shown that this activity could also depend on the short-term plasticity of the synaptic connections [37] and their ever-changing mutual innervation.

In tissue from the Parkinsonian rodent model, the striatal microcircuit is observed as overactive, not quite silent or with little activity as in control conditions. This excess in activity occurs without any excitatory drive or stimulus. However, a network state becomes dominant during the alternation of activity between neuronal ensembles attracting most active neurons and being more recurrent [8]. In this way, the circuit is metaphorically trapped by one network state, decreasing alternation and resembling what is seen in the patient who has trouble in changing or initiating a movement. Pharmacological bioassays in the striatum have been performed while observing the Parkinsonian overactivity. Adding L-DOPA [38] or nicotine [39] to the Parkinsonian striatal circuit reduced this activity and returned the circuit to resemble control conditions. To go beyond alternation and recurrence of network states, the dynamics of transitions between these states has been analyzed [9, 40], and a temporal sequence of these transitions was constructed using Eulerian paths—where every transition is traveled once—the paths that form the dynamics were then analyzed. In control conditions, more than a half of the sequences are closed forming reverberations. But in Parkinsonian and dyskinetic conditions, most transitions conformed open Eulerian paths [9]. In addition to the temporal dynamics of cell assemblies, neural network analysis was performed to compare control and pathological conditions.

4. Network analysis in neuroscience

Network analysis is a branch of discrete mathematics known as graph theory, which started in 1736 thanks to the mathematician Leonard Euler. Basically, a graph is a set of nodes and the links or edges between them. Nodes could be people, brain areas, neurons, etc., and links could be some relation between them: friendship, anatomical connections, synapses, action of modulators, etc. In the last 15 years, the interest included complex networks, which are characterized by irregular and complex structures evolving in time [41]. Complex networks may maintain their properties despite changes in scale: temporal or spatial [42]. To study cerebral connectivity, anatomical and functionally, this theoretical framework is being used in many areas of neuroscience: neuroanatomy, neurodevelopment, cognitive neuroscience, etc. [43, 44]. Sporns and Hagmann, simultaneously and independently, called "connectome" to the network of connections that make up a brain [45, 46]. This concept has been extended to include functional connectivity of any kind, obtaining functional connectomes [47]. Functional connectivity refers to the associations that relate the activity between the elements of the cerebral network, not necessarily anatomical, for example, the coactivity between cerebral areas, nucleus or neurons [9], their correlations [48] or coherence [49]. Network analysis in neuroscience has shown a hierarchical organization and scale-free connectivity at different scales: microcircuits [9, 50], larger circuits [51, 52], and the whole brain [49]. The characterization of functional connectomes using quantitative parameters allows compare the complexity of the neuronal interactions between control, pathological or pharmacological treated conditions.

5. Functional connectome of the striatal microcircuit

Network analysis at the microcircuit level started recently [9, 43, 51]. Here, we describe the analysis of the striatal microcircuit. The first step to get a functional connectome is to define the nodes and a specific functional connection between them. In the striatum, cell assemblies were analyzed at histological level by taking the neurons as the nodes and the coactivity between neurons as the functional links [9]. However, other functional links are being assayed and a consistency between different approaches is being observed (unpublished). In the present case, each neuron is functionally connected with other neurons when they are active during the same minimal time window. At the end of the recording the neural network or, more specifically, the functional connectome is obtained. The next step is to measure the parameters of the connectome to answer what kind of topology the network has and whether there are neurons with particular connections. To determine whether the network has random connectivity or regular connectivity, two main parameters are used: the characteristic path length (L) and the clustering coefficient (C) [41]. These two metrics were then compared with models of random and regular networks. A main observation was that the striatal connectome has neither random nor regular connectivity, but has properties of both at an intermediate point [9] known as "small-world" networks, which belong to the set of complex networks [53]. Other property found for the striatal microcircuit was free-scale, i.e., the same properties are maintained at different temporal and spatial scales. This property seen in the striatal microcircuit [9], has also been found in somatosensory, auditory, and primary motor cortices microcircuits [50, 51]. To determine the scale-free property, the distribution of connections P(k) was obtained. Next, we observed that this distribution could be fitted to a power law function indicating that it is a scale-free network [54]: there are few neurons with many connections and many neurons with few connections. In other words, there are some particular neurons that have the most connections in the network, so-called "hub neurons," that play a key role in the connectivity: they provide the physical substrate to have mutual innervation and connect different ensembles. Since Sherrington description, this property is necessary to alternate activity between ensembles. Even if a network is scale-free, it does not mean that has a modular organization as hypothesized for brain microcircuits [55–57]. Thus, a next question to answer was whether the connectome is constituted hierarchically, in a modular way. This was shown to be the case because the distribution of clustering coefficients C(k) of the nodes were also well fitted to a power law function [58]. Thus, a modular architecture has been seen in the striatal microcircuit [9], as well as in the somatosensory and auditory cortices microcircuits [51]. In summary, the striatal microcircuit connectome is a complex network, with "small-world" and scale-free properties forming hierarchical modules. In addition, network analysis allowed to describe with single neuron resolution some particular neurons identified by their connectivity as "hub neurons."

6. Key role of hub neurons

Since some neurons can be identified by their particular connectivity as hub neurons, the next step is to know what class of neurons they are. There are evidences that some hub neurons are interneurons (unpublished). The functional connectome in the striatum was observed in an area of about 1 mm^2 with hub neurons connecting many neurons at distances larger than 500 μm, while synapses between projection neurons can only be found at a distances less than 100 μm [16–18]. Indeed, only interneurons can extend their axons to connect neurons at distances up to 1 mm. This inference was confirmed by whole cell patch clamp recordings of some hub neurons identifying fast-spiking (PV), low-threshold spiking (LTS) and cholinergic interneurons (ACh) [9, 36]. Transgenic mice in which optogenetic stimulation activates a particular neural population [59] shows that hub neurons connect with different groups of neurons perhaps inducing the coactivity that underlies network states, and therefore, are responsible for their alternation. However, further experiments using transgenic animals and optogenetics are needed to identify the classes of neurons that form striatal modular circuits and under what conditions.

7. Pathological changes in the functional connectome

To know the role of cortical afferents in the striatal microcircuit, we used decorticated striatal slices. The decorticated striatal microcircuit preserves some active network states conforming temporal sequences, albeit alternation between ensembles is greatly reduced. In fact, network analysis revealed a loss of active hub neurons [9]. This result suggested that cortical afferents maintain privileged connections with striatal hub neurons, probably interneurons, to organize striatal activity.

Similarly, in the rodent model of Parkinson's disease, there is a significant loss of hub active neurons. Not strangely, the Parkinsonian striatal microcircuit shows less transitions between network states, confirming that one larger neuronal ensemble becomes dominant [8, 38], recruiting the majority of active neurons [9]. These results indicate that the majority of hub neurons are functionally eliminated during dopamine deprivation and a remaining set of hub neurons help to maintain the dominant state. This is supported by studies that suggest a breakdown of corticostriatal connectivity during Parkinson's disease [60, 61]. Other studies show potentiation of synaptic currents of some classes of interneurons [62, 63]. It is also known that drugs as L-DOPA or nicotine could return the microcircuit to control conditions [38, 39], implying that hub neurons are not physically eliminated during dopamine deprivation. The role of the interneurons has been recently addressed [9], since previous studies did not consider them [64].

In the L-DOPA-induced dyskinesia model, the microcircuit keeps showing a significant increase in activity with respect to the controls. In fact, more functional connections and even more hub neurons, and more transitions between network states correlate with the increase of prokinetic gamma rhythms described in dyskinetic subjects [65]. The "return" of hub neurons confirmed that they were not physically but only functionally removed during the Parkinsonian state. Their reappearance during dyskinesia indicates that they are necessary in the striatal microcircuit to produce movements. Nevertheless, the dyskinetic striatal microcircuit exhibited a loss of hierarchical modules [9]. This finding could be seen as a correlate of the excessive disordered movements present in dyskinetic subjects.

8. Primitive process in the striatal microcircuit

It is well known that pyramidal neurons connect preferentially to interneuron pools and not to the projections neurons or motoneurons in the spinal cord [66]. Thus, the present findings suggest a principle of general organization, which can explain how the same cell assemblies could be used in different behaviors depending on the activation of certain hub neurons by the cortical commands. According to Huyck [31, 67], any neural model at the microcircuit level should fulfill a primitive process: to have an input that selects the operators, apply operators on the operands, store results, and generate an output. In the striatum, the working hypothesis would be that input coming from the cortex selects the interneurons—operators—and apply their operations on the projections neurons—operands—the information is stored and striatal output is generated, the result of the whole operation: activation and inhibition of agonist and antagonist muscles in sequence (**Figure 1**). This hypothesis implies that cortical afferents organize groups of interneurons to induce the activity in a similar way as in the processes described by the cognitive theory of Allen Newel [31, 67]. Being the hub neurons the operators and the projections neurons the operands, the process of alternating network states, the sequences and the reverberations could underlie the actions of minimal motor routines [29]. Each microcircuit could be associated with others to produce different actions, depending on the group of operators activated by the cortex. This would explain the changes in the dynamics of the microcircuit and the functional relations between their neurons [68]. Now, there is technology to record several simultaneous neurons *in vivo* at the microcircuit level to study the functional connectome under different behaviors. Thus, the multiple combinations of connections being described at the cellular level may make sense.

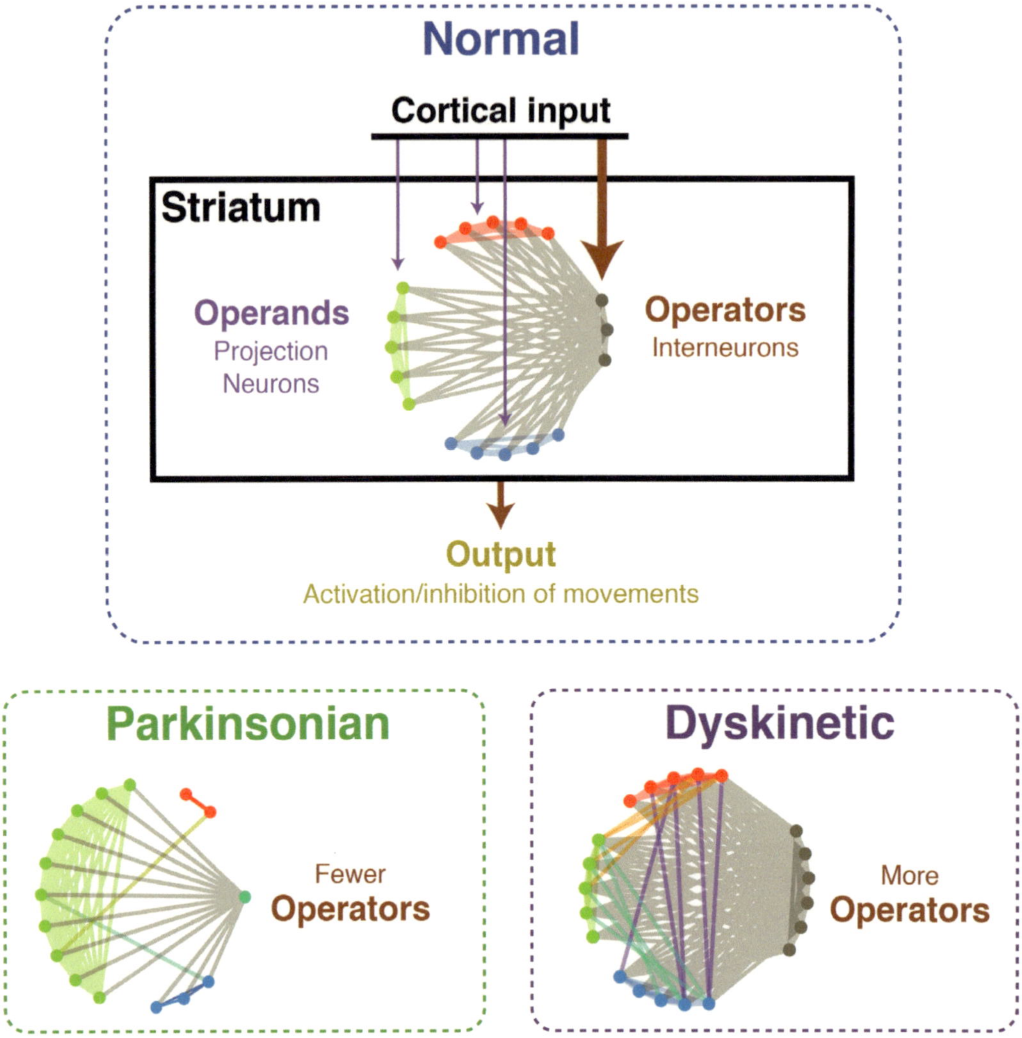

Figure 1. New model of cell assemblies activation in the striatal microcircuit.

9. Final conclusions

In this chapter, studies at the microcircuit histological level are remarked. There are many problems when jumping from the cellular/molecular level to the systems level without knowing what happens at microcircuit level when trying to understand how the brain works. The output seen at the systems level is the product of the microcircuits specific to each area, not of particular neurons or synapses; assumed in the cellular/molecular paradigm. To bridge the gap, analysis and perspectives from the microcircuit level are necessary [43, 69].

Using network analysis at the microcircuit level, it is observed that the striatal microcircuit has a set of highly connected hub neurons, which communicate efficiently with different neural groups. These groups underlie the neural states that alternate and reverberate. The structure of the striatal connectome has "small-world" properties, is scale-free and has a hierarchical modular organization, as other complex networks seen in nature. The cortical commands use the hub neurons to organize the dynamics of the circuit and given the distances between the neurons that conform a neuronal ensemble, it can be inferred that hub neurons should be long axon neurons, that is, interneurons. After striatal decortication or during the 6-OHDA model of Parkinson's disease hub neurons decrease significantly and as a consequence, the transitions between ensembles and circuit dynamics decrease, reflecting metaphorically hypokinesia and rigidity, and supporting previous studies that show a breakdown of corticostriatal communication in Parkinsonian subjects. In L-DOPA-induced dyskinesia, the opposite happens: the number of hub neurons and the transitions between ensembles increase. However, this occurs together with a loss of the hierarchical architecture. This also is reminiscent of the signs seen in dyskinetic subjects: uncoordinated involuntary movements. Finally, we conclude that the pathophysiology and pharmacology of the nervous system can be studied in living tissue at histological scale by using simultaneous recording and network analysis.

Author details

Jesús Pérez-Ortega and José Bargas*

*Address all correspondence to: jbargas@ifc.unam.mx

División de Neurociencias, Instituto de Fisiología Celular, Universidad Nacional Autónoma de México, Mexico City, Mexico

References

[1] Kalia LV, Lang AE. Parkinson's disease. Lancet. 2015;**386**:896-912

[2] Ascherio A, Schwarzschild MA. The epidemiology of Parkinson's disease: Risk factors and prevention. The Lancet Neurology. 2016;**15**:1257-1272

[3] Obeso JA, Olanow CW, Nutt JG. Levodopa motor complications in Parkinson's disease. Trends in Neurosciences. 2000;**23**:S2-S7

[4] Jenner P. Molecular mechanisms of L-DOPA-induced dyskinesia. Nature Reviews Neuroscience. 2008;**9**(9):665-677

[5] Ungerstedt U. 6-Hydroxy-dopamine induced degeneration of central monoamine neurons. European Journal of Pharmacology. 1968;**5**(1):107-110

[6] Schwarting R, Huston J. The unilateral 6-hydroxydopamine lesion model in behavioral brain research. Analysis of functional deficits, recovery and treatments. Progress in Neurobiology. 1996;**50**(2-3):275-331

[7] Simola N, Morelli M, Carta AR. The 6-Hydroxydopamine model of Parkinson's disease. Neurotoxicity Research. 2007;**11**(3-4):151-167

[8] Jáidar O, Carrillo-Reid L, Hernández A, Drucker-Colín R, Bargas J, Hernández-Cruz A. Dynamics of the Parkinsonian striatal microcircuit: Entrainment into a dominant network state. The Journal of Neuroscience. 2010;**30**(34):11326-11336

[9] Pérez-Ortega J, Duhne M, Lara-González E, et al. Pathophysiological signatures of functional connectomics in Parkinsonian and dyskinetic striatal microcircuits. Neurobiology of Disease. 2016;**91**:347-361

[10] Zesiewicz TA, Sullivan KL, Hauser RA. Levodopa-induced dyskinesia in Parkinson's disease: Epidemiology, etiology, and treatment. Current Neurology and Neuroscience Reports. 2007;**7**:302-310

[11] Bargiotas P, Konitsiotis S. Levodopa-induced dyskinesias in Parkinson's disease: Emerging treatments. Neuropsychiatric Disease and Treatment. 2013;**9**:1605-1617

[12] Obeso JA, Rodriguez-Oroz MC, Stamelou M, Bhatia KP, Burn DJ. The expanding universe of disorders of the basal ganglia. Lancet. 2014;**384**(9942):523-531

[13] Cenci MA, Lundblad M. Ratings of L-DOPA-induced dyskinesia in the unilateral 6-OHDA lesion model of Parkinson's disease in rats and mice. Current Protocols in Neuroscience. 2007;**Chapter 9**(October):Unit 9.25

[14] Graybiel AM. Building action repertoires: Memory and learning functions of the basal ganglia. Current Opinion in Neurobiology. 1995;**5**(6):733-741

[15] Gerfen CR, Bolam JP. The neuroanatomical organization of the basal ganglia. In: Steiner H, Tseng KY, editors. Handbook of Basal Ganglia Structure and Function. London: Elsevier; 2010. p. 3-28

[16] Czubayko U, Plenz D. Fast synaptic transmission between striatal spiny projection neurons. Proceedings of the National Academy of Sciences of the United States of America. 2002;**99**(24):15764-15769

[17] Taverna S, Ilijic E, Surmeier DJ. Recurrent collateral connections of striatal medium spiny neurons are disrupted in models of Parkinson's disease. Journal of Neuroscience. 2008;**28**(21):5504-5512

[18] Tunstall MJ, Oorschot DE, Kean A, Wickens JR. Inhibitory interactions between spiny projection neurons in the rat striatum. Journal of Neurophysiology. 2002;**88**(3): 1263-1269

[19] Grillner S. Biological pattern generation: The cellular and computational logic of networks in motion. Neuron. 2006;**52**(5):751-766

[20] Wilson C, Kawaguchi Y. The origins of two-state spontaneous membrane potential fluctuations of neostriatal spiny neurons. Journal of Neuroscience. 1996;**16**(7):2397-2410

[21] Kawaguchi Y, Wilson CJ, Augood SJ, Emson PC. Striatal interneurones: Chemical, physiological and morphological characterization. Trends in Neurosciences. 1995;**18**(12):527-535

[22] Tepper JM, Bolam JP. Functional diversity and specificity of neostriatal interneurons. Current Opinion in Neurobiology. 2004;**14**(6):685-692

[23] Ibáñez-Sandoval O, Tecuapetla F, Unal B, Shah F, Koós T, Tepper JM. A novel functionally distinct subtype of striatal neuropeptide Y interneuron. Journal of Neuroscience. 2011;**31**(46):16757-16769

[24] Albin RL, Young AB, Penney JB. The functional anatomy of basal ganglia disorders. Trends in Neurosciences. 1989;**12**(10):366-375

[25] Kravitz AV, Freeze BS, Parker PRL, et al. Regulation of Parkinsonian motor behaviours by optogenetic control of basal ganglia circuitry. Nature. 2010;**466**(7306):622-626

[26] Hebb DO. The Organization of Behavior. New York: Wiley; 1949

[27] Bakhurin KI, Mac V, Golshani P, Masmanidis SC. Temporal correlations among functionally specialized striatal neural ensembles in reward-conditioned mice. Journal of Neurophysiology. 2016;**115**(3):1SS521-1532

[28] Carrillo-Reid L, Miller J-EK, Hamm JP, Jackson J, Yuste R. Endogenous sequential cortical activity evoked by visual stimuli. Journal of Neurophysiology. 2015;**35**(23):8813-8828

[29] Cui G, Jun SB, Jin X, et al. Concurrent activation of striatal direct and indirect pathways during action initiation. Nature. 2013;**494**(7436):238-242

[30] Harris KD. Neural signatures of cell assembly organization. Nature Reviews Neuroscience. 2005;**6**(5):399-407

[31] Huyck CR. Cell assemblies as an intermediate level model of cognition. In: Wermter S, Austin J, Willshaw D, editors. Emergent Neural Computational Architectures Based on Neuroscience. Vol. 2036. Berlin: Springer; 2001. p. 383-397

[32] Lansner A. Associative memory models: From the cell-assembly theory to biophysically detailed cortex simulations. Trends in Neurosciences. 2009;**32**(3):178-186

[33] Markram H, Muller E, Ramaswamy S, et al. Reconstruction and simulation of neocortical microcircuitry. Cell. 2015;**163**(2):456-492

[34] Miller J-EK, Ayzenshtat I, Carrillo-Reid L, Yuste R. Visual stimuli recruit intrinsically generated cortical ensembles. Proceedings of the National Academy of Sciences. 2014;**111**(38):E4053-E4061

[35] Vergara R, Rick C, Hernández-López S, et al. Spontaneous voltage oscillations in striatal projection neurons in a rat corticostriatal slice. Journal of Physiology. 2003;**553**(Pt 1): 169-182

[36] Carrillo-Reid L, Tecuapetla F, Tapia D, et al. Encoding network states by striatal cell assemblies. Journal of Neurophysiology. 2008;**99**(3):1435-1450

[37] Carrillo-Reid L, Lopez-Huerta VG, Garcia-Munoz M, Theiss S, Arbuthnott GW. Cell assembly signatures defined by short-term synaptic plasticity in cortical networks. International Journal of Neural Systems. 2015;**25**(7):1550026

[38] Plata V, Duhne M, Pérez-Ortega JE, et al. Global actions of nicotine on the striatal microcircuit. Frontiers in Systems Neuroscience. 2013;7(November):78

[39] Plata V, Duhne M, Pérez-Ortega JE, Barroso-Flores J, Galarraga E, Bargas J. Direct evaluation of L-DOPA actions on neuronal activity of Parkinsonian tissue in vitro. BioMed Research International. 2013;**2013**:519184

[40] Carrillo-Reid L, Tecuapetla F, Vautrelle N, et al. Muscarinic enhancement of persistent sodium current synchronizes striatal medium spiny neurons. Journal of Neurophysiology. 2009;**102**(2):682-690

[41] Boccaletti S, Latora V, Moreno Y, Chavez M, Hwang D. Complex networks: Structure and dynamics. Physics Reports. 2006;**424**(4-5):175-308

[42] Marković D, Gros C. Power laws and self-organized criticality in theory and nature. Physics Reports. 2014;**536**(2):41-74

[43] Feldt S, Bonifazi P, Cossart R. Dissecting functional connectivity of neuronal microcircuits: Experimental and theoretical insights. Trends in Neurosciences. 2011;**34**(5):225-236

[44] Sporns O. Networks of the Brain. MIT Press; 2011. Cambridge, Massachusetts

[45] Sporns O, Tononi G, Kötter R. The human connectome: A structural description of the human brain. PLoS Computational Biology. 2005;**1**(4):e42

[46] Hagmann P. From diffusion MRI to brain connectomics [thesis]; 2005

[47] Biswal BB, Mennes M, Zuo X-N, et al. Toward discovery science of human brain function. Proceedings of the National Academy of Sciences. 2010;**107**(10):4734-4739

[48] Zuo X-N, Ehmke R, Mennes M, et al. Network centrality in the human functional connectome. Cerebral Cortex. 2012;**22**(8):1862-1875

[49] Sporns O, Betzel RF. Modular brain networks. Annual Review of Psychology. 2016;**67**(1):613-640

[50] Beggs JM, Plenz D. Neuronal avalanches in neocortical circuits. Journal of Neuroscience. 2003;**23**(35):11167-11177

[51] Sadovsky AJ, JN ML. Scaling of topologically similar functional modules defines mouse primary auditory and somatosensory microcircuitry. Journal of Neuroscience. 2013;**33**(35):14048-14060

[52] Sporns O, Bullmore ET. From connections to function: The mouse brain connectome atlas. Cell. 2014;**157**(4):773-775

[53] Watts DJ, Strogatz SH. Collective dynamics of "small-world" networks. Nature. 1998;**393**(6684):440-442

[54] Barabási A-L, Albert R. Emergence of scaling in random networks. Science. 1999;**286**(5439):509-512

[55] Eichenbaum HB, Davis JL. Biological neural networks. In: Eichenbaum HB, Davis JL, editors. Neuronal Ensembles: Strategies for Recording and Decoding. New York: Wiley-Liss; 1998. p. 1-15

[56] Kumar A, Rotter S, Aertsen A. Spiking activity propagation in neuronal networks: Reconciling different perspectives on neural coding. Nature Reviews Neuroscience. 2010;**11**(9):615-627

[57] Mountcastle VB. Perceptual Neuroscience: The Cerebral Cortex. Cambridge, MA: Harvard University Press; 1998

[58] Ravasz E, Barabasi A. Hierarchical organization in complex networks. Physical Review E. 2003;**67**(2):26112

[59] Boyden ES, Zhang F, Bamberg E, Nagel G, Deisseroth K. Millisecond-timescale, genetically targeted optical control of neural activity. Nature Neuroscience. 2005;**8**(9):1263-1268

[60] Hammond C, Bergman H, Brown P. Pathological synchronization in Parkinson's disease: Networks, models and treatments. Trends in Neurosciences. 2007;**30**(7):357-364

[61] Stephens B, Mueller AJ, Shering AF, et al. Evidence of a breakdown of corticostriatal connections in Parkinson's disease. Neuroscience. 2005;**132**:741-754

[62] Barroso-Flores J, Herrera-Valdez MA, Lopez-Huerta VG, Galarraga E, Bargas J. Diverse short-term dynamics of inhibitory synapses converging on striatal projection neurons: Differential changes in a rodent model of Parkinson's disease. Neural Plasticity. 2015;**2015**:1-13

[63] Dehorter N, Guigoni C, Lopez C, et al. Dopamine-deprived striatal GABAergic interneurons burst and generate repetitive gigantic IPSCs in medium spiny neurons. Journal of Neuroscience. 2009;**29**(24):7776-7787

[64] Huot P, Johnston TH, Koprich JB, Fox SH, Brotchie JM. The pharmacology of L-DOPA-induced dyskinesia in Parkinson's disease. Pharmacological Reviews. 2013;**65**(1):171-222

[65] Dupre KB, Cruz AV, McCoy AJ, et al. Effects of L-DOPA priming on cortical high beta and high gamma oscillatory activity in a rodent model of Parkinson's disease. Neurobiology of Disease. 2015;**86**:1-15

[66] Eichenbaum H. The Cognitive Neuroscience of Memory. Boston: Oxford University Press; 2002

[67] Newel A. Unified Theories of Cognition. Cambridge, MA: Harvard University Press; 1990

[68] Surmeier DJ, Carrillo-Reid L, Bargas J. Dopaminergic modulation of striatal neurons, circuits, and assemblies. Neuroscience. 2011;**198**:3-18

[69] Grillner S. Megascience efforts and the brain. Neuron. 2014;**82**(6):1209-1211

Section 2

Endocrine Pathophysiology

Chapter 4

Transthyretin in the Evaluation of Health and Disease in Human and Veterinary Medicine

Csilla Tóthová and Oskar Nagy

Additional information is available at the end of the chapter

http://dx.doi.org/10.5772/intechopen.68725

Abstract

Transthyretin (also known as prealbumin) is an important transport protein, which plays an essential role in the binding of thyroid hormones and retinol with varying affinities in mammalian, as well as avian species. The determination of transthyretin concentrations may be used as a diagnostic tool for some disease conditions in humans, but is more often used as a nutritional marker to assess protein-calorie malnutrition and as prognostic indicator in critically ill patients. Transthyretin has shorter half-life (2–3 days) than that of albumin and belongs to negative acute phase proteins. This may complicate the use of transthyretin as a nutritional marker and the interpretation of results in the diagnosis of diseases. Although some studies have been carried out to determine the usefulness of transthyretin in selected disease conditions and disorders also in animals, it is a relatively rarely used parameter to evaluate health state and illness in veterinary medicine. The usefulness of transthyretin in the diagnosis of diseases and evaluation of nutritional status in humans and animals are reviewed in this article, including the laboratory assays available to measure its concentrations and the possible clinical application of the results, as well as its usefulness as a prognostic indicator in some disease conditions.

Keywords: disease marker, nutritional state, prealbumin, serum proteins, transthyretin

1. Introduction

Transthyretin is an important transport protein of the blood, which was originally named prealbumin because it migrates faster than albumin, and is visible as a band anodic to the main albumin fraction on electrophoretic gels [1]. According to Hamilton and Benson [2], this property is attributed to human prealbumin, not to bovine. Kaneko [3] reported that prealbumin is not always visualized on electrophoretograms and may not exist in all animal species. In the 1980s, the name was changed to transthyretin (TTR) describing its ability to bind both thyroid hormones and retinol-binding protein (RBP) [4]. Moreover, transthyretin is one of the precursors, which may be found in amyloid deposits [5]. In humans, analyses of the concentrations of TTR in serum are recommended by some investigators as a screening marker for inflammation, malnutrition, or both [6]. In animals, there are only scarce literature data about this protein as a biomarker of health state and its use in the laboratory diagnosis [7].

2. Structure

Transthyretin is a small globular non-glycosylated tryptophan-rich protein of a homotetrameric structure, composed of four identical subunits with two thyroxine-binding sites per tetramer [8]. The binds for retinol-binding protein are placed at the surface of the molecule and do not interfere with thyroxin binding (**Figure 1**) [9]. Its molecular mass is of 54.98 kDa, which is small enough to penetrate the vascular wall and migrate into the extravascular space as easily as albumin or transferrin [10]. In some conditions, the transthyretin molecules may aggregate and form insoluble fibrillar deposits, which may be associated with amyloid diseases, predominantly senile systemic amyloidosis or neurodegenerative familial amyloidotic polyneuropathy [11, 12].

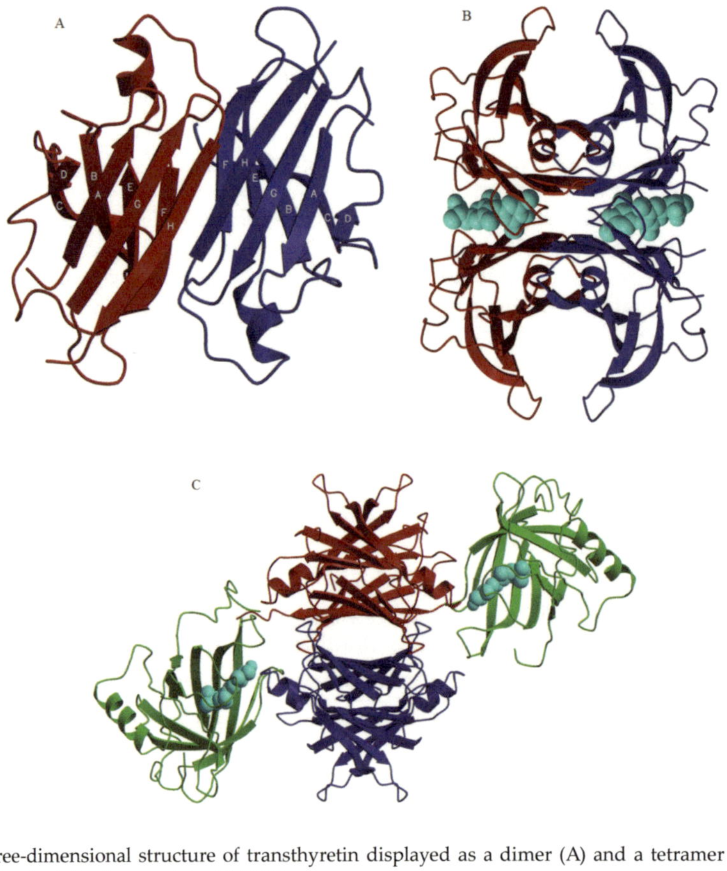

Figure 1. The three-dimensional structure of transthyretin displayed as a dimer (A) and a tetramer in complex with thyroxine (B) and retinol-binding protein (C) [103].

3. Functions

Transthyretin is a serum protein with multiple functional properties [13]. The main physio logical functions of TTR include the carriage of thyroid hormone and indirectly vitamin A, which may promote the maturation of lymphocytes [14, 15]. Although each monomer of the TTR molecule has two binding sites for thyroid hormones, the binding of one molecule of T3 or T4 may reduce the binding affinity for the second site [6]. Moreover, the binding affinity for T3 is lower compared with that for T4. Transthyretin binds and transports approximately 15–20% of thyroid hormones circulating in the serum and up to 80% of thyroxine in the central nervous system (CNS) [16]. About 70% of thyroid hormones are transported by thyroxin-binding globulin (TBG), which is the major serum transport protein in humans [17]. The remaining part of thyroid hormones is transported by albumin. These proteins are responsible for the transporting of thyroid hormones to cells and maintaining a large store of these hormones in the blood in a non-diffusible form [2]. Among animal species, the concentration of TBG in the dog is only 15% of those observed in humans [18]. Cats do not appear to have a high-affinity thyroid-binding protein such as TBG, but have only transthyretin and albumin [19]. Some other small molecules may bind in the thyroxine-binding sites of TTR, including some natural products, drugs or toxicants [20]. These interactions with TTR may be important when TTR becomes a major circulating thyroxine-binding protein, for example, in humans with complete or partial TBG deficiency, or when the concentration of thyroxine in the serum is markedly increased [21].

In addition to the binding and carriage of thyroid hormones, transthyretin has a more important function, that is, the transport of retinol (vitamin A) through its association with retinol-binding protein (RBP) from its main storage site in the liver to target cells [22]. Retinol is bound to RBP, and then RBP binds to transthyretin. This binding of RBP to TTR was suggested to prevent the extensive loss of RBP, which is of low molecular weight and would be rapidly eliminated from plasma by glomerular filtration if it were not complexed to transthyretin [23, 24]. Although each of the four monomers has a binding site for RBP, the tetramer binds only one molecule of RBP with high affinity, and possibly a second with lower affinity [25].

Moreover, transthyretin acts as a negative acute phase reactant, serum concentrations of which fall due to decreased synthesis in inflammation, trauma, tissue injury or stress [26].

4. Synthesis

Transthyretin is synthesized mainly by hepatic parenchymal cells and in the choroid plexus of the brain, which has the highest concentration of TTR in the body [27, 28]. In cerebrospinal fluid, it is the second most abundant protein, which may be involved in the pathogenesis of Alzheimer's disease, depression and lead intoxication [29]. Other tissues have been reported also to produce TTR, but in much lower concentrations [30]. Small amounts of TTR are also produced by retinal pigment epithelium and the pineal gland [31]. Transthyretin has also been found in adult pancreatic islet cells, enterochromaffin cells in the gastrointestinal mucosa, as well as kidney cells [32, 33]. Neoplastic tissues, including choroid plexus papillomas, glucagonomas and gut carcinomas, have been reported also to secrete transthyretin [33]. During fetal life, TTR is synthesized by the embryonic yolk sac endothelium [34]. Any alteration in energy-to-protein balance impairs the body mass reserves and causes early depression in the production of transthyretin [35].

The major sites of transthyretin degradation are the liver, muscles and skin, but a small amount of TTR may be catabolized by other tissues, including kidneys, adipose tissues, testes, as well as the gastrointestinal tract [36]. Transthyretin has a half-life in plasma of approximately 2 days, which is much shorter than that of albumin [37]. Transthyretin is therefore more sensitive to changes in protein-energy status, but its concentrations closely reflect the recent nutritional status rather than the overall nutritional support [38, 39].

5. Laboratory assays

Transthyretin is considered a more sensitive indicator of visceral protein status than albumin and transferrin because of its short half-life and low concentration in the body [40]. Conventionally, radial immunodiffusion and electroimmunodiffusion have been used for routine determination of transthyretin in humans [41]. Faster and more precise immunonephelometric and immunoturbidimetric assays have been developed also, which are easily applicable to many laboratory-automated equipments available in hospitals [6, 42]. Moreover, a sensitive enzyme immunoassay (enzyme-linked immunosorbent assay (ELISA)) for the determination of TTR values has been described, but this method is more time consuming and expensive compared with the above mentioned, and is more applicable, for example, for the estimation of TTR in the cerebrospinal fluid in nanogram amounts [43]. In veterinary medicine, species-specific ELISA is the most common analytical tool for the detection and quantification of transthyretin, utilizing monoclonal anti-TTR antibodies. In some avian species, for example, in budgerigars (*Melopsittacus undulatus*) transthyretin (prealbumin) constitutes as high as 75% of the total albumin concentration [44]. Therefore, it may be visualized and quantified easily by protein electrophoresis.

6. Factors influencing the concentrations of TTR

The concentration of TTR in serum is affected by many factors, including age, gender, as well as blood-drawing methods. In humans, the concentrations of transthyretin increase gradually after birth until they reached the adult values of 20–40 mg/dL [45]. A progressive increase of TTR concentrations with postnatal age was reported also by Kanakoudi et al. [46] in infants. Similarly, Cardoso and Falção [47] observed a marked increase of TTR concentrations in the period from birth till day 28 of age in preterm infants with very low birth weight. According to these authors, the serum concentrations of transthyretin in this important period of life are associated with the recent protein status, and reflect the balance between synthesis and degradation. Moreover, MacDonald et al. [48] stated that TTR values may predict future weight gain and concluded that if the serum concentrations of TTR remain stable or increase, it can be expect that the newborn is in reasonable nitrogen balance and will gain weight subsequently. According to Benvenga et al. [49], the concentrations of TTR progressively decrease after 50–60 years. Approximately from the year 60 of age, muscle mass undergoes stepwise shrinking leading to sarcopenia, which may be responsible for the aforementioned decrease in the concentrations of TTR [50, 51]. In animals, the influence of age on the concentrations of TTR during the growth and development is not well described. A marked increase of TTR values from 72.9 to 251.4 mg/L was observed by Tóthová et al. [7] in calves 1 day after colostrum intake with a consecutive gradual decrease till the end of the third month of life. Rona [52] described that bovine colostrum contains among other bioactive molecules a small amount of prealbumin (transthyretin). Thus, the increase of serum TTR concentrations observed in calves after colostrum intake may reflect the adequate nutrition, as well as its hepatic synthesis due to adequate protein and energy intake [14]. In neonatal rats, low concentrations of TTR were found in the immediate postnatal period, which increases at the time when the concentrations of both thyroxine and corticosterone increase [53]. On the other hand, there were no significant differences in the serum concentrations of TTR in three different age groups of pigs from 10 to 25 weeks [54].

The concentrations of transthyretin linearly increase after birth without marked sexual differences during infant growth [55]. During human puberty, major hormonal and metabolic alterations occur, which result in increased height, weight gain and a substantial redistribution of body tissues. While androgens promote the development of muscle mass in male teenagers, oestrogens contribute to minimal enlargement of the female musculature and stimulate the accretion of subcutaneous fat depots [56]. These differences lead to higher concentrations of TTR in male adolescents compared with values recorded in teenage girls [57]. Higher concentrations of TTR in males compared with females were found also by Benvenga et al. [49] and Gaggiotti et al. [58]. Studies dealing with the evaluation of gender-related differences in the concentrations of TTR in animals were not found.

Pregnancy, hormonal changes, physiological status and stress are other factors that may influence the concentrations of transthyretin. In humans, the concentrations of TTR were evaluated by Zhu et al. [59] during normal pregnancy. The values of TTR increased significantly in the third month of gestation and rapidly decreased following 20 weeks of gestation. Transthyretin was measured also in females with severe preeclampsia, showing significantly decreased TTR concentrations in these patients compared with the control group. Transthyretin is synthesized also by placental trophoblasts, which are critical to the normal fetal development. Thus, disorders caused by the production of TTR may result in fetal distress [60]. The aforementioned results indicated that TTR may be a reliable biomarker for the diagnosis of severe preeclampsia [59]. Similarly, Kalkunte et al. [61] suggested a relationship between reduced TTR production and preeclampsia. The importance, functional role and alterations in the concentrations of TTR during pregnancy in animals have not been reported. Our findings suggest no significant changes in TTR concentrations during the last week of pregnancy and early stages of lactation in dairy cows (unpublished data). However, further evaluations are needed to establish the values of transthyretin and its possible changes in pregnant and lactating cows, which may be useful for veterinary practitioners in the early diagnosis, prevention and finding therapeutic solutions in periparturient dairy cows.

In humans, for the measurement of concentrations of TTR, it was recommended to take blood samples after 15–20 min in the sitting position [6]. Lower values are expected in bedridden patients, while standing position prior to blood sampling may result in higher concentrations.

7. The usefulness of transthyretin in the human clinical practice

7.1. Nutritional marker

Transthyretin may be used as important diagnostic tool for various disease conditions in humans, but is more often used as an indicator of malnutrition [62]. Several studies have shown a correlation between the concentrations of TTR and nutritional status [63, 64]. According to Ingenbleek and Young [14], low TTR concentrations are associated with inadequate protein calorie consumption or malnutrition. However, TTR may not serve as a reliable nutritional marker in patients with high concentrations of C-reactive protein (CRP), because of the activation of inflammatory responses [65]. This may complicate the use of TTR as an indicator of nutritional status, since inflammatory processes can lead to the decrease of serum TTR concentrations (negative acute phase protein) [66]. The CRP/TTR ratio may be a useful index in these cases to differentiate inflammatory states from protein malnutrition [67]. Very high ratios (>20) are indicative of acute phase response rather than protein malnutrition, while mild inflammatory processes may be accompanied by approximately a 10-fold increase in the concentrations of CRP and in CRP/TTR index values [6]. However, an inflammatory and nutrition index in animals was not yet established.

Surprisingly, extreme cases of starvation, including anorexia nervosa, have not been associated with a decrease of TTR concentrations. Nova et al. [68] reported normal values of transthyretin in patients with anorexia nervosa, which were comparable to values found in controls and did not differ after nutritional intervention. Barbe et al. [69] stated also that transthyretin concentrations in the majority of anorectic patients did not differ from those in control subjects, even in the presence of severe cachexia, but increased after weight gain. On the other hand, Gendall et al. [70] found lower concentrations of TTR in women with bulimia nervosa. These contradictory data indicate that further studies are needed to determine the effect of the aforementioned generalized malnutrition states on the values of transthyretin.

7.2. Disease marker

As transthyretin (prealbumin) belongs to negative acute phase proteins, its serum concentrations may be affected by many disease conditions, including trauma, inflammatory diseases, infections or malignancy (**Table 1**). Patients with severe sepsis or multiple injuries often have very low concentrations of TTR, related to severe acute phase response [71]. Studies have suggested that TTR may be a sensitive marker for the diagnosis of patients with liver cell damage, liver cirrhosis or hepatocellular carcinoma, reflecting the impaired liver synthetic function [72, 73]. Hutchinson et al. [74] and Yasmin et al. [75] found significantly lower concentrations of TTR in various types of chronic liver diseases when compared with controls with no impairment of liver functions. Moreover, Liu et al. [72] reported significantly lower

TTR values in patients who died compared to survivors suggesting its role in predicting the prognosis of patients with decompensated liver cirrhosis.

Pneumonia in children caused by *Mycoplasma pneumonia* was also associated with lower TTR concentrations compared to a healthy control group [76]. Similarly, Luo et al. [77] recorded reduced TTR values in patients with tuberculosis and lung cancer, while the serum concentrations of TTR were lower in patients suffering from tuberculosis than in patients with lung cancer. Moreover, the changes in TTR values were in accordance with the therapeutic effects of anti-tuberculosis drugs, which may be useful by the monitoring of therapy in these patients. However, seeing that nutritional imbalance is very common in patients with tuberculosis and after chemotherapy in subjects with lung cancer, poor performance status should be taken into consideration when interpreting serum TTR values in these patients and should be further investigated.

The concentrations of transthyretin may be altered also by thyroid diseases, especially endemic goitre [6]. Low concentrations of TTR were found by Vergani et al. [78] in patients with untreated thyrotoxicosis, but the values recorded in the majority of cases with untreated hypothyroidism were within normal range. The concentrations of transthyretin were measured also by Ishida et al. [79] in patients with various thyroidal states. In patients with untreated hyperthyroidism, markedly low serum TTR values were found, but were normalized by treating with anti-thyroid drug. Similarly, the aforementioned authors observed markedly low TTR concentrations in patients with subacute thyroiditis, but in patients with hypothyroidism the TTR values were within the normal range.

Changes in the concentrations of TTR were evaluated also in subjects affected by protein-losing enteropathy, which is characterized by marked losses of serum proteins through the bowel wall into the gastrointestinal tract resulting in hypoproteinaemia [80]. Despite hypoproteinaemia, Takeda et al. [81] observed TTR values within the normal range in patients with protein-losing gastroenteropathy. This phenomenon may be explained by the slightly increased production of rapidly turned-over proteins (including TTR) by the liver in response to the gastrointestinal losses.

Alteration	Associated disease condition
Decrease	Inflammatory diseases, infections, trauma, malignancy Severe sepsis, multiple injuries Liver cell damage, liver cirrhosis, hepatocellular carcinoma, chronic liver diseases
	Thyroid diseases, endemic goitre Protein-losing enteropathy
	Chronic malnutrition
Increase	Dehydration Chronic renal failure, renal insufficiency Anti-inflammatory therapy, anabolic steroids Acute alcohol intoxication Hodgkin's lymphoma, pancreatic cancer

Table 1. Abnormalities in the serum concentrations of transthyretin and associated diseases (adapted from Ref. [6]).

Increased serum concentrations of transthyretin are typically associated with chronic renal failure, presumably due to the decreased tubular uptake and degradation of RBP [82]. Cano [83] stated also that chronic renal failure may result in an increase of serum TTR concentrations, but these elevated TTR values during renal insufficiency are secondary to the lack of RBP degradation in renal tubules and to the subsequent increase in TTR. The concentrations of TTR may rise also during corticosteroid therapy and administration of anabolic steroids, as well as in patients using anti-inflammatory agents [6, 84]. Young et al. [85] found increased concentrations of TTR in ill-surgical patients receiving anabolic steroids, which may enhance amino acid and water uptake by tissues and increase the utilization of fat. Increased TTR concentrations may be seen in acute alcohol intoxication, caused by the leakage of proteins from damaged hepatic cells [86]. Transthyretin was shown to be upregulated also in Hodgkin´s lymphoma and pancreatic cancer [11, 87].

7.3. Prognostic indicator

Several studies evaluated the significance of TTR as a prognostic biomarker and suggested that low concentrations may be associated with poor prognosis [88, 89]. Transthyretin was found as a prognostic factor for treatment outcomes and/or nutritional status of colon, oesophagus, ovarian and lung cancers [90–92]. In these studies, the concentrations of TTR correlated with response to treatment and clinical outcomes. Ho et al. [93] reported that low values of TTR may serve as prognostic factor for overall survival in cancer patients. However, the interpretation of its values in patients with systemic inflammatory response may be challenging. In these conditions, further clinical assessments and laboratory assays may be helpful, including markers of inflammation such as C-reactive protein, erythrocyte sedimentation rate or white blood cell number.

According to Cheng et al. [94], TTR has also been identified as a significant predictor of clinical outcomes after surgical intervention. Therefore, it may be used as part of the blood screening completed before surgery to determine pre-surgery health. Low TTR values before surgery may be associated with an increased risk of complications, including infections or pneumonia. Devakonda et al. [88] reported that surgery patients with low preoperative TTR values had significantly longer hospital duration of stay and longer intensive care unit duration of stay. Moreover, low concentrations of transthyretin were associated with higher rates of infectious complications, mortality and other surgical complications [95, 96].

8. The usefulness of transthyretin in veterinary medicine

Despite the physiological importance of transthyretin in health and as disease marker, there are only a few studies analysing its usefulness in the clinical and laboratory diagnosis of diseases in animals. Studies performed in dogs suggested that not only quantitative but also qualitative differences exist between human and canine TTR [97]. Transthyretin from dog plasma was of lower molecular mass compared to human TTR in samples subjected to sodium dodecyl-polyacrylamide gel electrophoresis with subsequent Western blot analysis [98]. Piechotta et al. [99] investigated the serum concentrations of TTR in dogs with nonthyroidal illness (including neoplasia, allergy, cardiac disease, gastrointestinal disease, parasitism and hepatic disease) and low T4 concentrations compared with those in healthy dogs and dogs with primary hypothyroidism. They found significantly decreased serum concentrations of TTR in dogs with nonthyroidal illness (24.8 mg/L) compared with its concentration in hypothyroid dogs (41.1 mg/L). On the other hand, significant differences in TTR values were not found between hypothyroid and healthy dogs, or between dogs with nonthyroidal illness and healthy dogs. In the study presented by Raila et al. [100], low concentration of TTR was found in a young dog with chronic renal failure, probably caused by its increased urinary excretion. Changes in the serum concentrations of TTR were observed also in rats during protein-energy malnutrition [62]. The mean value of transthyretin in healthy pig serum obtained by Campbell et al. [54] was 302 ± 8 mg/L, but following *Streptococcus suis* type 2 infection the concentrations markedly decreased. In horses, transthyretin was identified using immunodiffusion technique, but the study was performed many years ago [101]. Establishing a quantitative method, such as an enzyme immunoassay, to measure the concentrations of TTR may be useful also in horses. In cattle, there are very little published reports about the usefulness of transthyretin in the diagnosis of diseases. Our preliminary results suggest lower concentrations of TTR in diarrhoic calves at the age of 1 month compared with healthy animals at the same age. Similarly, *Mycobacterium avium paratuberculosis* seropositive cows showed lower TTR values than those obtained in healthy cattle (unpublished data). Chang et al. [102] have isolated and sequenced transthyretin not only in humans and other mammalian species but also in birds, including emu, chicken, ostrich and pigeon. This study showed that TTR has greater than 98% homology and has a very similar binding pattern across species. However, additional studies should be done to determine the effect of various diseases on the serum concentrations of TTR in animals.

9. Conclusions

Presented data suggest that transthyretin may contribute to the evaluation of health state and diagnosis of some diseases also in animals. Changes in serum concentrations of TTR may be indicative of inadequate nutrient intake and may serve as an additional diagnostic tool for clinicians in the evaluation of some pathological conditions. It may be used as an integral part of the overall health assessment or in hospitalized animals to evaluate their nutritional status during the treatment and recovery. Low serum TTR concentrations may be considered a sign of increased risk of malnutrition, requiring further nutritional assessment.

Acknowledgement

This work was supported by Scientific Grant Agency of Ministry of Education SR Nos. 1/0154/15 and 1/0486/17.

Author details

Csilla Tóthová* and Oskar Nagy

*Address all correspondence to: tothova@uvm.sk

Clinic of Ruminants, University of Veterinary Medicine and Pharmacy, Košice, Slovakia

References

[1] Harris RI, Kohn J. The pre-albumin fraction: A useful parameter in the interpretation of routine protein electrophoresis. Journal of Clinical Pathology. 1974;**27**:986-989

[2] Hamilton JA, Benson MD. Transthyretin: A review from a structural perspective. CMLS Cell & Molecular Life Science. 2001;**58**:1491-1521

[3] Kaneko JJ. Serum proteins and the dysproteinemias. In: Kaneko JJ, editor. Clinical Biochemistry of Domestic Animals. 5th ed. London, UK: Academic Press; 1997. pp. 117-138

[4] Goodman DS, Peters T, Robbins J, Schwick G. Prealbumin becomes transthyretin. Journal of Biological Chemistry. 1981;**256**:12-14

[5] Skinner M, Cohen AS. The prealbumin nature of the amyloid protein in familial amyloidotic polyneuropathy (FAP). Biochemical and Biophysical Research Communications. 1981;**99**:1326-1332

[6] Johnson AM, Merlini G, Sheldon J, Ichibara K. Clinical indications for plasma protein assay: Transthyretin (prealbumin) in inflammation and malnutrition. Clinical Chemistry and Laboratory Medicine. 2007;**45**:419-426

[7] Tóthová C, Nagy O, Nagyová V, Kováč G. The concentrations of selected blood serum proteins in calves during the first three months of life. Acta Veterinaria Brno. 2016;**85**:33-40

[8] Foss TR, Wiseman RL, Kelly JW. The pathway by which the tetrameric protein transthyretin dissociates. Biochemistry. 2005;**44**:15525-15533

[9] Monaco HL, Rizzi M, Coda A. Structure of a complex of two plasma proteins: Transthyretin and retinol-binding protein. Science. 1995;**268**:1039-1041

[10] Ingbar SH. Pre-albumin: A thyroxin binding protein of human plasma. Endocrinology. 1958;**63**:256-259

[11] Saraiva MJM. Transthyretin mutations in hyperthyroxinemia and amyloid diseases. Human Mutations. 2001;**17**:493-503

[12] Morais-de-Sá E, Pereira PJB, Saraiva MJM, Damas AM. The crystal structure of transthyretin in complex with diethylstilbestrol: A promising template for the design of amyloid inhibitors. Journal of Biological Chemistry. 2004;**279**:53483-53490

[13] Buxbaum JN, Reixach N. Transthyretin: The servant of many masters. Cell & Molecular Life Science. 2009;**66**:3095-3101

[14] Ingenbleek Y, Young V. Transthyretin (prealbumin) in health and disease: Nutritional implications. Annual Review of Nutrition. 1994;**14**:495-533

[15] Aliyazicioglu Y, Deger O, Karahan C, Yildirmis S, Kucukoduk S. Reference values of cord blood transferrin, ceruloplasmin, alpha-1 antitrypsin, prealbumin, and alpha-2 macroglobulin concentrations in healthy term newborns. Turkish Journal of Pediatrics. 2007;**49**:52-54

[16] Hagen GA, Elliot WJ. Transport of thyroid hormones in serum and cerebrospinal fluid. Journal of Clinical Endocrinology. 1973;**37**:415-422

[17] Robbins J, Cheng S-Y, Gershengorn MC, Glinoer D, Cahnmann HJ, Edelnoch H. Thyroxine transport proteins in plasma: Molecular properties and biosynthesis. Recent Progress in Hormone Research. 1978;**34**:477-519

[18] Larsson M, Pettersson T, Carlstrom A. Thyroid hormone binding in serum of 15 vertebrate species: Isolation of thyroxine-binding globulin and prealbumin analogs. General and Comparative Endocrinology. 1985;**58**:360-375

[19] Bigler B. Thyroxine binding serum proteins in the cat as compared to dog and man. Schweiz Arch Tierheilkd. 1976;**118**:559-562

[20] Baures PW, Oza VB, Peterson SA, Kelly JW. Synthesis and evaluation of inhibitors of transthyretin amyloid formation based on the non-steroidal anti-inflammatory drug, flufenamic acid. Bioorganic & Medicinal Chemistry. 1999;**7**:1339-1347

[21] Munro SL, Lim CF, Hall JG, Barlow JW, Craik DJ, Topliss DJ, Stockigt JR. Drug competition for thyroxin binding to transthyretin (prealbumin): Comparison with effects on thyroxine-binding globulin. Journal of Clinical Endocrinology & Metabolism. 1989;**68**:1141-1147

[22] Kanai M, Raz A, Goodman D. Retinol binding protein: The transport protein for vitamin A in human plasma. Journal of Clinical Investigation. 1968;**47**:2025-2044

[23] Goodman DS, Raz A. Extraction and recombination studies of the interaction of retinol with human plasma retinol-binding protein. Journal of Lipid Research. 1972;**13**:338-347

[24] Davis JT, Ong DE. Synthesis and secretion of retinol-binding protein by cultured rat sertoli cells. Biology of Reproduction. 1992;**47**:528-533

[25] Monaco HL. The transthyretin-retinol-binding protein complex. Biochimica et Biophysica Acta. 2000;**1482**:65-72

[26] Gabay C, Kushner I. Acute-phase proteins and other systemic responses to inflammation. New England Journal of Medicine. 1999;**340**:448-454

[27] Felding P, Fex G. Cellular origin of prealbumin in the rat. Biochimica et Biophysica Acta. 1982;**716**:446-449

[28] Schreiber G. The evolution of transthyretin synthesis in the choroid plexus. Clinical Chemistry and Laboratory Medicine. 2002;**40**:1200-12010

[29] Ando Y. Transthyretin: It's miracle function and pathogenesis. Rinsho Byori. 2009;**57**: 228-235

[30] Tormey WP, O'Brien PA. Clinical associations of an increased transthyretin band in routine serum and urine protein electrophoresis. Annals in Clinical Biochemistry. 1993;**30**:550-554

[31] Ong DE, Davis JT, O'Day WT, Bok D. Synthesis and secretion of retinol-binding protein and transthyretin by cultured retinal pigment epithelium. Biochemistry. 1994;**33**: 1835-1842

[32] Wakasugi S, Maeda S, Shimada K. Structure and expression of the mouse prealbumin gene. Journal of Biochemistry (Tokyo). 1986;**100**:49-58

[33] Jacobsson B. In situ localization of transthyretin-mRNA in the adult human liver, choroid plexus and pancreatic islets and in endocrine tumours of the pancreas and gut. Histochemistry. 1989;**91**:299-304

[34] Gray HDA, Gray ES, Horne CHW. Sites of prealbumin production in the human fetus using indirect immunoperoxidase technique. Wirchows Archives. 1985;**406**:463-473

[35] Ingenbleek Y, Bernstein LH. Plasma transthyretin as a biomarker of lean body mass and catabolic states. Advances in Nutrition. 2015;**6**:572-580

[36] Makover A, Moriwaki H, Ramakrishnan R, Saraiva MJM, Blaner WS, Goodman DS. Plasma transthyretin: Tissue sites of degradation and turnover in the rat. Journal of Biological Chemistry. 1988;**263**:8598-8603

[37] Socolow EL, Woeber KA, Purdy RH, Holloway MT, Ingbar SH. Preparation of I131-labeled human serum prealbumin and its metabolism in normal and sick patients. Journal of Clinical Investigation. 1965;**44**:1600-1609

[38] Ingenbleek Y, Young VR. Significance of prealbumin in protein metabolism. Clinical Chemistry and Laboratory Medicine. 2002;**40**:1281-1291

[39] Guerra LT, Rosa AR, Romani RF, Gurski RR, Schirmer CC, Kruel CD. Serum transferrin and serum prealbumin as markers of response to nutritional support in patients with esophageal cancer. Nutrition Hospital. 2009;**24**:241-242

[40] Hamlin CR, Pankowsky DA. Turbidimetric determination of transthyretin (prealbumin) with a centrifugal analyzer. Clinical Chemistry. 1987;**33**:144-146

[41] Benson MD, Dwulet FE. Identification of carriers of a variant plasma prealbumin (transthyretin) associated with familial amyloidotic polyneuropathy, Type I. Journal of Clinical Investigation. 1985;**75**:71-75

[42] Jacob RA, Gorman N. Automated rate-immunonephelometric determination of serum prealbumin (transthyretin). Clinical Chemistry. 1983;**29**:564-566

[43] Vatassery GT, Quach HT, Smith WE, Benson BA, Eckfeldt JH. A sensitive assay of transthyretin (prealbumin) in human cerebrospinal fluid in nanogram amounts by ELISA. Clinica Chimica Acta. 1991;**197**:19-25

[44] Cray C, Tatum LM. Applications of protein electrophoresis in avian diagnostics. Journal of Avian Medicine and Surgery. 1998;**12**:4-10

[45] Stabilini R, Vergani C, Agostoni A, Agostoni RPV. Influence of age and sex on prealbumin levels. Clinica Chimica Acta. 1968;**20**:358-359

[46] Kanakoudi F, Drossou V, Tzimouli V, Diamanti E, Konstantinidis T, Germenis A, Kremenopoulos G. Serum concentrations of 10 acute-phase proteins in healthy term and preterm infants from birth to age 6 months. Clinical Chemistry. 1995;**41**:605-608

[47] Cardoso LEMB, Falção MC. Nutritional assessment of very low birth weight infants: Relationships between anthropometric and biochemical parameters. Nutrition Hospital. 2007;**22**:322-329

[48] MacDonald MG, Mullett MD, Seshia MMK. Avery′s Neonatology: Pathophysiology & Management of the Newborn. 6th ed. Philadelphia: Lippincott Williams & Wilkins; 2005. pp. 380-413

[49] Benvenga S, Bartalena L, Antonelli A, Li Calzi L, Di Pasquale G, Trimarchi F, Pinchera A. Radioimmunoassay for human thyroxine-binding prealbumin. Annals in Clinical Laboratory Science. 1986;**16**:231-240

[50] Ingenbleek Y, De Visscher M. Hormonal and nutritional status: Critical conditions for endemic goiter epidemiology? Metabolism. 1979;**28**:9-19

[51] Gallagher D, Visser M, De Meersman RE, Sepúlveda D, Baumgartner RN, Pierson RN, Harris T, Heymsfield SB. Appendicular skeletal muscle mass: Effects of age, gender and ethnicity. Journal of Applied Physiology. 1997;**83**:229-239

[52] Rona ZP. Bovine colostrum emerges as immune system modulator. American Journal of Natural Medicine. 1998;**3**:19-23

[53] Thomas T, Schreiber G. Acute-phase response of plasma protein synthesis during experimental inflammation in neonatal rats. Inflammation. 1985;**9**:1-7

[54] Campbell FM, Waterston M, Andresen LO, Sorensen NS, Heegaard PM, Eckersall PD. The negative acute phase response of serum transthyretin following *Streptococcus suis* infection in the pig. Veterinary Research. 2005;**36**:657-664

[55] Vahlquist A, Rask L, Peterson PA, Berg T. The concentrations of retinol-binding protein, prealbumin, and transferrin in the sera of newly delivered mothers and children of various ages. Scandinavian Journal of Clinical Laboratory Investigation. 1975;**33**:569-575

[56] Veldhuis JD, Roemmich JN, Richmond EJ, Rogol AD, Lovejoy JC, Sheffield-Moore M, Mauras N, Bowers CY. Endocrine control of body composition in infancy, childhood and puberty. Endocrine Reviews. 2005;**26**:114-146

[57] Bienvenu J, Jeppson JO, Ingenbleek Y. Transthyretin & retinol-binding protein. In: Ritchie RF, Nawolotskaia O, editors. Serum Proteins in Clinical Medicine. Scarborough: Foundation for Blood Research; 1996. pp. 9.011-9.018

[58] Gaggiotti G, Orlandoni P, Ambrosi S, Onorato G, Piloni S, Amadio L, Spazzafumo L, La Rocca R. The influence of age and sex on nutritional parameters in subjects aged 60 years and over. Archives of Gerontology and Geriatrics. 1995;**20**:117-128

[59] Zhu L, Chen Y, Liu C, Deng H, Zhang N, Wang S, Zhang Z. Transthyretin as a novel candidate biomarker for preeclampsia. Experimental and Therapeutic Medicine. 2014;**7**:1332-1336

[60] McKinnon B, Li H, Richard K, Mortimer R. Synthesis of thyroid binding proteins transthyretin and albumin by human trophoblast. Journal of Clinical Endocrinology & Metabolism. 2005;**90**:6714-6720

[61] Kalkunte SS, Neubeck S, Norris WE, Cheng S-B, Kostadinov S, Hoang DV, Ahmed A, von Eggeling F, Shaikh Z, Padbury J, Berg G, Olofsson A, Markert UR, Sharma S. Transthyretin is dysregulated in preeclampsia, and its native form prevents the onset of disease in a preclinical mouse model. American Journal of Pathology. 2013;**183**:1425-1436

[62] Henze A, Rohn S, Gericke B, Raila J, Schweigen FJ. Structural modifications of serum transthyretin in rats during protein-energy malnutrition. Rapid Communications in Mass Spectrometry. 2008;**22**:3270-3274

[63] Brugler L, Stankovic A, Bernstein L, Scott F, O'Sullivan-Maillet J. The role of visceral protein markers in protein calorie malnutrition. Clinical Chemistry and Laboratory Medicine. 2002;**40**:1360-1369

[64] Shenkin A. Assessment of nutritional status—Implications for nutritional support and hospitalization. Plasma Protein Monitor. 2005;**1**:9-11

[65] Davis CJ, Sowa D, Keim KS, Kinnare K, Peterson S. The use of prealbumin and C-reactive protein for monitoring nutrition support in adult patients receiving enteral nutrition in an urban medical center. JPEN Journal of Parenteral and Enteral Nutrition. 2012;**36**:197-204

[66] Kaysen GA. Effects of inflammation on plasma composition and endothelial structure and function. Journal of Renal Nutrition. 2005;**15**:94-98

[67] Ferard G, Gaudias J, Bourguignat A, Ingenbleek Y. C-reactive protein to transthyretin ratio for the early diagnosis and follow-up of postoperative infection. Clinical Chemistry and Laboratory Medicine. 2002;**40**:1334-1338

[68] Nova E, Lopez-Vidriero I, Varela P, Toro O, Casas JJ, Marcos AA. Indicators of nutritional status in restricting-type anorexia nervosa patients: A 1-year follow-up study. Clinical Nutrition. 2004;**23**:1353-1359

[69] Barbe P, Bennet A, Stebenet M, Perret B, Louvet JP. Sex-hormone-binding globulin and protein-energy malnutrition indexes as indicators of nutritional status in women with anorexia nervosa. American Journal of Clinical Nutrition. 1993;**57**:319-322

[70] Gendall KA, Bulik CM, Joyce PR. Visceral protein and hematological status of women with bulimia nervosa and depressed controls. Physiology & Behavior. 1999;**66**:159-163

[71] Clark MA, Hentzen BT, Plank LD, Hill GI. Sequential changes in insulin-like growth factor 1, plasma proteins, and total body protein in severe sepsis and multiple injury. Journal of Parenteral and Enteral Nutrition. 1996;**20**:363-370

[72] Liu F, Cai LY, Zhong L, Chen C, Xu F, Zhao ZX, Chen XM. Model for end-stage liver disease combined with serum prealbumin to predict the prognosis of patients with decompensated liver cirrhosis. Journal of Digestive Diseases. 2010;**11**:352-357

[73] Saito M, Seo Y, Yano Y, Miki A, Yoshida M, Azuma T. Short-term reductions in non-protein respiratory quotient and prealbumin can be associated with the long-term deterioration of liver function after transcatheter arterial chemoembolization in patients with hepatocellular carcinoma. Journal of Gastroenterology. 2012;**47**:704-714

[74] Hutchinson DR, Halliwell RP, Smith MG, Parke DW. Serum „prealbumin" as an index of liver function in human hepatobiliary disease. Clinica Chimica Acta. 1981;**114**:69-74

[75] Yasmin MY, Aziz B, Nazim M, Madhavan RK. Prealbumin rather than albumin is a more sensitive indicator of acute liver disease. Malaysian Journal of Pathology. 1993;**15**:147-150

[76] Hua SL, Jiang XJ. The clinical value of serum albumin and prealbumin levels in children with lobar pneumonia caused by *Mycoplasma pneumonia*. American Journal of Respiratory and Critical Care Medicine. 2016;**193**:A6735

[77] Luo H, Zhu B, Gong L, Yang J, Jiang Y, Zhou X. The value of serum prealbumin in the diagnosis and therapeutic response of tuberculosis: A retrospective study. PLoS ONE. 2013;**8**:e79940

[78] Vergani C, Stabilini R, Agostoni A. Thyroxine-binding prealbumin in thyrotoxicosis and hypothyroidism. Clinical Chemistry. 1969;**15**:216-218

[79] Ishida M, Kajita Y, Ochi Y, Hachiya T, Miyazaki T, Yoshimura M, Ijichi H. Measurement of serum thyroxine binding prealbumin in various thyroidal states by radioimmunoassay. Endocrinology Japan. 1982;**29**:607-613

[80] Ungaro R, Babyatsky MW, Zhu H, Freed JS. Protein-losing enteropathy in ulcerative colitis. Case Reports in Gastroenterology. 2012;**6**:177-182

[81] Takeda H, Ishihama K, Fukui T, Fujishima S, Orii T, Nakazawa Y, Shu HJ, Kawata S. Significance of rapid turnover proteins in protein-losing gastroenteropathy. Hepatogastroenterology. 2003;**50**:1963-1965

[82] Kopple JD, Mehrotra R, Suppasyndh O, Kalantar-Zadeh K. Observations with regard to the National Kidney Foundation K/DOQI clinical practice guidelines concerning serum transthyretin in chronic renal failure. Clinical Chemistry and Laboratory Medicine. 2002;**40**:1308-1312

[83] Cano NJ. Metabolism and clinical interest of serum transthyretin (prealbumin) in dialysis patients. Clinical Chemistry and Laboratory Medicine. 2002;**40**:1313-1319

[84] Oppenheimer JH, Werner SC. Effect of prednisone on thyroxine-binding proteins. Journal of Clinical Endocrinology. 1966;**26**:715-721

[85] Young GA, Yule AG, Hill GL. Effects of an anabolic steroid on plasma amino acids, proteins, and body composition in patients receiving intravenous hyperalimentation. JPEN Journal of Parenteral and Enteral Nutrition. 1983;**7**:221-225

[86] Staley MJ, Naidoo D, Pridmore SA. Concentrations of transthyretin (prealbumin) and retinol-binding protein in alcoholics during alcohol withdrawal. Clinical Chemistry. 1984;**30**:1887

[87] Kuszajewski M, Clontz A. Prealbumin is best for nutritional monitoring. Nursing. 2005;**35**:70-71

[88] Devakonda A, George L, Raoof S, Esan A, Saleh A, Bernstein LH. Transthyretin as a marker to predict outcome in critically ill patients. Clinical Biochemistry. 2008;**41**:1126-1130

[89] Bae HJ, Lee HJ, Han DS, Suh YS, Lee YH, Lee HS, Cho JJ, Kong SH, Yang HK. Prealbumin levels as a useful marker for predicting infectious complications after gastric surgery. Journal of Gastrointestinal Surgery. 2011;**15**:2136-2144

[90] Mahlck C-G, Granvist K. Plasma prealbumin in women with epithelial ovarian carcinoma. Gynecologic and Obstetric Investigation. 1994;**37**:135-140

[91] Byström P, Berglund Å, Nygren P, Wernroth L, Johansson B, Larsson A, Glimelius B. Evaluation of predictive markers for patients with advanced colorectal cancer. Acta Oncologica. 2012;**51**:849-859

[92] Kelly P, Paulin F, Lamont D, Baker L, Clearly S, Exon D, Thompson A. Pre-treatment plasma proteomic markers associated with survival in oesophageal cancer. British Journal of Cancer. 2012;**106**:955-961

[93] Ho S-Y, Guo H-R, Chen HHW, Peng C-J. Nutritional predictors of survival in terminally ill cancer patients. Journal of the Formosan Medical Association. 2003;**102**:544-550

[94] Cheng V, Inaba K, Haltmeier T, Gutierrez A, Siboni S, Benjamin E, Lam L, Demetriades D. Serum transthyretin is a predictor of clinical outcomes in critically ill trauma patients. Surgery. 2015;**158**:438-444

[95] Zago LB, Dupraz H, Weisstaub A, Godoy MF, Slobodianik NH, Gasali F, Dirube C, Torino F, Rio ME. Indices of protein status as predictors of complications in low risk surgical patients of hernias and lithiasis. Nutrition Research. 2000;**20**:203-213

[96] Yang HT, Yim H, Cho YS, Kim D, Hur J, Kim JH, Lee BC, Seo DK, Kim HS, Chun W. Prediction of clinical outcomes for massively-burned patients via serum transthyretin levels in the early postburn period. Journal of Trauma Acute Care Surgery. 2012;**72**:999-1005

[97] Fex G, Laurell CB, Thulin E. Purification of prealbumin from human and canine serum using a two-step affinity chromatographic procedure. European Journal of Biochemistry. 1977;**75**:181-186

[98] Forterre S, Raila J, Forterre F, Brunnberg L, Schweigert FJ. Characterisation of transthyretin and retinol-binding protein in plasma and cerebrospinal fluid in dogs. The Veterinary Journal. 2006;**171**:451-455

[99] Piechotta M, Raila J, Rick M, Beyerbach M, Hoppen H-O. Serum transthyretin concentration is decreased in dogs with nonthyroidal illness. Veterinary Clinical Pathology. 2012;**41**:110-113

[100] Raila J, Aupperle H, Raila G, Schoon HA, Schweigert FJ. Renal pathology and urinary protein excretion in a 14-month-old Bernese mountain dog with chronic renal failure. Journal of Veterinary Medicine Series A. 2007;**54**:131-135

[101] Ek N. Identification of the Pr prealbumin proteins in horse serum. Acta Veterinaria Scandinavica. 1977;**18**:458-470

[102] Chang L, Munro SL, Richardson SJ, Schreiber G. Evolution of thyroid hormone binding by transthyretins in birds and mammals. European Journal of Biochemistry. 1999;**259**:534-542

[103] Wojtczak A, Cody V, Luft JR, Panqborn W. Structures of human transthyretin complexed with thyroxine at 2.0 A resolution and 3′,5′-dinitro-N-acetyl-L-thyronine at 2.2 A resolution. Acta Crystallographica Section D Biological Crystallography. 1996;**52**:758-765

Chapter 5

The Intricate Relationship between Diabetes, Diet and the Gut Microbiota

Gratiela G. Pircalabioru, Ariana Picu, Laura Petcu, Marcela Popa and Mariana Carmen Chifiriuc

Additional information is available at the end of the chapter

http://dx.doi.org/10.5772/intechopen.70602

Abstract

The most recent World Health Organization report revealed that the number of adults suffering from diabetes has almost quadrupled since 1980 to 422 million, thus drawing attention to the urgent need to step up prevention and treatment of this disease. This chronic ailment is often associated with serious complications such as increased risk of heart disease, stroke and kidney failure. In 2012 alone, diabetes lead to 1.5 million deaths. This dramatic rise is mainly due to the increased prevalence of type 2 diabetes and factors driving it include overweight and obesity. Novel studies in this area have advanced our understanding regarding the complex relationship between diet, gut microbiota and diabetes. Despite no clear microbiota signature is associated with diabetes, patients harbour a reduction of butyrate-producing species (*Faecalibacterium prausnitzii, Roseburia intestinalis)* as well as an increase in opportunistic pathogens. Furthermore, the functions of the gut microbiome (i.e., vitamin metabolism, transport of sugars, carbohydrate metabolism, short chain fatty acid (SCFA) synthesis, etc.) are also different in patients with type 2 diabetes, a fact that may significantly alter the course of disease. Diet is one of the most decisive factors that have an impact on the gut microbiome. Nutritional interventions using prebiotics (i.e., inulin-type fructans), polyphenols and arabinoxylans have been employed for the treatment of diabetes. Besides the shifts produced by these dietary components in the microbiome composition, it is worth mentioning their impact on host physiology through modulation of gut peptide production and glucose metabolism. The information presented within this chapter summarizes the most recent advances in the study of the microbiome-diet-diabetes interplay and analyses how these novel findings can be used in order to establish new therapeutic approaches for those with diabetes.

Keywords: diabetes, obesity, microbiota, diet, prebiotics, gut physiology

1. Diabetes: the "silent killer"

Diabetes mellitus (DM) is defined as "a heterogeneous syndrome characterized by a complex disorder in regulating the body's energy metabolism, which also affects the use of carbohydrates, lipids and proteins" [1]. Several processes are involved in the evolution of diabetes pathology ranging from autoimmune pancreatic β cells destruction that induces insulin deficiency, up to anomalies, which causes insulin resistance. Increased blood glucose levels (≥126 mg/dL), blood glucose at 2 h after 75 g oral glucose (≥200 mg/dL), HbA1c (≥6.5%), or all of them characterize diabetes mellitus simultaneously. The American Diabetes Association (ADA) has classified diabetes mellitus into several types: (i) type 1 DM (T1D)—characterized by the destruction of pancreatic β cells; (ii) type 2 DM (T2D)—characterized by a progressive deficiency of insulin secretion on a background of pre-existing insulin resistance; (iii) gestational DM—diabetes diagnosed during pregnancy; and (iv) other specific types of diabetes due to other causes such as genetic defects of β pancreatic cells, genetic defects in the action of insulin, diseases of exocrine pancreas, endocrinopathies, diabetes induced by drugs or chemicals, etc. Type 1 diabetes (T1D) also known as juvenile diabetes or insulin-dependent diabetes mellitus is a very common autoimmune disorder in children and adolescents, and it is caused by the cellular-mediated autoimmune destruction of pancreatic β-cells, leading to an absolute insulin deficiency, which interferes with glucose metabolism [2]. T1D has two variants: (i) type I A is due to the destruction of the pancreatic cells under the influence of immune factors, in which case autoantibodies to islet cells can be detected in serum and (ii) type I B in which the pancreatic β-cell lysis occurs in the absence of an obvious anti-pancreatic mechanism [3]. Patients with this type of diabetes are usually young (under 30 years), have normal weight and require continuous insulin administration for survival. T1D symptoms are usually present with the onset of hyperglycaemia and include polyphagia, polydipsia, polyuria, weight loss, paraesthesia, recurrent infections and ketoacidosis tendency. The T1D prevalence of 1:300 is increasing worldwide, and it represents 5–10% of all diabetes mellitus cases [4]. The main cause of T1D is genetic predisposition with the human leucocyte antigen (HLA) DR3-DQ2 and DR4-DQ8 haplotypes as the most prevalent variants involved, which are common for other autoimmune diseases such as celiac disease [5]. Besides genetic predisposition, other factors such as infections, birth delivery mode, diet and the use of antibiotics have all been linked to T1D development [6], but the mechanisms linking them to T1D development are not clear.

DM type 2 (T2D) comprises a heterogeneous group of conditions characterized by varying degrees of insulin resistance or inappropriate insulin secretion and elevated plasma glucose (hyperglycaemia). Hyperglycaemia of this type of diabetes is due to genetic or metabolic defects of insulin synthesis and/or secretion, which once identified have become particularly important in discovering new effective therapeutic means. Pre-diabetes stages (IFG and IGT) typically precede T2D [7]. T2D appears at the age of 40 or above and is not associated with autoimmune aetiology but with metabolic syndrome involving hypertension, atherosclerotic cardiovascular disease, low high density lipoprotein cholesterol (HDLc), high circulating level of low density lipoprotein cholesterol (LDLc), decreased fibrinolysis, increased plasma lipopolysaccharide (LPS) due to alteration of mucosal permeability, obesity and especially visceral or abdominal type of obesity (visceral fat tissue is more metabolically active than the subcutaneous adipose tissue), producing pro-inflammatory adipokines and peripheral insulin resistance. According to the ADA guidelines of 2016: "Standards of medical care in diabetes" (Diabetes Care), the criteria for the diagnosis of T2D refer to: (i) Glucose concentration in venous blood (fasting plasma glucose) ≥126 mg/dL (7.0 mmol/L) in at least two consecutive determinations, measured after at least 8 h of fasting; (ii) Glucose concentration in venous blood 2 h after oral glucose tolerance test—OGTT—(ingestion of 75 g of anhydrous glucose dissolved in water) ≥200 mg/dL (11.1 mmol/L); (iii) HbA1C ≥48 mmol/mol determined in the medical laboratory by the National Glycohemoglobin Standardization Program (NGSP) and standardized by DCCT (Diabetes Control and Complications Trial); and (iv) Glucose concentration in venous blood ≥200 mg/dL (11.1 mmol/L) randomly determined in hyperglycaemic individuals. Some potential risk factors for T2D are family history and race. Specifically, Hispanic, Asian American, or Indian Americans are at greater risk to develop T2D. Age is another risk factor worth considering, as individuals who are 40–45 years old or older have a greater risk for developing the condition. Diabetic patients have an increased incidence of cardiovascular disease, atherosclerosis, peripheral arteriopathy and cerebrovascular disease. Long-term complications of diabetes include retinopathy with possible loss of vision, nephropathy followed in time by renal insufficiency, peripheral neuropathy with risk of leg ulceration and amputation. Neuropathy autonomously induces gastrointestinal, genitourinary, cardiovascular and sexual dysfunction. Like most other conditions, the earlier that diabetes is detected, the more successfully it can be managed. There is no cure for type 2 diabetes, but it can be very well managed if identified early. The latest data released by a group of WHO experts provide an alarming prognosis of the diabetes epidemic. It is estimated that by 2025, there will be 324 million people with diabetes. Thus, the prevalence will increase from 2.8% (2000) to 4.3% (2025). The T2D epidemic is considered one of the worst in the history of humankind. What is alarming, however, is that at the time of T2D diagnosis, a large percentage of people already have chronic complications and/or morbid associations. The WHO predictions for 2030 place T2D as the seventh cause of death worldwide. Epidemiological data revealed an increased prevalence for both obesity and T2D in developed countries, suggesting the role of diet and lifestyle in the pathogenesis of these two diseases [1]. Recently, it has been shown that overeating saturated fats and refined sugars can lead to dyslipidemia and insulin resistance. Thus, T2D prevalence is directly proportional to the energy intake of saturated fatty acids [8]. Currently, type 2 diabetes is most commonly encountered in most cases associated with overweight or obesity in adults. WHO classifies obesity grades by the formula: Body Mass Index (BMI) = weight/height^2 in: (i) Overweight—BMI 25–29.9 kg/m^2; (ii) Grade I obesity—BMI 30–34.9 kg/m^2; (iii) Grade II obesity—BMI 35–39.9 kg/m^2; and (iv) Grade III obesity—BMI > 40 kg/m^2. In T2D, the most common type of obesity is the central or abdominal type [9]. An increased prevalence of T2D in the predominantly abdominal distribution of adipose tissue was reported independent of the degree of obesity [10]. On the other hand, there are studies that show that obesity is not sufficient or mandatory for the appearance of T2D. In support of this hypothesis, there are several arguments: the presence of T2D in a normal weight phenotype, the existence of populations with high prevalence of obesity, but the low prevalence of T2D, the predominance of obesity in females, in contrast to that of T2D that does not differ between genders and finally data according to which in most populations studied most obese individuals do not have T2D [1]. Cross-sectional studies have failed to determine a causal relationship between T2D and obesity or a common factor triggering both diseases, but prospective and longitudinal studies have provided some evidence of the direct role of obesity in T2D pathogenesis. Prospective studies on the populations of Japan, Sweden and the Pima Indians show that the central distribution of body adiposity is a major risk factor for the emergence of T2D, regardless of the degree of obesity [11]. However, these studies only suggest that insulin synthesis or deficiency obesity and defects predispose to T2D but offer little data on the duration of these anomalies or their interaction [1]. There is increasing evidence that adipose tissue has a limited capacity to store the energy surplus [12] and that overstressed adipocytes suffer a process of apoptosis or necrosis, precipitating an inflammatory response which contribute to the development of insulin resistance [13].

The specificity of obesity in T2D is also the infiltration of adipose tissue with monocytes and activated macrophages leading to the synthesis of pro-inflammatory cytokines (IL-6 and TNF-α). Because of changes induced in the adipose tissue (lipolysis and lipids products), hepatic lipid synthesis (especially of very low-density lipoproteins-VLDL and triglycerides) occurs. Due to the changes in lipid metabolism, T2D is also characterized by dyslipidemia (elevated triglycerides, LDL-C levels and low HDLc) [14].

2. The gut microbiota-evolution, composition and functions

The gut microbiota is a dynamic system composed of tens of trillions of microorganisms, which carry out essential functions for the human host. The first composition of the microbiota is acquired at birth when microorganisms from the mother and the environment rapidly colonize the neonatal gastrointestinal tract. Thus, the delivery mode is a keystone factor which determines whether the newborn is colonized by *Lactobacillus*, *Prevotella* or *Sneathia* spp. from the birth canal or by *Staphylococcus* sp. and *Propionibacterium* spp. coming from the skin of the mother and other participants in the caesarean section [15].

Subsequently birth, diet becomes the main modulator of the microbiota composition. In line with this, breastfeeding babies harbour a distinct microbiota from formula-fed babies. While breastfeeding enhances the prevalence of lactic acid bacteria, infant formulas promote the enrichments of species like *Staphylococcus aureus* and *Bacteroides* spp. Until 3 years of age, the microbiota is highly influenced by diet and disease and, in time, its composition becomes very similar to one of the adults [16]. At around 7 years old, 90% of the microbiota is composed of bacteria from the phyla Bacteroidetes and Firmicutes, while the remaining 10% is made of Proteobacteria, Tenericutes and Cyanobacteria [17]. A study by Arumugam et al. proposed the existence of three gut enterotypes for the entire world population: *Bacteroides*, *Rumincoccus* and *Prevotella* [18]. Furthermore, these enterotypes were linked to dietary patterns [19]. For instance, the *Prevotella* enterotype was found to be more prevalent in case of individuals that had a diet rich in fibre and low in fat, whereas the *Bacteroides* enterotype was characteristic for people eating a diet dominated by animal fat and protein. In addition, recent studies have investigated school-age children from different regions of the world and highlighted the role of age, diet, geographical localization and traditions in shaping the microbiota. Children from Mexico,

Indonesia, Thailand and Malawi have a diet with a low level of animal protein and fat and a high content of plant polysaccharides and fibre, which translate into a microbiota rich in *Prevotella*. Conversely, children from Japan, the United States, Italy and China have a Western diet rich in fat, animal protein and low in fibre and thus have a microbiota dominated by *Bacteroides* [17]. However, the enterotype hypothesis was recently challenged by Knights et al. who showed that enterotypes can vary widely and continuously over time within an individual [20].

The gastrointestinal (GI) tract of a healthy host is home to 10^2 microbial cells within the stomach into the duodenum and jejunum, whereas the distal ileum harbours around 10^8 microbial cells. However, the highest microbial level (around 10^{12} cells) resides in the highly anaerobic environment of the colon. Since most of these microbes are not cultivatable, the advent of culture-independent sequencing has provided a valuable insight into the composition of the microbiota in health and disease conditions. Despite the large volume of data generated by sequencing technologies, our understanding of the functional properties of these microorganisms comes from germ-free animals. Thus, animals, which were born and reared under sterile conditions, have provided strong evidence regarding the role of microbiota in shaping immunity, host metabolism and even social development. Unlike animals reared under specific pathogen-free (SPF) conditions, germ-free animals were shown to have a defective development of the immune system with impaired development of the gut-associated lymphoid tissue, with fewer and smaller Peyer's patches [21].

3. The immunity-diet-microbiota interplay in type 1 diabetes

The microbiota modulates the immune response of the host even before birth as suggested by the fact that the intrauterine environment is not completely sterile. Indeed, there is evidence that the placenta harbours a low-abundance commensal microbiota similar to the oral microbiota [22]. Thus, the foetus is exposed to antigens against which it has to develop immunological tolerance. Following birth, diet represents the crucial factor guiding microbiota composition as well as immunity. Dietary antigens correlated with T1D are modulated by feeding regimens (breast milk vs infant formula) and the introduction of solid foods (particularly of wheat). While infant formula has been historically associated with T1D, breast milk has beneficial immunomodulatory effects in the neonatal gut. Within this line of thought, studies in mice showed that sIgA transferred passively in breast milk promotes gut homeostasis and prevents bacterial translocation [23].

Studies in Finnish and American children revealed that fat and protein intake from milk products promote a risk of advanced β-cell autoimmunity and consequently progression to T1D [24]. Patients with T1D and latent autoimmune diabetes of adults were shown to have elevated titres of anti-β-casein antibodies. Several bovine β-casein variants have a Pro-Gly-Pro-Ile-Pro motif in their sequence, which is also present in the glucose transporter GLUT2. Hence, a plausible explanation for pancreatic damage is a cross reactivity of the immune system initially targeted against the dietary antigen in milk.

T1D is similar in terms of its genetic HLA-associated risk with celiac disease and T1D children have an altered T-cell reactivity against wheat antigens in the gut [25]. Consequently, diets high in gluten are considered an important culprit for microbiota changes and T1D development [26]. Thus, introduction of gluten-containing foods between 3 and 7 months of age can significantly decrease the risk of T1D autoimmunity [27].

Gluten is a well-known trigger for celiac disease and recently for T1D due to its effects on gut permeability. As a consequence of the impaired gut barrier, gliadin peptides move across the epithelium into the lamina propria where they are detected by dendritic cells. Dendritic cells recognize gliadin peptides and migrate to other sites including the pancreatic lymph nodes where they activate autoreactive T cells [27].

4. The microbiota in type 1 diabetes

The involvement of the intestinal microbiota in the pathophysiology of T1D was highlighted by several animal studies. Valuable insights into the role of microbiota in diabetes pathogenesis were obtained using diabetes prone animals, specifically non-obese diabetic (NOD) mice and bio-breeding diabetes prone (BB-DP) rats.

Initial studies showed that NOD mice with chronic viral infection were characterized by a lower diabetes incidence [28]. Mycobacteria infection and stimulation with bacterial antigens lowered the incidence of diabetes development in NOD mice suggesting that a germ-free niche augments the risk of diabetes development [29]. However, this is not the case since recent studies suggested that rather certain microbes (i.e., *Bacillus cereus*) were modulating the risk of diabetes development [30].

Within a study by Brugman et al., the use of BB-DP rats and fluorescence in situ hybridization targeted against the 16S rRNA of *Clostridium*, *Lactobacillus* and *Bacteroides* showed that rats that developed diabetes harboured higher levels of *Bacteroides* [31]. Further investigations revealed that BB-DP rats had a microbiota with lower levels of *Lactobacillus* and *Bifidobacterium* when compared to diabetes-free rats. More recently, Patterson et al. used the streptozocin (STZ)-induced T1D rat model to offer information regarding diabetes onset and progression in terms of microbial shifts [32].Thus, T1D was linked to a shift in the Bacteroidetes:Firmicutes ratio, whereas later T1D progression was characterized by an enrichment of lactic acid bacteria (i.e., *Lactobacillus, Bifidobacterium)*. In addition, STZ-induced T1D rats exhibited a reduced microbial diversity 1 week after disease onset, and this diminished diversity was maintained throughout the study.

Importantly, the integrity of the intestinal epithelium plays a pivotal role in the functioning of the immune system by regulating the passage of antigens to dendritic cells. A compromised barrier epithelium is associated with increased gut permeability, which favours the exposure to antigens and may subsequently lead to autoimmunity. T1D prone rats were shown to have increased gut permeability and diminished levels of the tight junction protein claudin [33]. Furthermore, upregulation of the protein zonulin which regulates tight junctions increased intestinal permeability and the prevalence of diabetes in BB-DP rats [34]. Within this line of thought, a study using the BB-DP rat model hypothesized that administration of *Lactobacillus johnsonii N6.2* delayed diabetes development via regulation of gut integrity, specifically by increasing the tight junction protein claudin-1 [35].

MyD88 is an adapter protein downstream of multiple toll-like receptors involved in sensing of microorganisms. The knock out of this protein in the NOD mouse was shown to protect against diabetes. Importantly, heterozygous MyD88KO/+ NOD mice, which normally develop disease, are protected from diabetes when colonized from birth with the intestinal microbiota of a MyD88-KO NOD donor mouse [36]. Thus, disease progression in the NOD mouse is partially determined by an exacerbated innate immune response to commensal microbiota, and changes in the composition of the microbiota may diminish this response and counteract disease.

Considerable effort has been made in the last years in order to provide more information regarding the composition of the diabetogenic microbiota in humans. As expected, the pattern of bacterial abundance is distinct between different studies due to variations caused by ethnicity, geography and age. Despite these variations, all studies have shown *Bacteroides* as a main driver for T1D-associated dysbiosis. Indeed, there is a direct relation between the abundance of *Bacteroides* and T1D-associated autoantibodies [37, 38]. However, another study found no difference in *Bacteroides* levels when analysing children with anti-islet cell autoimmunity versus healthy controls [39].

Dysbiosis was linked to autoimmunity and subsequent progression to T1D. Importantly, the appearance of β-cell autoimmunity precedes the onset of hyperglycemia for over 15 years [40]. Therefore, targeting the microbiota could potentially postpone T1D development in children with β-cell autoimmunity.

Recently, Kostic et al. highlighted specific features of the T1D microbiome [38]. The study investigated 33 infants from Finland and Estonia who were genetically predisposed to diabetes and observed a relative 25% reduction in alpha-diversity in T1D patients compared to non-converters and seroconverters (positive for at least two of the autoantibodies analysed including insulin autoantibodies, islet cell antibodies, islet antigen-2 antibodies and glutamic acid carboxylase antibodies). Microbiota shifts were evident in T1D children but not in the seroconverters without disease. T1D subjects were shown to harbour an enrichment of "pathobionts that is of commensal bacteria able to become pathogens such as Rikenellaceae, *Blautia* and the *Ruminococcus* and *Streptococcus* genera." Furthermore, the authors observed a depletion of bacteria such as *Lachnospiraceae* and *Veillonellaceae*, which are commonly under abundant in inflammatory conditions (**Figure 1**).

A healthy gut microbiota is enriched with butyrate producers (i.e., *Faecalibacterium*) which determine elevated production of mucin and increased tight junction assembly which all determine an elevated epithelial integrity (**Figure 1**). A niche with high mucin production favours the enrichment of mucin degrading bacteria such as *Akkermansia muciniphila.* T1D subjects were reported to be colonized by lower levels of butyrate producing microorganisms such as *Roseburia* and *Faecalibacterium* and of mucin degrading bacteria such as *Akkermansia* and *Prevotella* [37, 41, 42]. In addition, the Bacteroidete: Firmicutes ratio was proposed as an early marker for autoimmune diseases since a higher level of Bacteroidetes was evident in children who developed T1D [43].

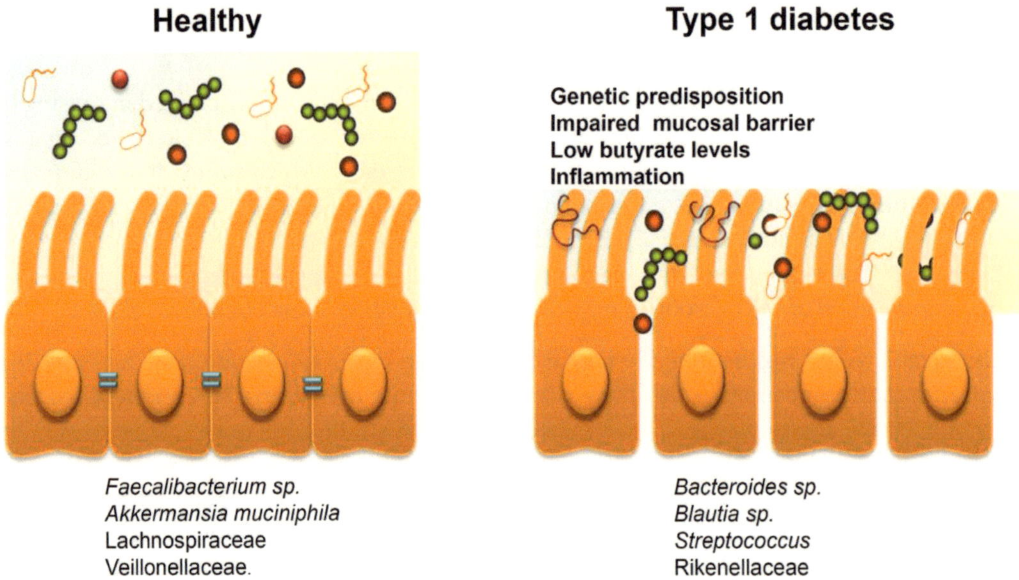

Figure 1. The microbiota in type 1 diabetes. Individuals with type 1 diabetes have an impaired gut barrier function with a thinner mucus layer and increased intestinal permeability. Their microbiota is enriched in *Bacteroides, Blautia, Streptococcus and Rikenellaceae* but low in butyrate producers such as *Faecalibacterium prausnitzii* and mucin degraders such as *Akkermansia muciniphila*.

5. Diet and type 2 diabetes

Food intake has been strongly associated to diabetes and obesity not only in terms of quantity but also in terms of quality of diet. The food shortage and famine during the two World Wars has significantly decreased the diabetes mortality in countries around Europe. However, in countries like the United States of America and Japan, where there was no shortage of food, there was no change in diabetes mortality [44]. Almost two decades ago, the role of diet in T2D was suggested by the observation that diabetes was prevalent among rich people who had an easier access to food such as refined sugar, flour and oil [45]. While in the past it was considered a disease of the rich, nowadays T2D is more prevalent among those with a lower income. Many studies have shown a strong correlation between high intake of sugars and development of T2D. A study by Ludwig et al. analysed 500 ethnically diverse children for a period of 19 months and reported that the frequency of obesity increased for each additional serving of carbonated soft drinks consumed [46]. Several prospective studies revealed link between fat intake and subsequent risk of developing T2DM. A diabetes study involving more than a thousand subjects without a prior diagnosis of diabetes which were investigated for a period of 4 years reported a relationship among T2D, impaired glucose tolerance and fat intake [47, 48]. The high levels of fructose corn syrup used for the manufacturing soft drinks increase the blood glucose levels and the body mass index, thus suggesting that the intake of soft drinks is linked with obesity and T2D [49]. In addition, diet soft drinks were reported to contain glycated chemicals, which significantly enhance insulin resistance [50]. Whereas high consumption of sweets, red meat and fried foods lead to an increased risk of insulin resistance and T2DM [51], a diet rich in fruits and vegetables may prevent disease development [52]. In addition, interventional studies revealed that high carbohydrate and high monounsaturated fat diets improved insulin sensitivity [53], whereas increased intake of white rice leads to an increased risk of T2D in Japanese women [54].

6. Popular diets and their impact on the microbiota

The most popular diets include omnivore, vegetarian, gluten-free, vegan, Western and Mediterranean. All of these dietary regimes have been studied regarding their role in shaping the microbiota. A gluten-free diet was associated with a decrease in *Bifidobacterium* and *Lactobacillus*, while populations of pathobionts (potentially unhealthy microbes), such as *Escherichia coli* and total *Enterobacteriaceae,* increased in parallel to reductions in polysaccharide intake after beginning the diet [55]. In another study by Bonder et al., a short-term gluten-free diet lead to reductions in *Ruminococcus bromii* and *Roseburia faecis* and an increase in *Victivallaceae* and *Clostridiaceae* [56].

The Western diet which is low in fibre but high in animal protein and fat was associated with a decrease in the total bacterial load and with lower levels of beneficial commensals such as *Bifidobacterium* and *Eubacterium* sp. [19, 57]. Importantly, consumption of a Western diet has also been linked with the generation of cancer-promoting nitrosamines [58]. Both vegan and vegetarian diets are high in fermentable plant-based foods. When comparing a vegan or a vegetarian diet to an omnivorous diet, it was reported that vegan and vegetarian individuals had lower abundance of *Bacteroides* and *Bifidobacterium species* [59].

The traditional Mediterranean diet consists of vegetables, olive oil, cereals, legumes, nuts, moderate consumption of poultry, fish and wine and a low consumption of dairy products, red meat and refined sugars [60]. Among the different diets, the Mediterranean diet is regarded as a healthy balanced diet due to its beneficial content of monounsaturated and polyunsaturated fatty acids, elevated vegetable protein content and high levels of antioxidants and fibre. The Mediterranean diet was associated with a high abundance of *Lactobacillus, Bifidobacterium* and *Prevotella,* and a decrease in *Clostridium* [61]. Furthermore, those consuming a Mediterranean diet exhibited increased levels of short chain fatty acids (SCFAs) and low urinary trim ethylamine oxide, which is associated with elevated cardiovascular risk [62]. The effects mediated by the Mediterranean diet include weight loss, improvement of the lipid profile and the decrease of inflammation.

7. Diet-microbiota interactions shape the risk of type 2 diabetes

Diet represents the main modulator of the composition and metabolism of the gut microbiota. The main macronutrients represented by proteins, carbohydrates and fats have a crucial impact on the microbiome. The role of dietary protein in shaping the microbiota has been described since 1977 when individuals who consumed a diet rich in beef harboured elevated levels of *Bacteroides* and *Clostridia* and low levels of *Bifidobacterium adolescentis* compared to those who had a meatless diet [63]. Several studies have recently used different forms of protein including vegetarian pea protein, whey protein and animal protein (meats, eggs and cheese) and correlated protein consumption with microbial diversity [61]. Conversely, the consumption of animal-based protein positively correlated with the abundance of bile-tolerant anaerobes such as *Alistipes, Bacteroides* and *Bilophila* [64]. Even though it may promote a greater weight loss, a protein-rich diet can also be detrimental. Thus, individuals on a high protein/low carbohydrate diet had a microbiota with diminished levels of *Roseburia* and *Eubacterium rectale* and low levels of butyrate in their feces [65]. Similarly, patients with inflammatory bowel disease (IBD) had a similar microbiota signature, with low levels of *Roseburia* and decreased butyrate levels [66]. In addition, elevated intake of red meat has been linked to elevated levels of the proatherogenic trimethylamine-N-oxide (TMAO) [62]. Animal studies have shown that high protein consumption increases the levels of insulin-like growth factor 1 (IGF-1), which are known to be correlated with a high risk of diabetes and overall mortality. Indeed, proteins of vegetarian origin have been linked to a lower mortality in comparison with animal-derived proteins [67].

In addition to high protein content, animal-based diets are also high in fat. The well-known Western diet, which is nowadays the main culprit for obesity and diabetes development, is high in saturated and trans fats and low in mono and polyunsaturated fats [61]. While consumption of high saturated and trans fat diets increases cholesterol levels and is associated with a risk of cardiovascular disease, mono and polyunsaturated fats decrease the risk of chronic disease [68]. Human studies have revealed that a high-fat diet increases the abundance of total anaerobic microorganisms and the levels of *Bacteroides* as well [19, 57]. The consumption of different types of fat has different effects on the microbiome. Consumption of a low fat diet promotes the overabundance of *Bifidobacterium* and leads to a reduction of fasting glucose and total cholesterol. Conversely, a high saturated fat diet determined the establishment of a microbiota enriched in *Faecalibacterium prausnitzii*, and a diet high in monounsaturated fat was correlated to a reduced total bacterial load and reduced cholesterol [69].

Animal studies revealed that a high fat diet promotes a microbiota with less *Lactobacillus intestinalis* and with more *Clostridiales, Bacteroides* and *Enterobacteriales.* In addition, the abundance of *L. intestinalis* was negatively correlated with fat mass and body weight [70]. Studies in mice compared the effects of different type of lipids on the microbiota. Thus, lard-fed mice harboured elevated *Bacteroides* and *Bilophila* whereas mice fed with fish oil had increased lactic acid bacteria (*Lactobacillus* and *Streptococcus*), increased *Verrucomicrobia* (*A. muciniphila*) and *Actinobacteria* (*Bifidobacterium* and *Adlercreutzia*). In addition, lard-fed mice had white adipose tissue inflammation and impaired insulin sensitivity compared to fish oil-fed mice [71].

Among all the dietary macronutrients, carbohydrates are the most studied. Based on their ability to be degraded enzymatically in the small intestine, carbohydrates are either digestible (i.e., starch and sugars including glucose, lactose, fructose and sucrose) or non-digestible (resistant starch and fibre). Upon degradation, digestible carbohydrates release glucose into the bloodstream and lead to an insulin response [61]. Humans who were fed high levels of glucose, fructose and sucrose in the form of dates had a microbiota enriched in *Bifidobacteria,* and low in *Bacteroides* [72, 73]. Moreover, the addition of lactose to the aforementioned diet replicated the same bacterial shifts but it also decreased the levels of *Clostridia* species [74].

Recently, a subject of debate in the field of carbohydrates and their role in shaping the microbiota is represented by the use of artificial sweeteners. Artificial sweeteners such as saccharin, sucralose and aspartame were intended to be a healthier, no-calorie food additive for replacing natural sugar. However, recent work by Suez et al. showed that artificial sweeteners are more prone to induce glucose intolerance than consumption of sucrose or glucose. The effects exhibited by artificial sweeteners were attributed to the induction of microbiota changes characterized by increased abundance of *Bacteroides* and decreased *Lactobacillus reuteri* [75]. Conversely, the use of natural sugars such as fructose, sucrose and glucose promoted microbiota shifts exactly opposed the ones induced by the use of artificial sweeteners.

Unlike digestible carbohydrates, non-indigestible carbohydrates are not digested in the small bowel but rather reach the colon where they undergo fermentation by commensal microbiota leading to SCFAs production such as butyrate, propionate and acetate. Butyrate is an important energy source for intestinal epithelial cells and a modulator of enterocyte differentiation, proliferation and restitution. Loss of microbial producers of SCFA can alter the communication between host epithelium and resident bacteria, thus contributing to the development of colitis. For instance, *F. prausnitz ii* is depleted not only in IBD patients [66] but also in diabetics.

Dietary fibres are essential for intestinal health and have been designated as prebiotics, that is non-digestible dietary constituents that benefit host health via selective stimulation of the growth and/or activity of certain microorganisms [76]. Prebiotics can originate from a multitude of sources including inulins, unrefined wheat, unrefined barley, raw oats, soybeans and non-digestible oligosaccharides such as fructooligosaccharides (FOS), galactooligosaccharides (GOS), fructans, polydextrose, xylooligosaccharides(XOS) and arabinooligosaccharides (AOS) [77]. A low fibre diet has been associated with a reduced bacterial abundance [78] and high consumption of these non-digestible carbohydrates resulted in an increase in microbiota gene richness in obese patients [79]. Many studies revealed that a diet rich in non-digestible carbohydrates targets the microbiota by increasing probiotic bacteria such as bifidobacteria and lactic acid bacteria. Indeed, diets rich in whole grain and wheat bran led to an increase of intestinal *Bifidobacteria* and *Lactobacilli* [80, 81]. FOS , polydextrose- and AOS-based prebiotics were shown to reduce *Clostridium* and *Enterococcus* species. In addition, resistant starch and whole grain barley increased the abundance of *Ruminococcus, E. rectale* and *Roseburia* [61].

8. The microbiota in type 2 diabetes

Genetics, lifestyle and increased bodyweight all contribute to the development of type 2 diabetes. Around 80% of individuals with T2D are overweight thus suggesting an important role of diet and microbiota in the pathophysiology of this disease. The link between microbiota and T2D first became evident in studies on germ-free mice. Thus, colonization of germ-free animals with microbiota harvested from conventionally raised mice lead to a significant increase in body fat and insulin resistance [82]. A following study showed that germ-free mice were resistant to diet-induced obesity [83].

Subsequently, several studies have documented the microbiota shifts associated with T2D. After analysing a cohort of Chinese patients with T2D, Qin et al. showed that the diabetic microbiome is low in butyrate-producing bacteria such as Clostridiales sp., *F. prausnitzii, Roseburia intestinalis* and *E. rectal* [84]. Moreover, the T2D intestinal niche contained opportunistic pathogens including the sulfate-reducing *Desulfovibrio, Bacteroides caccae* and *E. coli*. In line with these findings, a study in Scandinavian post-menopausal women revealed decreased levels of *F. praunitzii* and *R. intestinalis* in T2D compared with individuals having impaired glucose tolerance. In addition, both Chinese and Scandinavian T2D cohorts exhibited elevated *Lactobacillus* levels. Obesity and impaired glucose metabolism were reported to have an altered ratio between Bacteroidetes and Firmicutes [85]; however, neither the Chinese nor the Scandinavian study found this microbiota change.

The Chinese study revealed an increase of *E. coli* in T2D patients and another Danish study showed that Proteobacteria levels were elevated in T2D [86]. These Gram-negative bacteria could potentially be involved in the pathophysiology of T2D. Specifically, the lipopolysaccharides (LPS) released by these bacteria could promote a subclinical proinflammation, which is typical to both diabetes and obesity. Recent studies revealed that T2D is characterized by elevated endotoxemia. Indeed, mice receiving high fat (HF) diet until they developed diabetes had endotoxemia, increased intestinal permeability and a distinct microbiots [87]. In addition, the term of metabolic infection has emerged in order to describe the role of the microbiome in endotoxemia-associated inflammation together with insulin resistance in T2D. Endotoxin of microbial origin could play a role in the insulin resistance associated with T2D since blood levels of bacterial DNA (mostly Proteobacteria) were shown to be increased in prediabetes.

One caveat of the currently available human studies is the lack of information regarding the role of antidiabetic medication in altering the microbiota. The first-line drug of choice for type 2 diabetes treatment is represented by metformin. In the Swedish study, the diabetic patients received metformin treatment and their microbiota was enriched in Enterobacteriaceae and had low levels of *Eubacterium* and *Clostridium*. In mice-fed a high-fat diet, metformin was shown to affect both the host glucose metabolism as well as the microbiota by increasing the levels of *Akkermansia* [88]. Recently, metformin treatment has also been shown to alter the microbiota composition in T2D patients by increasing *Escherichia* sp. and decreasing the abundance of *Intestinibacter* sp. (**Figure 2**) [89].

http://dx.doi.org/10.5772/intechopen.70602

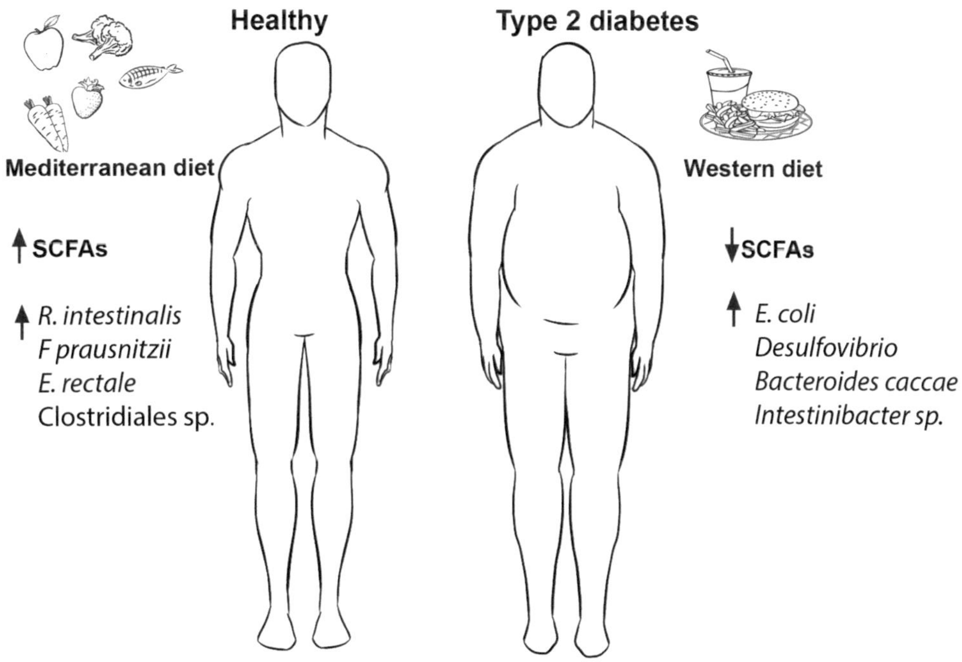

Figure 2. The microbiota in type 2 diabetes. Overweight and obese individuals consuming an unhealthy diet such a Western diet are prone to develop type 2 diabetes. While healthy individuals consuming a balanced diet with a high content of monounsaturated and polyunsaturated fatty acids, elevated vegetable protein content, and high levels of antioxidants and fibre harbour a microbiota rich in *R. intestinalis, F. prausnitz ii, E. rectale, Lactobacillus* sp. and Clostridiales, individuals with type 2 diabetes have a microbiota characterized by higher levels of *Desulfovibrio* sp., *Bacteroides* sp. and *Intestinibacter* sp.

9. Probiotic interventions

Due to their anti-inflammatory, hypoglycaemic, insulinotropic, antioxidative and satietogenis properties, probiotics can be employed as a treatment for T2D. The insulinotropic effect of genetically engineered *Escherichia coli Nissle 1917* for GLP-1 was investigated in Caco-2 cells; it was observed that the probiotic strain stimulated the epithelial cells leading to the secretion of insulin corresponding to blood insulin concentration of 164 pmol/ml to 164 nmol/ml [90]. In addition, Paszti-Gere et al. reported that oxidative stress causing damage to insulin-secreting ß-cells was counteracted by metabolites of *Lactobacillus plantarum* 2142. Specifically, the spent culture supernatant of *L. plantarum 2142* decreased the oxidative stress-induced overexpression of pro-inflammatory cytokines IL-8 and TNF-α in IPEC-J2 cell line [91]. The multiple mechanisms of probiotics in T2D treatment have emerged from studies by using animal models. Oral administration (0.05%) or diet supplementation (0.1%) of heat-killed *L. casei* in different mouse models including KK-Ay mice, NOD mice and Alloxan induced diabetic mice reduced the plasma glucose level and diabetes development [92, 93]. Feeding neonatal STZ-induced diabetic (n-STZ) rats with a diet containing *Lactobacillus rhamnosus GG* for a period of 9 weeks determined a lower blood haemoglobin level and an improved glucose tolerance in comparison to the control group receiving a conventional diet. The *L. rhamnosus GG* treatment group had a serum insulin level significantly higher than the control group at 30 min after glucose loading [94]. Furthermore, feeding VSL#3 lowered β-cell destruction and inflammation in NOD mice, and this effect was accompanied by increased IL-10 secretion in pancreas, Peyer's patches and spleen. In a separate study, the feeding of a probiotic containing *Lactobacillus acidophilus NCDC14* and *L. casei NCDC19* significantly lowered free fatty acids, the blood glucose and glycosylated haemoglobin, and trigycerides in fructose-induced diabetic rats [95]. The feeding of the same probiotic to STZ-induced rats suppressed the STZ-induced oxidative damage in pancreatic tissues by inhibiting lipid peroxidation, generation of nitric oxide and improved the antioxidant potential of glutathione, superoxide dismutase, and catalase and glutathione peroxidase. These data suggest that oral administration of the probiotic significantly ameliorated the risk factors such as dyslipidemia, hyperglycemia and oxidative stress in diabetic rats [96]. Probiotic pre-treatment with a mixture containing *Bifidobacterium lactis, L. acidophilus* and *L. rhamnosus* lowered the blood glucose and improved the bioavailability of gliclazide, a second-generation sulphonylurea used for treating non-insulin dependent diabetes mellitus T2D in alloxan induced diabetic rats [97]. The antidiabetic effects against insulin resistance of different probiotics can also be due to increased liver natural killer T (NKT) cells. NKT cells are involved in regulating the inflammatory process in the liver which is the main organ responsible for inflammation-mediated insulin resistance. Depletion of liver NKT enhanced the production of pro-inflammatory cytokines, and HFD was known to induce depletion of hepatic NKT cells leading to insulin resistance. HFD-induced depletion of NKT cells in male C57BL-6 mice was significantly improved by administration of the VSL#3 probiotic. This probiotic treatment also leads to weight loss, and improved insulin resistance and inflammation by modulating TNF-*α* expression and reducing NF-kB binding activity [98]. Treatment with *L. plantarum* DSM 15313 and *L. reuteri* GMNL-263 was reported to lower the blood glucose and glycosylated haemoglobin, in HFD-fed C57BL/6 J mice and STZ-induced diabetic rats [99, 100]. DCs from NOD mice were stimulated with three different strains of lactobacilli including *L. casei*, *L. reuteri* and *L. plantarum* for a period of 24 h. Out of the strains tested, *L. casei* was found to induce DCs to generate the highest level of IL-10 and the lowest level of IL-12 expression. When the *L. casei*-stimulated DCs were transferred to NOD mice, they showed a significant delay in diabetes incidence [101]. *Bifidobacterium longum* CGMCC NO. 2107 added as a supplemed in HFD was shown to reduce the metabolic endotoxin (LPS) plasma concentrations and to improve intestinal inflammation [102]. Amar et al. analysed the effect probiotic treatment has on mucosal dysbiosis, bacterial translocation and glucose metabolism [103]. The results obtained revealed that the bacterial translocation was prevented in mice lacking the microbial pattern recognition receptors Nod1 or CD14. Nevertheless, it was increased in Myd88 deficient mice and ob/ob mouse under the same conditions. In addition, the administration of *Bifidobacterium animalis* subsp. *lactis 420* reduced the bacterial translocation to mesenteric adipose tissue, decreasing the expression of major pro-inflammatory cytokines TNF-a, IL-1b and IL-6 in mesenteric adipose tissue, liver and muscle. In addition, *B. animalis* subsp. *lactis 420* also improved the insulin sensitivity and fasting hyperinsulinaemia in HFD fed mice [103].

Since there are a few reports in this area, the knowledge regarding the efficacy of probiotic administration in diabetic human subjects is quite limited. Consumption of probiotic yoghurt was shown to improve the antioxidant status and lipid profile in T2D patients. Several randomized, double blind, placebo-controlled clinical trials evaluated the effects of probiotic administration on antioxidant status, blood glucose and lipid profile in T2D. The patients with T2D mellitus enrolled in these studies were divided into two groups: the probiotic intervention group consumed 300 g/d of probiotic yoghurt containing 10^6 cfu/mL *L. acidophilus La5* and 10^6 cfu/mL *B. lactis Bb12*, whereas the control group consumed 300 g/d of conventional yoghurt during a period of 6 weeks. The probiotic treatment cohort exhibited a significant decrease in fasting blood glucose as well as an increase in the activities of the erythrocyte superoxide dismutase and glutathione peroxidase. In addition, the total cholesterol: high-density lipoprotein (HDL)-C and LDL-C: HDL-C ratios were decreased in the probiotic-treated patients compared to the control [104, 105]. Another randomized, double-blind, placebo-controlled study was performed on 20 elderly diabetic volunteers aged 50–60 years, over for a period of 30 days to study the effect of a symbiotic drink (a preparation with a combination of both probiotics and prebiotics) on glycaemia and cholesterol levels. The symbiotic group that consumed 10^8 cfu/mL *Bifidobacterium bifidum*, 10^8 cfu/mL of *L. acidophilus*, and 2 g oligofructose harboured a significantly increased HDL cholesterol, and a decrease in fasting glycemia but, importantly, no significant changes were observed in the placebo group [106]. Recently, in a study by Shao et al., 67 diabetic patients with gastrointestinal cancer were randomized into the probiotic treatment group (33 patients receiving enteral nutrition with probiotics, glutamine and fish oil) and the control group (34 patients receiving regular enteral nutrition). Fasting blood glucose and insulin were recorded on the day before surgery and post-operative days 3 and 7. Insulin resistance index (HOMA-IR) was calculated as well by using the homeostasis model assessment (HOMA) for both groups, and the supplementary data on incidence of nosocomial infections, intestinal function recovery time and length of hospitalization were also recorded [107].

The enteral nutrition with probiotics, glutathione and fish oil was associated with a low fasting insulin and insulin resistance index compared to the control group. The length of hospital stay was significantly decreased from 21 to 17 days in the treatment group. Nevertheless, no significant differences in nosocomial infection and intestinal function recovery were observed between the two groups. The role of maternal probiotic-supplemented dietary counseling during pregnancy on colostrum adiponectin concentration in neonatal nutrition, metabolism and immunity was analysed in a randomized, placebo-controlled study by Luoto et al. [108]. Specifically, 256 pregnant women were randomized into three groups: dietary intervention with probiotics (diet/ *L. rhamnosus GG* and *B. lactis*), with placebo (diet/placebo) and a control cohort (control/placebo). Dietary intake was analysed by food records at each pregnancy trimester, and subsequently colostrum samples were collected after birth for the analysis of adiponectin concentration. An improved adiponectin concentration is a parameter of neonatal metabolic homeostasis and is also an indicator of reduced chances of gestational diabetes. Probiotic treatment increased the colostrum adiponectin concentration compared to the control (12.7 ng/ml vs. 10.2 ng/ml). Nevertheless, other studies state that probiotic use does not provide a benefit for the diabetic host. For instance, a randomized, double-blinded clinical trial using the commercial probiotic *L. acidophilus NCFM* in a group of 45 men for a timeframe of 4 weeks revealed that there were no changes in the expression of baseline inflammatory markers and in the systemic inflammatory response following probiotic treatment [109].

10. Prebiotics: a useful tool for the management of diabetes

Prebiotics were initially defined as "a non-digestible food ingredient that beneficially affects the host by selectively stimulating the growth and/or activity of one or a limited number of bacteria in the colon, and thus improves host health" [110]. Later, prebiotics were designated as selectively fermented ingredients that allow certain changes in the composition and/or activity of the gastrointestinal microbiota that confer benefits upon host well-being and health [111]. Prebiotic substances need to meet certain criteria such as: (i) fermentation by the commensal microbiota; (ii) selective stimulation of the growth and/or activity of probiotic bacteria; and (iii) resistance to gastric pH, hydrolysis by the host enzymes and gastrointestinal absorption [112]. The currently known prebiotics which achieve the aforementioned criteria include non-digestible carbohydrates, fructooligosaccharides, galactooligosaccharides and lactulose. Prebiotics, such as fructooligosaccharides and inulin, undergo digestion by probiotics such as bifidobacteria and stimulate their growth [113, 114]. Besides their involvement in stimulating the expansion of probiotics, prebiotics also stimulate immunity, inhibit pathogen growth and produce vitamins. In addition, prebiotics were suggested to promote cell differentiation, cell-cycle arrest and apoptosis of transformed colonocytes by epigenetic modifications and by decreasing the transformation of bile acids [110]. Prebiotics administration may have a regulatory role in modulating endogenous metabolism since the SCFAs obtained as an end product of the carbohydrate metabolism improve glucose tolerance. SCFAs also decrease glucagon levels and activate glucagon-like peptide1 (GLP-1), which can stimulate the elevation of insulin production and elevate insulin sensitivity [115, 116]. SCFAs were shown to have an important role in T2DM patients because they promote secretion of GLP-1, a hormone that inhibits glucagon secretion, decreases hepatic gluconeogenesis and improves insulin sensitivity [117].

Prebiotics were also suggested to lead to hypercholesterolemia by lowering cholesterol absorption and by the generation of SCFAs upon selective fermentation by commensal microbiota [118]. A daily intake of 20 g of the prebiotic inulin significantly lowered serum triglycerides compared to the control group. Inulin treatment also decreased serum LDL-cholesterol and increased serum HDL-cholesterol [119]. Moreover, normolipidemic individuals consuming 18% of inulin on a daily basis without any other dietary restrictions exhibited a decrease in total plasma cholesterol and triacylglycerols as well as an increased fecal concentration of Lactobacillus-lactate [120]. The inclusion of inulin in the diet of rats increased the excretions of fecal lipids and cholesterol compared to that of the control group due to a reduced cholesterol absorption [121]. Other prebiotics including resistant starches and their derivatives, oligodextrans, lactose, lactoferrin-derived peptides and N-acetylchitooligosaccharides were also shown to have hypocholesterolaemic effects in T2DM patients who are at high risk of developing cardiovascular complications [112]. A diet enriched with arabinoxylan and resistant starch consumed by adults with metabolic syndrome leads to a reduction in the total species diversity of the faecal associated intestinal microbiota and an increase in *Bifidobacterium* and butyrate levels [122].

Clinical trials reported that dietary polyphenols increase the population of *Bifidobacterium* sp. in the gut [123]. Daily consumption of red wine polyphenols for a period of 4 weeks significantly increased the levels of *Bifidobacterium, Prevotella, Bacteroides, Bacteroides uniformis, Eggerthella lenta, Enterococcus,* and *Blautia coccoides-E. rectale* groups compared with baseline, but there was no control drink for comparison [124]. Meta-analyses of acute or short-term, randomized controlled trials revealed that chocolate or cocoa-reduced insulin and fasting insulin after glucose challenge and improved insulin resistance with no effect on fasting glucose and glycated haemoglobin (HbA1c) [125].

Consumption of dark chocolate containing 500 mg polyphenols for a period of 4 weeks reduced blood pressure (BP), fasting glucose and insulin resistance in lean and overweight females compared to 20 g of placebo dark chocolate with negligible polyphenol content [126]. Drinking cocoa flavanols (902 mg) for 12 weeks also improved insulin sensitivity in overweight and obese individuals compared to a low-flavanol cocoa drink [127]. In contrast, daily consumption of 25 g dark chocolate for 8 weeks did not ameliorate fasting glucose, insulin and HbA1c levels in hypertensive diabetic subjects compared to those consuming 25 g of white chocolate [128]. Given the conflicting results obtained, current data are insufficient to use cocoa polyphenols for glycaemic control.

Cinnamon contains several polyphenols such as procyanidin, cinnamtannin trans-cinnamic acid and flavones (cinnamaldehyde and trans-cinnamaldehyde) and catechin, and several studies have shown the positive effects of cinnamon on glycaemic control [123]. Two clinical studies reported positive effects of cinnamon on fasting blood glucose levels, but no significant changes of HbA1c, LDL, HDL, total cholesterol or TG [129, 130]. Other studies reported no significant changes in fasting glucose, lipids, HbA1c, or insulin levels in 43 subjects with T2D receiving 1 g of cinnamon daily for 3 months [131], 25 postmenopausal women with T2D taking 1.5 g of cinnamon daily for 6 weeks [132], in 11 healthy subjects taking cinnamon (3 g) daily for 4 weeks [133], and in 72 adolescents with T1D taking 1 g of cinnamon daily [134]. A randomized, placebo-controlled, double-blind clinical trial of 58 subjects with T2D found that intake of 2 g daily of cinnamon for 12 weeks significantly reduced HbA1c, systolic blood and diastolic blood pressure [135]. Whole grains including wheat, soy, rye and flaxseed and nuts such as almonds, pecans and hazelnuts are an important source of polyphenols [136]. Whole grain intake is associated with a reduced risk of T2D, but the mechanism of the protection is not well understood [137]. Extra virgin olive oil and olive leafs are another source of polyphenols such as oleuropein and hydroxytyrosol, and they are suggested to have beneficial effects in T2D [138]. The Mediterranean diet supplemented with virgin olive oil or nuts harboured anti-inflammatory effects by decreasing chemokines, interleukin-6 (IL-6) and adhesion molecules, and T-lymphocytes and monocytes [139]. A study of 3541 patients with high cardiovascular risk revealed that a Mediterranean diet rich in extra virgin oil leads to a 40% reduction in the risk of T2D compared with the control group [140].

Supplementation with olive leaf polyphenols improved insulin sensitivity and pancreatic β-cells secretory capacity after oral glucose challenge in overweight, middle-aged men at the risk of developing metabolic syndrome [141, 142]. Supplementation with a 500 mg olive leaf extract tablet for 14 weeks in subjects with T2D significantly lowered HbA1c and fasting insulin but had no effects on postprandial insulin levels [142, 143].

Red wine, berries, grape skins, rhubarb roots, red wine and peanuts, and the roots of rhubarb are sources of resveratrol, a polyphenol naturally synthesized by plants in response to infection and injury. Resveratrol supplementation in obese men for a period of 30 days reduced glucose, insulin, insulin resistance index and leptin, and decreased inflammatory markers (TNF-α, leukocytes). Even though resveratrol supplementation also decreased adipose tissue lipolysis and plasma fatty acid and glycerol in the postprandial state [144], the study lacked some of the necessary controls therefore more investigations are needed in order to state that resveratrol has antidiabetic effects.

11. Conclusions and perspectives

The diet-microbiota-diabetes trio is a hot research topic at the moment, and it still requires further investigation. Even though several studies highlight the benefits associated to the consumption of probiotics in the management of diabetes, their use is hindered by the insufficient information regarding their mechanisms of action. Furthermore, additional human studies are still needed in order to get a better understanding of the role held by the ethnicity and diet in shaping the diabetic microbiome. Finally, future studies combining microbiota analysis, metabolomics, proteomics as well as treatment regimens will provide valuable information regarding the pathomechanisms of diabetes and potentially ways to prevent the onset of disease.

Acknowledgements

This work was supported by the Research Grant PN III - P2-2.1-BG-2016-0369-116/2016.

Author details

Gratiela G. Pircalabioru[1*], Ariana Picu[1,2], Laura Petcu[1,2], Marcela Popa[1] and Mariana Carmen Chifiriuc[1]

*Address all correspondence to: gratiela87@gmail.com

1 Research Institute of the University of Bucharest, ICUB, Bucharest, Romania

2 National Institute of Diabetes Nutrition and Metabolic Diseases (NIDNMD) "Prof. N.C. Paulescu", Bucharest, Romania

References

[1] Ionescu C. Tratat de Diabet Paulescu. Targoviste: Academiei Romane; 2004. p. 243-244, 734-750, 755-777, 895-1067

[2] A. D. Association. Standards of medical care in diabetes—2015: Summary of revisions. Diabetes Care. 2015;**38**(1):S4

[3] Grigore Mihaescu CC. Immunology and Immunopathology. Editura Medicala; Bucharest, Romania. 2015

[4] Pettitt DJ, Talton J, Dabelea D, Divers J, Imperatore G, Lawrence JM, Liese AD, Linder B, Mayer-Davis EJ, Pihoker C, et al. Prevalence of diabetes in U.S. Youth in 2009: The search for diabetes in youth study. Diabetes Care. 2014;402-408

[5] Kantarova D, Buc M. Genetic susceptibility to type 1 diabetes mellitus in humans. Physiological Research. 2007;**56**:255-266

[6] Atkinson MA, Eisenbarth GS. Type 1 diabetes: New perspectives on disease pathogenesis and treatment. Lancet. 2001;**358**(9277):221-222

[7] Kasper D et al. Harrison's Principles of Internal Medicine. McGraw-Hill; NewYork, USA. 2015

[8] Le Roith D, Taylor SI, Olefsy JM. Diabetes Mellitus. A Fundamental and Clinical Text. Lippincot, Williams and Wilkins; Philadelphia, Pennsylvania, United States. 2000

[9] Feldman R, Sender AJ, Siegelaub AB. Difference in diabetic and nondiabetic fat distribution patterns by skinfold measurements. Diabetes. 1969;**18**:478-486

[10] Hartz AJ, Rupley DC, Rimm AA. The association of girth measurements with disease in 32,856 women. American Journal of Epidemiology. 1984;**119**:71-80

[11] Lillioja S, Mott DM, Spraul M. Insulin resistance and insulin secretory dysfunction as precursors of non-insulin-dependant diabetes mellitus: Prospective studies of Pima Indians. The New England Journal of Medicine. 1993;**329**:1988-1992

[12] Gray SL, Vidal-Puig AJ. Adipose tissue expandability in the maintenance of metabolic homeostasis. Nutrition Reviews. 2007;**65**(6 Pt 2):S7-S12

[13] Cinti S, Mitchell G, Barbatelli G. Adipocyte death defines macrophage localization and function in adipose tissue of obese mice and humans. Jounral of Lipid Research. 2005;2347-2355

[14] Longo DL, Fauci AS, Dennis L, Kasper LS, Hauser J, Jameson JL, Loscalzo J. Harrison's Principle of Internal Medicine. Vol. I. McGraw-Hill; New York City, New York, United States. 2011

[15] Dominguez-Bello MG, Costello EK, Contreras M, et al. Delivery mode shapes the acquisition and structure of the initial microbiota across multiple body habitats in newborns. Proc Natl Acad Sci USA. 2010;**107**(26):11971-11975

[16] Power SE, O'Toole PW, Stanton C, et al. Intestinal microbiota, diet and health. British Journal of Nutrition. 2014;**111**(3):387-402

[17] Mejía-León ME, de la Barca AM. Diet, microbiota and immune system in type 1 diabetes development and evolution. Nutrients. 2015;**7**(11):9171-9184

[18] Arumugam M, Raes J, Pelletier E, et al. Enterotypes of the human gut microbiome. Nature. 2011;**473**(7346):174-180

[19] Wu GD, Chen J, Hoffmann C, et al. Linking long-term dietary patterns with gut microbial enterotypes. Science. 2011;**80**:105-108

[20] Knights D, Ward TL, McKinlay CE, Miller H, Gonzalez A, McDonald D, Knight R. Rethinking 'enterotypes'. Cell Host & Microbe. 2014;**16**:433-437

[21] Macpherson AJ, Harris NL. Interactions between commensal intestinal bacteria and the immune system. Nat Rev Immunol. 2004;**4**:1626-1632

[22] Aagaard K, Ma J, Antony KM, et al. The placenta harbors a unique microbiome. Science Translational Medicine. 2014;**6**(237):237ra65

[23] Rogier EW, Frantz AL, Bruno ME, Wedlund L, Cohen DA, Stromberg AJ, Kaetzel CS. Secretory antibodies in breast milk promote long-term intestinal homeostasis by regulating the gut microbiota and host gene expression. Proc Natl Acad Sci USA. 2014;**111**:3074-3079

[24] Virtanen SM, Nevalainen J, Kronberg-Kippilä C, Ahonen S, Tapanainen H, Uusitalo L, Takkinen H-M, Niinistö S, Ovaskainen M-L, Kenward MG, et al. Food consumption and advanced β cell autoimmunity in young children with HLA-conferred susceptibility to type 1 diabetes: A nested case-control design. The American Journal of Clinical Nutrition. 2012;**95**:471-478

[25] Vaarala O. Is the origin of type 1 diabetes in the gut? Immunology and Cell Biology. 2012;**90**(3):271-276

[26] Davis-Richardson A, Triplett E. A model for the role of gut bacteria in the development of autoimmunity for type 1 diabetes. Diabetologia. 2015;**6**(10):1386-1393

[27] Larsen J, Weile C, Antvorskov JC, Engkilde K, Nielsen SMB, Josefsen K, Buschard K. Effect of dietary gluten on dendritic cells and innate immune subsets in BALB/c and NOD mice. PLoS One. 2015;**10**(3):e0118618

[28] Oldstone MB. Prevention of type I diabetes in nonobese diabetic mice by virus infection. Science. 1988;**80**:500-502

[29] Boerner BP, Sarvetnick NE. Type 1 diabetes: Role of intestinal microbiome in humans and mice. Annals of the New York Academy of Sciences. 2011;**1243**:103-118

[30] King C, Sarvetnick N. The incidence of type-1 diabetes in NOD mice is modulated by restricted flora not germ-free conditions. PLoS One. 2011;**6**(2):e17049-e17052

[31] Brugman S, Klatter FA, Visser JT, et al. Antibiotic treatment partially protects against type 1 diabetes in the bio-breeding diabetes-prone rat. Is the gut flora involved in the development of type 1 diabetes? Diabetologia. 2006;**49**(9):2105-2108

[32] Patterson E, Marques TM, O'Sullivan O, et al. Streptozotocin-induced type-1-diabetes disease onset in Sprague-Dawley rats is associated with an altered intestinal microbiota composition and decreased diversity. Microbiology. 2015;**161**(Pt 1):182-193

[33] Neu J, Reverte CM, Mackey AD, et al. Changes in intestinal morphology and permeability in the biobreeding rat before the onset of type 1 diabetes. Journal of Pediatric Gastroenterology and Nutrition. 2005;**40**(5):589-595

[34] Watts T, Berti I, Sapone A, et al. Role of the intestinal tight junction modulator zonulin in the pathogenesis of type I diabetes in BB diabetic-prone rats. Proceedings of the National Academy of Sciences of the United States of America. 2005;**102**(8):2916-2921

[35] Valladares R, Sankar D, Li N, et al. Lactobacillus johnsonii N6.2mitigates the development of type 1 diabetes in BB-DP rats. PLoS One. 2010;**5**(5):e10507-e10516

[36] Wen L, Ley RE, Volchkov PY, et al. Innate immunity and intestinal microbiota in the development of type 1 diabetes. Nature. 2008;**455**(7216):1109-1113

[37] De Goffau MC, Luopajärvi K, Knip M, Ilonen J, Ruohtula T, Härkönen T, Orivuori L, Hakala S, Welling GW, Harmsen HJ, et al. Fecal microbiota composition differs between children with β-cell autoimmunity and those without. Diabetes. 2013;**62**(4):1238-1244

[38] Kostic AD, Gevers D, Siljander H, Vatanen T, Hyötyläinen T, Hämäläinen A-M, Peet A, Tillmann V, Pöhö P, Mattila I, et al. The dynamics of the human infant gut microbiome in development and in progression toward type 1 diabetes. Cell Host & Microbe. 2015;**17**(2):260-273

[39] Endesfelder D et al. Compromised gut microbiota networks in children with anti-islet cell autoimmunity. Diabetes. 2014;**63**:2006-2014

[40] Ziegler AG, Rewers M, Simell O, Simell T, Lempainen J, Steck A, Winkler C, Ilonen J, Veijola R, Knip M, et al. Seroconversion to multiple islet autoantibodies and risk of progression to diabetes in children. Journal of the American Medical Association. 2013; **309**(23):2473-2479

[41] Murri M, Leiva I, Gomez-Zumaquero JM, Tinahones F, Cardona F, Soriguer F, Queipo-Ortuno MI. Gut microbiota in children with type 1 diabetes differs from that in healthy children: A case-control study. BMC Medicine. 2013;**309**(23):2473-2479

[42] Brown CT, Davis-Richardson AG, Giongo A, Gano KA, Crabb DB, Mukherjee N, Casella G, Drew JC, Ilonen J, Knip M, et al. Gut microbiome metagenomics analysis suggests a functional model for the development of autoimmunity for type 1 diabetes. PLoS One. 2011;**11**:e25792

[43] Giongo A, Gano KA, Crabb DB, Mukherjee N, Novelo LL, Casella G, Drew JC, Ilonen J, Knip M, Hyoty H, et al. Toward defining the autoimmune microbiome for type 1 diabetes. ISME Journal. 2011;**5**(1):82-91

[44] Lumey LH, Van Poppel FW. The Dutch famine of 1944-45: Mortality and morbidity in past and present generations. Social History of Medicine. 1994;**7**(2):229-246

[45] Seidell JC. Dietary fat and obesity: An epidemiologic perspective. The American Journal of Clinical Nutrition. 1998;**67**(3 Suppl):546S-550S

[46] Ludwig DS, Peterson KE, Gortmaker SL. Relation between consumption of sugar-sweetened drinks and childhood obesity: A prospective, observational analysis. Lancet. 2001; **357**(9255):505-508

[47] Lundgren H, Bengtsson C, Blohmé G, Isaksson B, Lapidus L, Lenner RA, et al. Dietary habits and incidence of noninsulin-dependent diabetes mellitus in a population study of women in Gothenburg, Sweden. The American Journal of Clinical Nutrition. 1989; **49**(4):708-712

[48] Marshall JA, Hamman RF, Baxter J. High-fat, low-carbohydrate diet and the etiology of non-insulin-dependent diabetes mellitus: The San Luis valley diabetes study. American Journal of Epidemiology. 1991;**134**(6):590-603

[49] Nseir W, Nassar F, Assy N. Soft drinks consumption and nonalcoholic fatty liver disease. World Journal of Gastroenterology. 2010;**16**(21):2579-2588

[50] Amin TT, Al-Sultan AI, Ali A. Overweight and obesity and their association with dietary habits, and sociodemographic characteristics among male primary school children in Al-Hassa, Kingdom of Saudi Arabia. Indian Journal of Community Medicine. 2008;**33**(3): 172-181

[51] Panagiotakos DB, Tzima N, Pitsavos C, C. C, Papakonstantinou E, Zampelas A, et al. The relationship between dietary habits, blood glucose and insulin levels among people without cardiovascular disease and type 2 diabetes: The ATTICA study. The Review of Diabetic Studies. 2005;**2**(4):208-215

[52] Villegas R, Shu XO, Gao YT, Yang G, Elasy T, Li H, et al. Vegetable but not fruit consumption reduces the risk of type 2 diabetes in Chinese women. Journal of Nutrition. 2008;**138**(3):574-580

[53] Krawagh AM, Alzahrani AM, Naser TA. Diabetes complications and their relation to glycemic control among patients attending diabetic clinic at king khalid national guard hospital in Jeddah, Saudi Arabia. Saudi Journal of Internal Medicine. 2012;**1**(1):29-33

[54] Nanri A, Mizoue T, Noda M, Takahashi Y, Kato M, Inoue M, et al. Rice intake and type 2 diabetes in Japanese men and women: The Japan public health center-based prospective study. The American Journal of Clinical Nutrition. 2010;**92**(6):1468-1477

[55] Sanz Y. Effects of a gluten-free diet on gut microbiota and immune function in healthy adult humans. Gut Microbes. 2010;**1**(3):135-137

[56] Bonder MJ, Tigchelaar EF, Cai X, Trynka G, Cenit MC, Hrdlickova B, et al. The influence of a short-term gluten-free diet on the human gut microbiome. Genome Medicine. 2016;**8**:45. doi: 10.1186/s13073-016-0295-y

[57] Drasar BS, Crowther JS, Goddard P, Hawksworth G, Hill MJ, Peach S, et al. The relation between diet and the gut microflora in man. Proceedings of the Nutrition Society. 2007; **32**(2):49-52

[58] Park JE, Seo JE, Lee JY, Kwon H. Distribution of seven N-nitrosamines in food. Toxicology Research. 2015;**31**(3):279-288

[59] Wu GD, Compher C, Chen EZ, Smith SA, Shah RD, Bittinger K, et al. Comparative metabolomics in vegans and omnivores reveal constraints on diet-dependent gut microbiota metabolite production. Gut. 2014;**1**:63-72

[60] Lopez-Legarrea P, Fuller NR, Zulet MA, Martinez JA, Caterson ID. The influence of Mediterranean, carbohydrate and high protein diets on gut microbiota composition in the treatment of obesity and associated inflammatory state. Asia Pacific Journal of Clinical Nutrition. 2014;**23**(3):360-368

[61] Singh RK et al. Influence of diet on the gut microbiome and implications for human health. Journal of Translational Medicine. 2017;**15**:73

[62] DeFilippis F, Pellegrini N, Vannini L, Jeffery IB, La Storia A, Laghi L, et al. High-level adherence to a Mediterranean diet beneficially impacts the gut microbiota and associated metabolome. Gut. 2015:gutjnl-2015. Gut. 2016;**65**:1812-1821

[63] Hentges DJ, Maier BR, Burton GC, Flynn MA, Tsutakawa RK. Effect of a high-beef diet on the fecal bacterial flora of humans. Cancer Research. 1977;**37**(2):568-571

[64] David LA, Maurice CF, Carmody RN, Gootenberg DB, Button JE, Wolfe BE, et al. Diet rapidly and reproducibly alters the human gut microbiome. Nature. 2014;**505**(7484):559-563

[65] Russell WR, Gratz SW, Duncan SH, Holtrop G, Ince J, Scobbie L, et al. High-protein, reduced-carbohydrate weight-loss diets promote metabolite profiles likely to be detrimental to colonic health. The American Journal of Clinical Nutrition. 2011;**93**(5):1062-1072

[66] Machiels K, Joossens M, Sabino J, De Preter V, Arijs I, Eeckhaut V, et al. A decrease of the butyrate-producing species Roseburia hominis and *Faecalibacterium prausnitzii* defines dysbiosis in patients with ulcerative colitis. Gut. 2014;**63**(8):1275-1283

[67] Levine ME, Suarez JA, Brandhorst S, Balasubramanian P, C. C., Madia F, et al. Low protein intake is associated with a major reduction in IGF-1, cancer, and overall mortality in the 65 and younger but not older population. Cell Metabolism. 2014;**19**(3):407-417

[68] Stamler J, Daviglus ML, Garside DB, Dyer AR, Greenland P, Neaton JD. Relationship of baseline serum cholesterol levels in 3 large cohorts of younger men to long-term coronary, cardiovascular, and all-cause mortality and to longevity. Journal of the American Medical Association. 2004;**284**(3):311-318

[69] Fava F, Gitau R, Griffin BA, Gibson GR, Tuohy KM, Lovegrove JA. The type and quantity of dietary fat and carbohydrate alter faecal microbiome and short-chain fatty acid excretion in a metabolic syndrome 'at-risk' population. International Journal of Obesity. 2013;**37**(2):216-223

[70] Lecomte V, Kaakoush NO, Maloney CA, Raipuria M, H. K, Mitchell HM, et al. Changes in gut microbiota in rats fed a high fat diet correlate with obesity-associated metabolic parameters. PLoS One. 2015;**10**(5):e0126931

[71] Caesar R, Tremaroli V, Kovatcheva-Datchary P, Cani PD, Bäckhed F. Crosstalk between gut microbiota and dietary lipids aggravates WAT inflammation through TLR signaling. Cell Metabolism. 2015;**22**(4):658-668

[72] Parvin S. Nutritional analysis of date fruits (*Phoenix dactylifera* L.) in perspective of Bangladesh. American Journal of Life Sciences. 2015;**3**(4):274

[73] Eid N, Enani S, Walton G, Corona G, Costabile A, Gibson G, et al. The impact of date palm fruits and their component polyphenols, on gut microbial ecology, bacterial metabolites and colon cancer cell proliferation. Journal of Nutrition Science. 2014;**3**:e46

[74] Francavilla R, Calasso M, Calace L, Siragusa S, N. M., Vernocchi P, et al. Effect of lactose on gut microbiota and metabolome of infants with cow's milk allergy. Pediatric Allergy and Immunology. 2012;**23**(5):420-427

[75] Suez J, Korem T, Zeevi D, Zilberman-Schapira G, Thaiss CA, Maza O, et al. Artificial sweeteners induce glucose intolerance by altering the gut microbiota. Nature. 2014; **514**(7521):181-186

[76] de Vrese M, Schrezenmeir J. Probiotics, prebiotics, and synbiotics. Advances in Biochemical Engineering/Biotechnology. 2008;**111**:1-66

[77] Pandey KR, Naik SR, Vakil BV. Probiotics, prebiotics and synbiotics – A review. The Journal of Food Science and Technology. 2015;**52**(12):7577-7587

[78] Halmos EP, Christophersen CT, Bird AR, Shepherd SJ, Gibson PR, Muir JG. Diets that differ in their FODMAP content alter the colonic luminal microenvironment. Gut. 2015;**64**(1):93-100

[79] Cotillard A, Kennedy SP, Kong LC, Prifti E, Pons N, Le Chatelier E, et al. Dietary intervention impact on gut microbial gene richness. Nature. 2013;**500**(7464):585-588

[80] Costabile A, Klinder A, Fava F, Napolitano A, Fogliano V, Leonard C, Gibson GR, Tuohy KM. Whole-grain wheat breakfast cereal has a prebiotic effect on the human gut microbiota: A double-blind, placebo-controlled, crossover study. British Journal of Nutrition. 2008;**99**(1):110-120

[81] Carvalho-Wells AL, Helmolz K, Nodet C, Molzer C, Leonard C, McKevith B, et al. Determination of the in vivo prebiotic potential of a maizebased whole grain breakfast cereal: A human feeding study. British Journal of Nutrition. 2010;**104**(9):1353-1356.

[82] Bäckhed F, Ding H, Wang T, et al. The gut microbiota as an environmental factor that regulates fat storage. Proceedings of the National Academy of Sciences of the United States of America. 2004;**101**(44):15718-15723

[83] Bäckhed F, Manchester JK, Semenkovich CF, et al. Mechanisms underlying the resistance to diet-induced obesity in germ-free mice. Proceedings of the National Academy of Sciences of the United States of America. 2007;**104**(3):979-984

[84] Qin J, Li Y, Cai Z, et al. A metagenome-wide association study of gut microbiota in type 2 diabetes. Nature. 2012;**490**(7418):55-60

[85] Turnbaugh PJ, Ley RE, Mahowald MA, et al. An obesity-associated gut microbiome with increased capacity for energy harvest. Nature. 2006;**444**(7122):1027-1031

[86] Larsen N, Vogensen FK, van den Berg FW, Nielsen DS, Andreasen AS, Pedersen BK, Al-Soud WA, Sørensen SJ, Hansen LH, Jakobsen M. Gut microbiota in human adults with type 2 diabetes differs from non-diabetic adults. PLoS One. 2010;**5**(2):e9085

[87] Serino M, Luche E, Gres S, et al. Metabolic adaptation to a high-fat diet is associated with a change in the gut microbiota. Gut. 2012;**61**(4):543-553

[88] Shin NR, Lee JC, Lee HY, et al. An increase in the *Akkermansia* spp. population induced by metformin treatment improves glucose homeostasis in diet-induced obese mice. Gut. 2014;**63**(5):727-735

[89] Forslund K et al. Disentangling type 2 diabetes and metformin treatment signatures in the human gut microbiota. Nature. 2015;**528**(7581):262-266

[90] Duan F, Curtis KL, March JC. Secretion of insulinotropic proteins by commensal bacteria: Rewiring the gut to treat diabetes. Applied and Environmental Microbiology. 2008;**74**(23):7437-7438

[91] Paszti-Gere E, Szeker K, Csibrik-Nemeth E, Csizinszky R, Marosi A, Palocz O, Farkas O, Galfi P. Metabolites of *Lactobacillus plantarum* 2142 prevent oxidative stressinduced overexpression of proinflammatory cytokines in IPEC-J2 cell line. Inflammation. 2012;**35**(4):1487-1499

[92] Matsuzaki T, Yamazaki R, Hashimoto S, Yokokura T. Antidiabetic effect of an oral administration of *Lactobacillus casei* in a non-insulin dependent diabetes mellitus (NIDDM) model using KK-Ay mice. Endocrine Journal. 1997;**44**(3):357-365

[93] Matsuzaki T, Takagi A, Ikemura H, Matsuguchi T, Yokokura T. Intestinal Microflora: Probiotics and Autoimmunity. Journal of Nutrition. 2007;**137**(3 Suppl 2):798S-802S

[94] Tabuchi M, Ozaki M, Tamura A, et al. Antidiabetic effect of Lactobacillus GG in streptozotocin-induced diabetic rats. Bioscience, Biotechnology, and Biochemistry. 2003;**67**(6):1421-1424

[95] Yadav H, Jain S. Antidiabetic effect of probiotic dahi containing *Lactobacillus acidophilus* and *Lactobacillus casei* in high fructose fed rats. Nutrition. 2007;**23**(1):62-68

[96] Yadav H, Jain S. Oral administration of dahi containing probiotic *Lactobacillus acidophilus* and *Lactobacillus casei* delayed the progression of streptozotocin-induced diabetes in rats. Dairy Research. 2008;**75**(2):1-7

[97] Al-Salami H, Butt G, Tucker I, Skrbic R, Golocorbin-Kon S, Mikov M. Probiotic pretreatment reduces gliclazide permeation (ex vivo) in healthy rats but increases it in diabetic rats to the level seen in untreated healthy rats. Archives of Drug Information 2008;**1**(1):35-41

[98] Ma X, Hua J. Probiotics improve high fat diet-induced hepatic steatosis and insulin resistance by increasing hepatic NKT cells. Journal of Hepatology. 2008;**49**(5):821-830

[99] Andersson U, Bränning C, Ahrné S, et al. Probiotics lower plasma glucose in the high-fat fed C57BL/6 J mouse. Beneficial Microbes. 2010;**1**:189-196

[100] Lu YC, Yin LT, Chang WT, Huang JS. Effect of *Lactobacillus reuteri* GMNL-263 treatment on renal fibrosis in diabetic rats. Journal of Bioscience and Bioengineering. 2010;**110**(6):709-715

[101] Manirarora JN, Parnell SA, Hu YH, Kosiewich MM, Alard P. NOD dendritic cells stimulated with lactobacilli preferentially produce IL-10 versus IL-12 and decrease diabetes incidence. Clinical and Developmental Immunology. 2011;**2011**:1-12

[102] Chen JJ, Wang R, Li XF, Wang RL. *Bifidobacterium longum* supplementation improved high-fat-fed-induced metabolic syndrome and promoted intestinal Reg I gene expression. Experimental Biology and Medicine. 2011;**236**:823-831

[103] Amar J, Chabo C, Waget A, et al. Intestinal mucosal adherence and translocation of commensal bacteria at the early onset of type 2 diabetes: Molecular mechanisms and probiotic treatment. EMBO Molecular Medicine. 2011;**3**:559-572

[104] Ejtahed HS, Mohtadi-Nia J, H., Rad A, et al. Effect of probiotic yogurt containing *Lactobacillus acidophilus* and *Bifidobacterium lactis* on lipid profile in individuals with type 2 mellitus. Journal of Dairy Science. 2011;**94**:3288-3294

[105] Ejtahed HS, Mohtadi-Nia J, Homayouni-Rad A, Niafar M, Asghari-Jafarabadi M, Mofid V. Probiotic yogurt improves antioxidant status in type 2 diabetic patients. Nutrition. 2012;**28**:539-543

[106] Moroti C, Souza Magri L, de Rezende Costa M, Cavallini DC, Sivieri K. Effect of the consumption of a new symbiotic shake on glycemia and cholesterol levels in elderly people with type 2 diabetes mellitus. Lipids in Health and Disease. 2012;**11**(1):29

[107] Shao F, Yang CG, Liu X, Yang DG. Application of microbiological and immunological enteral nutrition in patients with gastrointestinal cancer complicated with diabetes mellitus. Chinese Journal of Gastrointestinal Surgery. 2012;**15**:476-479

[108] Luoto R, Laitinen K, Nermes M, Isolauri E. Impact of maternal probiotic-supplemented dietary counseling during pregnancy on colostrum adiponectin concentration: A prospective, randomized, placebo-controlled study. Early Human Development. 2012;**88**:339-344

[109] Andreasen AS, Larsen N, Skovsgaard T, et al. Effects of *Lactobacillus acidophilus* NCFM on insulin sensitivity and the systemic inflammatory response in human subjects. British Journal of Nutrition. 2010;**104**:1831-1838

[110] Gibson GR, Roberfroid M. Dietary modulation of the human colonic microbiota: Introducing the concept of prebiotics. Journal of Nutrition. 1995;**125**(6):1401-1412

[111] Roberfroid M. Prebiotics: The concept revisited. American Society of Nutrition. 2007; **137**(3 Suppl 2):830S-837S

[112] Gibson GR, Probert HM, Loo JV, Rastall RA, Roberfroid MB. Dietary modulation of the human colonic microbiota: Updating the concept of prebiotics. Nutrition Research Reviews. 2004;**17**(2):259-275

[113] Przemyslaw J, Tomasik PT. Probiotics and Prebiotics. Cereal Chemistry. 2003;**80**(2): 113-117

[114] Pourghassem GB, Dehghan P, Aliasgharzadeh A, Asghari Jafar-abadi M. Effects of high performance inulin supplementation on glycemic control and antioxidant status in women with type 2 diabetes. Journal of Diabetes & Metabolism. 2013;**37**(2):140-148

[115] Parnell JA, Reimer RA. Prebiotic fibres dose-dependently increase satiety hormones and alter bacteroidetes and firmicutes in lean and obese JCR:LA-cp rats. British Journal of Nutrition. 2012;**107**(4):601-613

[116] Everard A, Lazarevic V, Derrien M, Girard M, Muccioli GG, Neyrinck AM, Possemiers S. van Holle A, Francois P, de Vos WM, et al. Responses of gut microbiota and glucose and lipid metabolism to prebiotics in genetic obese and diet-induced leptin-resistant mice. Diabetes. 2011;**60**(11):2775-2786

[117] Ahren B, Schmitz O. GLP-1 receptor agonists and DPP-4 inhibitors in the treatment of type 2 diabetes. Hormone and Metabolic Research. 2004;**36**(11-12):867-876

[118] Kim M, Shin HK. The water-soluble extract of chicory influences serum and liver lipid concentrations, cecal short-chain fatty acid concentrations and fecal lipid excretion in rats. Journal of Nutrition. 1998;**128**(10):1731-1736

[119] Causey JL, Feirtag JM, Gallaher DD, Tungland BC, Slavin JL. Effects of dietary inulin on serum lipids, blood glucose and the gastrointestinal, environment in hypercholesterolemic men. Nutrition Research. 2000;**20**(2):191-201

[120] Brighenti F, Casiraghi MC, Canzi E, Ferrari A. Effect of consumption of a ready-to-eat breakfast cereal containing inulin on the intestinal milieu and blood lipids in healthy male volunteers. European Journal of Clinical Nutrition. 1999;**53**(9):726-733

[121] Dikeman CL, Murphy MR, Fahey GC Jr. Dietary fibers affect viscosity of solutions and simulated human gastric and small intestinal digesta. Journal of Nutrition. 2006; **136**(4):913-919

[122] Hald S, Schioldan AG, Moore ME, Dige A, Lærke HN, Agnholt J, Bach Knudsen KE, Hermansen K, Marco ML, Gregersen DJ. Effects of arabinoxylan and resistant starch on intestinal microbiota and short-chain fatty acids in subjects with metabolic syndrome: A randomised crossover study. PLoS One. 2016;**11**:e0159223

[123] Kim YA, Keogh JB, Clifton PM. Polyphenols and glycemic control. Nutrients. 2016;**8**: pii: E17. DOI: 10.3390/nu8010017

[124] Queipo-Ortuno MI, Boto-Ordonez M, Murri M, Gomez-Zumaquero JM, Clemente-Postigo M, Estruch R, Cardona Diaz F, Andres-Lacueva C, Tinahones F. Influence of red wine polyphenols and ethanol on the gut microbiota ecology and biochemical biomarkers. American Journal of Clinical Nutrition. 2012;**95**(6):1323-1334

[125] Hooper L, Kay C, Abdelhamid A, Kroon PA, Cohn JS, Rimm EB, Cassidy A. Effects of chocolate, cocoa, and flavan-3-ols on cardiovascular health: A systematic review and meta-analysis of randomized trials. American Journal of Clinical Nutrition. 2012;**95**(3):740-751

[126] Almoosawi S, Tsang C, Ostertag LM, Fyfe L, Al-Dujaili EA. Differential effect of polyphenol-rich dark chocolate on biomarkers of glucose metabolism and cardiovascular risk factors in healthy, overweight and obese subjects: A randomized clinical trial. Food & Function. 2012;**3**(10):1035-1043

[127] Davison K, Coates AM, Buckley JD, Howe PR. Effect of cocoa flavanols and exercise on cardiometabolic risk factors in overweight and obese subjects. International Journal of Obesity. 2008;**32**(8):1289-1296

[128] Rostami A, Khalili M, Haghighat N, Eghtesadi S, Shidfar F, Heidari I, Ebrahimpour-Koujan S, Eghtesadi M. High-cocoa polyphenol-rich chocolate improves blood pressure in patients with diabetes and hypertension. ARYA Atherosclerosis. 2015;**11**(1):21-29

[129] Khan A, Safdar M, Ali Khan MM, Khattak KN, Anderson RA. Cinnamon improves glucose and lipids of people with type 2 diabetes. Diabetes Care. 2003;**26**(12):3215-3218

[130] Mang B, Wolters M, Schmitt B, Kelb K, Lichtinghagen R, Stichtenoth DO, Hahn A. Effects of a cinnamon extract on plasma glucose, hba, and serum lipids in diabetes mellitus type 2. European Journal of Clinical Investigation. 2006;**36**(5):340-344

[131] Blevins SM, Leyva MJ, Brown J, Wright J, Scofield RH, Aston CE. Effect of cinnamon on glucose and lipid levels in non insulin-dependent type 2 diabetes. Diabetes Care. 2007; **30**(9):2236-2237

[132] Vanschoonbeek K, Thomassen BJ, Senden JM, Wodzig WK, van Loon LJ. Cinnamon supplementation does not improve glycemic control in postmenopausal type 2 diabetes patients. Journal of Nutrition. 2006;**136**(4):977-980

[133] Tang M, Larson-Meyer DE, Liebman M. Effect of cinnamon and turmeric on urinary oxalate excretion, plasma lipids, and plasma glucose in healthy subjects. American Journal of Clinical Nutrition. 2008;**87**(5):1262-1267

[134] Altschuler JA, Casella SJ, MacKenzie TA, Curtis KM. The effect of cinnamon on A1C among adolescents with type 1 diabetes. Diabetes Care. 2007;**30**(4):813-816

[135] Akilen R, Tsiami A, Devendra D, Robinson N. Glycated haemoglobin and blood pressure-lowering effect of cinnamon in multi-ethnic type 2 diabetic patients in the UK: A randomized, placebo-controlled, double-blind clinical trial. Diabetes Medicine. 2010; **27**(10):1159-1167

[136] Perez-Jimenez J, Neveu V, Vos F, Scalbert A. Identification of the 100 richest dietary sources of polyphenols: An application of the phenol-explorer database. European Journal of Clinical Nutrition. 2010;**64**(Suppl 3):S112-S120

[137] Ye EQ, Chacko SA, Chou EL, Kugizaki M, Liu S. Greater whole-grain intake is associated with lower risk of type 2 diabetes, cardiovascular disease, and weight gain. Journal of Nutrition. 2012;**142**(7):1304-1313

[138] Cardona F, Andres-Lacueva C, Tulipani S, Tinahones FJ, Queipo-Ortuno MI. Benefits of polyphenols on gut microbiota and implications in human health. Journal of Nutritional Biochemistry. 2013;**24**(8):1415-1422

[139] Estruch R. Anti-inflammatory effects of the mediterranean diet: The experience of the PREDIMED study. Proceedings of the Nutrition Society. 2010;**69**(3):333-340

[140] Salas-Salvado J, Bullo M, Estruch R, Ros E, Covas MI, Ibarrola-Jurado N, Corella D, Aros F, Gomez-Gracia E, Ruiz-Gutierrez V, et al. Prevention of diabetes with mediterranean diets: A subgroup analysis of a randomized trial. Annals of Internal Medicine. 2014;**160**(1):1-10

[141] Shiomi Y et al. GCMS-based metabolomic study in mice with colitis induced by dextran sulfate sodium. Inflammatory Bowel Disease. 2011;**17**:2261-2274

[142] De Bock M, Derraik JG, Brennan CM, Biggs JB, Morgan PE, Hodgkinson SC, Hofman PL, Cutfield WS. Olive (olea europaea l.) leaf polyphenols improve insulin sensitivity in middle-aged overweight men: A randomized, placebo-controlled, crossover trial. PLoS One. 2013;e57622

[143] Wainstein J, Ganz T, Boaz M, Bar Dayan Y, Dolev E, Kerem Z, Madar Z. Olive leaf extract as a hypoglycemic agent in both human diabetic subjects and in rats. Journal of Medicinal Food. 2012;605-610

[144] Timmers S, Konings E, Bilet L, Houtkooper RH, van de Weijer T, Goossens GH, Hoeks J, van der Krieken S, Ryu D, Kersten S, et al. Calorie restriction-like effects of 30 days of resveratrol supplementation on energy metabolism and metabolic profile in obese humans. Cell Metabolism. 2011;612-622

Section 3

Structural Pathophysiology

Chapter 6

Hypophosphatasia: A Systemic Skeletal Disorder Caused by Alkaline Phosphatase Deficiency

Hideo Orimo

Additional information is available at the end of the chapter

http://dx.doi.org/10.5772/intechopen.70597

Abstract

Hypophosphatasia (HPP) is an inherited systemic bone disease caused by the deficiency of tissue-nonspecific alkaline phosphatase (TNAP). HPP is classified into six forms and the symptoms of HPP vary depending on the form. The pathophysiology of HPP is basically due to a defect of bone mineralization. TNAP is encoded by the *ALPL* gene, and the TNAP protein expressed in bone, kidney, liver, and neuronal cells and is linked to the cell membrane via a glycosylphosphatidylinositol anchor. TNAP is an ectoenzyme hydrolyzing phosphate compound such as inorganic pyrophosphate. TNAP plays an important role in mineralization of hard tissues. Defect of mineralization process causes hypomineralization of hard tissues, which leads to rickets or osteomalacia and dental manifestations. In addition, hypomineralization of the ribs results in respiratory failure in the severe forms, which is the main cause of death. Inheritance of HPP is autosomal recessive, but autosomal dominant cases have been reported in the milder forms. To date, a total of 335 mutations in the *ALPL* gene have been reported, and mutation sites are scattered throughout the gene. Recent development of enzyme replacement therapy has opened up a new vista on the treatment of this previously untreatable disease.

Keywords: hypophosphatasia, alkaline phosphatase, mineralization, bone, enzyme replacement therapy

1. Introduction

Hypophosphatasia (HPP; Online Mendelian Inheritance in Man (OMIM) #241500,241,510, 146,300) is an inherited systemic bone disease that is due to a deficiency of tissue-nonspecific alkaline phosphatase (TNAP) [1–3]. The first case of HPP was reported by the Canadian pediatrician John Campbell Rathbun in 1948 as a new developmental anomaly [4]. That case was an infantile form, and the patient's mutations were identified 50 years later using DNA of the surviving parents as a compound heterozygote of p.A114T and p.D294A [5]. Since then, a total of 335 mutations in the gene for TNAP (the *ALPL* gene) have been reported [6]. The symptoms of HPP vary and are classified into six HPP forms [1, 2]. The pathophysiology of HPP is basically due to a defect of bone mineralization. In severe forms, the patients show skeletal manifestations and respiratory failure derived from costal bone insufficiency, whereas in the mildest forms, they show only dental manifestations [1]. Recent development of enzyme replacement therapy (ERT) has opened up a new vista on the treatment of this previously untreatable disease [7].

2. TNAP: gene, structure of the protein, and its function as an enzyme

There are four human alkaline phosphatase (ALP) isoenzymes (**Table 1**): TNAP, placental alkaline phosphatase (PLAP), intestinal alkaline phosphatase (IAP), and germ cell ALP [8, 9]. The latter three ALPs are tissue-specific and are expressed in the placenta, intestine, and germ cells (embryonic and cancer cells), respectively [9]. TNAP, also known as the liver/bone/kidney (LBK) alkaline phosphatase, is expressed ubiquitously; liver, bone, kidney, neuronal cells, and white blood cells in particular are tissues that show marked expression [10].

Human TNAP is encoded by the *ALPL* gene that is located on the short arm of chromosome 1 (1p36.1–34). The coding region of the gene is approximately 1.5 kb in length, and it is extended over more than 50 kb of genomic DNA [11]. The *ALPL* gene consists of 12 exons of which exons 2–12 are coding exons and there exist two alternative noncoding exons 1 (bone type and liver type) [12, 13]. The promoter region of the gene includes a TATA box, an Sp1 binding site, and a retinoic acid responsive element (RARE) [14, 15].

Common name	Protein name	Gene	Chromosomal location	Sites of expression	Function
Tissue-nonspecific (liver/bone/kidney)	TNAP (TNSALP)	*ALPL*	1p36.1–34	Ubiquitous	Mineralization entrance of pyridoxal phosphate into the neuronal cells
Intestinal	IAP	*ALPI*	2q34–37	Intestine	Degradation of LPS* lipid absorption
Placental	PLAP (PAP)	*ALPP*	2q34–37	Placenta	Degradation of LPS* (?)
Germ cell (placental like)	–	*ALPP2*	2q34–37	Germ cells Cancer cells	

*Lipopolysaccharides.

Table 1. Isoenzymes of human ALP.

Retinoic acid regulates the expression of TNAP via RARE [15], whereas another fat-soluble vitamin, active vitamin D (1,25-dihydroxycholecalciferol), regulates the expression of TNAP by modification of the stability of TNAP mRNA [16]. Furthermore, phosphates derived from ALP enzymatic activity are considered to regulate TNAP expression [17]. Epigenetic regulation by methylation of some of the promoter regions of the gene has been reported [18]. However, the precise regulatory mechanism of the *ALPL* gene regulation, especially its tissue-specific regulation, is not known. On the other hand, the genes encoding tissue-specific ALPs are located on the long arm of chromosome 2 and have a more compact gene structure [19–22].

The TNAP protein, which has a molecular weight of approximately 80 kDa, is linked to the outer cell membrane through a glycosylphosphatidylinositol (GPI) anchor [9]. The TNAP protein is initially synthesized as a 66 kDa peptide, and then *O*- and *N*-glycosides are attached in the endoplasmic reticulum. Eventually, TNAP is localized on the outer membrane of the cells via a GPI anchor [23]. This GPI anchor is added after hydrophobic amino acid residues at the C-terminus are eliminated. The GPI anchor consists of an ethanolamine phosphate, three residues of mannose, a glucosamine, and a phosphatidylinositol [9]. The precise amino acid residue in TNAP to which the GPI anchor is added has not been elucidated, whereas it is known to be an aspartate residue (D484) in PLAP [24, 25]. An active enzyme consists of a dimer and acts as an ectoenzyme. Approximately 58% of the amino acid residues in human TNAP sequences are conserved among mammalian ALPs [26]. On the other hand, approximately 90% of the amino acid residues are conserved among mammalian TNAPs, which allow prediction of missense mutations responsible for HPP [26]. Since the three dimensional structure of TNAP has not been solved, a simulation model based on human PLAP or mouse IAP is used to discuss TNAP structure [27–29]. The active site of the enzyme comprises a catalytic serine residue (S92 in the human PLAP), two Zn^{2+}-binding sites, and an Mg^{2+}-binding site. Ca^{2+} is also necessary as a cofactor. The crown domain is characteristic of mammalian ALPs and is considered to interact with extracellular proteins including collagen [30]. There are also isoforms of TNAP itself that depend on the tissue origin. Since these isoforms have different *O*-linked sugar chains, they show different patterns on the electrophoresis. [9, 31].

The systematic name of ALP is orthophosphoric-monoester phosphohydrolase [alkaline optimum] (EC 3.1.3.1) that hydrolyzes monophosphate esters, and the optimal pH is between 8 and 10 [9]. Inorganic pyrophosphate (PPi) and pyridoxal 5′-phosphate (PLP) are considered to be natural substrates of the enzyme [32]. PPi is an inhibitor of hydroxyapatite formation, which is essential for bone mineralization. PLP is an active vitamin B_6 and is necessary in neuronal cells for the biosynthesis of γ-aminobutyric acid (GABA), which acts as an inhibitory neurotransmitter. PLP on the outside of neuronal cells must be dephosphorylated by TNAP at the cell membrane before it can enter the neuronal cells, and it is then be rephosphorylated within the neuronal cells [32, 33]. In laboratory testing, ALP enzymatic activity is usually estimated using *p*-nitrophenylphosphate as an artificial substrate [9].

3. Molecular process of mineralization and the role of TNAP in mineralization

Biomineralization in hard tissues including bone occurs in a two-step process [34]. Hypertrophic chondrocytes, osteoblasts, and odontocytes in the bone and dental tissues bud matrix vesicles (MVs) from the cell membrane [2, 35]. MVs are 50–200 nm in diameter and are enclosed by a membrane. MVs are a type of extracellular vesicles; however, the difference between MVs and exosomes, which are secreted by cells in the nonmineralized condition, is unclear [36]. TNAP is one of the most abundant proteins on the membrane of an MV [34]. The other proteins that are abundant in MVs are annexins A2, A5, and A6, Ca^{2+}-ATPase, nucleotide pyrophosphatase phosphodiesterase 1 (NPP1), Pit-1 (a sodium-phosphate cotransporter), and PHOSPHO1, all of which have important roles in mineralization [9, 34]. Biologically, mineralization is defined as the deposition of hydroxyapatite ($Ca_{10}(PO_4)_6(OH)_2$) crystals among the collagen fibers. If this process is insufficient, extracellular spaces are not mineralized, which leads to the formation of an abnormal soft tissue called osteoid tissue. In the first step of the mineralization, hydroxyapatite is formed in an MV. The membrane lipids of the MV provide a source of phosphate; of these lipids, phosphatidylcholine and phosphatidylethanolamine are hydrolyzed by phospholipase C (PLC), yielding phosphocholine (PCho) and phosphoethanolamine (PEA), respectively [37]. Subsequently, PCho and PEA are hydrolyzed by PHOSPHO1, a cytosolic phosphatase abundant in MVs [38]. The phosphate transporter, Pit-1, provides another source of phosphate. On the other hand, calcium is incorporated into MVs via an annexin calcium channel, which consists of annexins A2, A5, and A6 [34, 35]. When the concentration of calcium phosphate rises beyond the solubility of calcium phosphate, hydroxyapatite crystal formation begins. Subsequently, hydroxyapatite crystals penetrate the MV membrane and elongate in the extracellular space [34, 35]. For the elongation of hydroxyapatite, calcium and phosphate should be provided by the extracellular space. Although calcium ions may be abundant in this milieu, phosphate is provided mainly by the TNAP on the MV membrane, which hydrolyzes PPi to yield inorganic phosphate (Pi) [2, 8, 34]. This hydrolysis by TNAP has dual roles; it supplies a source of phosphate for hydroxyapatite formation and degrades an inhibitor of hydroxyapatite formation (PPi). Ultimately, formed hydroxyapatite crystals deposit among collagen fibers, and mineralization is complete (**Figure 1**). Although the crown domain of TNAP can bind collagen and is suggested to have a role in hydroxyapatite deposition, it has not been elucidated whether TNAP plays a direct role in hydroxyapatite deposition.

Extracellular PPi is formed by NPP1 on the MV membrane by hydrolysis of ATP and also provided by a membrane transporter of PPi, ANKH (the human homolog of ANK, the mouse progressive ankylosis gene product). Therefore, mineralization is regulated by the balance of the activities of these three molecules: TNAP, NPP1, and ANKH [9, 39, 40], Experiments using mice with knockout of these three genes showed that loss of activity of NPP1 or ANKH leads to hypercalcification (ectopic calcification of aorta and/or vertebrae and joints), whereas that of TNAP causes hypomineralization [41].

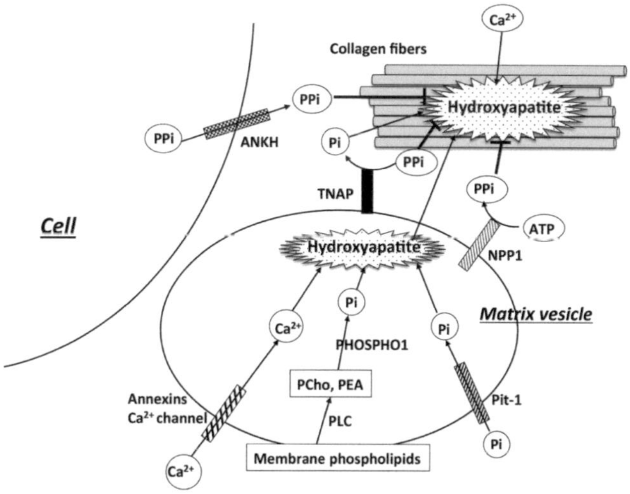

Figure 1. Mineralization process focusing on the matrix vesicle.

4. Clinical features of HPP including laboratory tests

HPP is classified into six forms depending on the onset age and the clinical severity (**Table 2**): perinatal (lethal) form, perinatal benign form, infantile form, childhood form, adult form, and odontohypophosphatasia [3]. The perinatal form occurs in utero and exhibits the most severe manifestations. Patients are stillborn or die during the early postnatal period. They show hypomineralization of the cranial bone and shortened and deformed limbs during gestation, which are easily revealed by ultrasonic examination. The hypomineralization of bones causes a membranous cranium and early craniosynostosis as well as musculoskeletal disorder after birth. The ribs are also hypomineralized, leading to respiratory failure after birth, which often requires respiratory aid. Failure of respiratory management often causes respiratory infections, which are the main cause of death. Epileptic seizures sometimes occur due to a deficit of PLP in neuronal cells, since PLP needs TNAP to enter neuronal cells. A deficit of PLP in neuronal cells causes a decrease in the inhibitory neurotransmitter GABA, leading to epileptic seizures. The perinatal benign form is a recently reported form [42]. Although the symptoms are recognized in gestation, prognosis is good and nonlethal. The infantile form occurs before 6 months of age and also shows severe manifestations. Patients display rickets and deformity of ribs and limbs, and fail to thrive. They also exhibit respiratory failure due to hypomineralization of the ribs, which requires respiratory aid. Recent progress in respiratory management elongates their lifespan. In addition, they often show hypercalcemia and hypercalciuria, leading to nephrocalcinosis. The childhood form shows manifestations after 6 months of age, whose symptoms are milder and not life-threatening. Patients show deformity of limbs, delayed walking, waddling gait, and muscle weakness. Craniosynostosis and

Form	Inheritance pattern	Onset	Symptoms	Prognosis
Perinatal	AR	In utero	Deformity of extremities	Lethal
			Membranous cranium	
			Respiratory failure	
			Epileptic seizures	
Perinatal benign	AR or AD	In utero	Rickets	Benign
Infantile	AR	After birth	Rickets, Craniosynostosis	Mostly lethal
		Before 6 months of age	Respiratory failure	
			Failure to thrive	
			Epileptic seizures	
			Premature loss of deciduous teeth	
Childhood	AR or AD	After 6 months of age	Rickets	Benign
			Musculoskeletal weakness	
			Premature loss of deciduous teeth	
Adult	AR or AD	Middle age	Osteomalacia	Benign
			Stress fractures	
Odontohypophosphatasia	AR or AD		Premature loss of deciduous teeth	Benign
			Dental caries	

AR: autosomal recessive, AD: autosomal dominant.

Table 2. Clinical features of hypophosphatasia.

high intracranial pressure sometimes occur. These patients also show premature loss of deciduous teeth due to failure of cementum formation [43]. Radiologically, childhood form patients exhibit a characteristic tongue-like radiolucent projection from the rachitic growth plate into the metaphysis due to a focal bone defect at the ends of long bones [1, 3]. The adult form occurs during middle age. Although the natural history of the adult form has not been well characterized, patients sometimes have a history of rickets and/or premature loss of deciduous teeth [44]. In the adult form, osteomalacia develops with pain associated with often recurring metatarsal stress fractures. In some patients, calcium pyrophosphate dehydrate crystals are deposited on articular cartilage due to an increase in concentrations of endogenous PPi [1]. Odontohypophosphatasia manifests only dental symptoms such as premature loss of deciduous teeth without skeletal symptoms due to rickets or osteomalacia.

http://dx.doi.org/10.5772/intechopen.70597

General
Failure to thrive
Poor feeding
Weakness
Skeletal
Hypomineralization
Rickets/osteomalacia
Short, deformed limbs
Membranous cranium
Craniosynostosis
Deformed ribs
Skeletal pain
Short statue
Muscular
Muscle weakness
Gait disturbances; delayed walking, waddling gait
Neuronal
Epileptic seizures (pyridoxine dependent)
Irritability
Respiratory
Respiratory failure
Renal
Nephrocalcinosis
Dental
Premature loss of deciduous teeth
Dental caries
Blood examination
Reduced serum ALP
Elevated plasma PPi, PLP and PEA
Elevated plasma Ca^{2+}
Urinalysis
Elevated urine PEA
Elevated urine Ca^{2+}

Different presentation of symptoms is exhibited depend on the forms.

Table 3. Signs and symptoms of HPP.

A common histopathological feature of HPP is hypomineralization of bone and teeth [1]. Extracellular hydroxyapatite crystals are reduced, although mineralization occurs within the MV, because PHOSPHO1 acts in the MV. Elongation of hydroxyapatite is impaired. Osteoid tissues are increased in bone, which contains nonmineralized extracellular matrix, and they cause rickets or osteomalacia [45].

For all forms, a characteristic laboratory finding is low serum alkaline phosphatase activity, in which the bone isozyme is reduced [1]. In addition, the natural enzyme substrates, plasma PPi and PLP are elevated. Urine PEA is also elevated, although it is doubtful whether this compound is a natural substrate of TNAP. However, because urine PEA is easy to evaluate by using high-performance liquid chromatography (HPLC), the measurement of PEA is widely used for the diagnosis [2]. The combination of low ALP activity with elevated PPi or PEA is strong evidence for HPP. In some milder cases, however, an increase in PEA is not shown, and, in some cases, PEA is slightly elevated in carriers [46]. Signs and symptoms of HPP are summarized in **Table 3**.

5. Genetic aspect of HPP

5.1. Inheritance of HPP

HPP is an autosomal recessive inherited disease [1]. Carriers usually do not exhibit any manifestations. Sometimes, however, carriers show subnormal serum ALP activity and slightly higher urine PEA values [2, 46]. The penetrance differs among forms. In some milder cases, an autosomal dominant cases have been reported [47, 48], and the dominant negative effect accounts for some autosomal dominant cases [48]. In addition, different severity of the symptoms within the same family has been reported [49, 50], suggesting the involvement of epigenetic mechanisms.

5.2. Prevalence of HPP

The prevalence of HPP was estimated as 1 in 100,000 live births in the Toronto area in Canada, where the first case was found [51]. In Manitoba, Canada, the prevalence is higher in the Mennonite group, being 1 in 2500, according to a founder effect of a particular mutation [52]. In Europe, the prevalence of severe cases is estimated as 1 in 300,000 [53], whereas in Japan it is 1 in 450,000 for patients who have the c.1559delT allele [46]. This particular allele is a severe allele and is characteristic of Japanese families (46.8% of Japanese patients with HPP have this deletion allele) [46].

5.3. Genetic diagnosis

When HPP is suspected, collection of the family history and the making of a pedigree are important for genetic counseling [54]. Clinical diagnosis can be done by laboratory biochemical examinations and ultrasonic and radiographic findings. Definitive diagnosis is performed by genetic testing. Genomic DNA of the patient is amplified, and the nucleotide sequences are determined. Polymerase chain reaction-single-strand conformation polymorphism (PCR-SSCP), PCR-denaturing gradient gel electrophoresis (PCR-DGGE), and high-resolution melting curve analysis (HRM) methods used to be employed for this purpose, but direct nucleotide sequencing may be the most effective current method of analysis. Once the mutation of the proband is determined, the inheritance can be pursued by testing the parents' DNA, which makes it possible to give a genetic counseling, because the inheritance pattern of HPP is basically Mendelian inheritance [54, 55]. However, as mentioned above, the same mutation can result in different phenotypes in some families. In addition, a rare case of paternal uniparental isodisomy has been reported [56]. Once a genetic diagnosis is established, enzymatic activity and mineralization activity can be evaluated [57]. An expression plasmid containing the mutant cDNA is transfected into U2OS cells, which are osteoblast-like cells that lack ALP activity. The cells are then cultured for an appropriate period, and enzymatic activity is estimated. For the mineralization assay, the transfected cells are cultured in a mineralization medium that contains β-glycerophosphate as an artificial substrate for TNAP, with or without ascorbic acid. After about 5 days of culture, mineralization is estimated by Alizarin Red S staining [57].

5.4. Prenatal diagnosis

Prenatal diagnosis by ALP enzymatic assay or by immunological detection using amniotic fluid and chorionic villus has been reported, but their diagnostic value is low [3] because of contamination of fetal intestinal ALP and maternal ALP. HPP can be diagnosed using ultrasonography and radiography during the second trimester, but the differential diagnosis is complicated. DNA-based diagnosis using chorionic villus is accurate if information about the nucleotide sequences within the family has been obtained [54, 58]. However, prediction of the prognosis of the disease is not easy, because of the fact that the same mutations can cause different phenotypes even in the same family. In addition, ethical considerations including genetic counseling are very important when prenatal genetic diagnosis is performed [54].

6. Mutations in the *ALPL* gene

To date, a total of 335 mutations in the *ALPL* gene have been reported [6]. The TNAP gene mutations' databases (http://www.sesep.uvsq.fr/03_hypo_mutations.php) of the University of Versailles-Saint Quentin en Yvelines provide up-to-date information regarding mutations [55]. Almost all of these mutations are located within the exons, although some mutations are in the promoter region, exon-intron boundaries and introns. In addition, over 70% of the mutations are missense mutations, 11% are small deletions, 6% are splicing mutations, 5% are nonsense mutations, 3% are small insertions, and 3% are large deletions [6]. Only one regulatory mutation has been reported [59]. Many of the patients are compound heterozygotes. Generally, the interaction between the mutant alleles determines the phenotypes of the patients. Residual activities of mutant TNAPs influence the enzymatic activity and the mineralizing activity of the compound heterozygotes. However, the relationships of genotype and phenotype are rather complicated, and the phenotypes are not always estimated from the combination of the genotypes. Mutation sites are scattered throughout the gene, but there are some "hot spots." In Caucasian patients, p.E191K (a moderate allele with a dominant negative effect) and p.D378V (a severe allele) are frequent mutations [60, 61], whereas c.1559delT (pL520RfsX86; a severe allele) and p.F327L (a moderate allele) are frequent in Japanese patients [62, 63]. c.1559delT also has founder effects, and the frequency of c.1559delT is mentioned above [46, 62].

7. Structure and function of mutant TNAP

Mutation sites of TNAP proteins are classified by its domain structure [30]. Severe phenotypes are associated with the mutations that are located in the active site and its vicinity, the homodimer interface, the crown domain, and the calcium-binding domain. Mutations in the active site valley (the entry site of the substrate into the active site) resulted in less severe phenotypes [30]. Mutations in the other regions of the protein are inclined to show residual enzymatic activity and are, therefore, milder phenotypes.

Because most of the patients are compound heterozygotes, the residual activity and phenotype are determined by the interaction of two mutant proteins [55]. In some cases, especially in autosomal dominant cases, dominant negative mechanisms are suggested, in which cases the mutant proteins affect the function of the wild-type enzymes [48]. Those interactions have not been precisely elucidated and need to be explored in more detail in order to reveal the genotype–phenotype interrelationships and pathophysiology of HPP.

8. Treatment of HPP based on the pathophysiology of the disease

There have been several trials for the treatment of HPP. Respiratory aid somehow succeeds in saving life in the perinatal and the infantile forms, although it is a symptomatic treatment. Other symptomatic treatments are diet therapies, including calcium restriction and vitamin D supplementation, and surgical operations for bone fractures and craniosynostosis [1]. In terms of treatment based on the pathophysiology of HPP, ERT has been attempted. Whyte et al. used the serum of Paget's disease patients who exhibited a high level of TNAP for enzyme replacement [64]. Infusion of PLAP has also been attempted based on the observation that, when the patients with mild forms become pregnant, which causes a high serum ALP level according to an increase in PLAP, they sometimes show improvement of symptoms. Those ERT attempts, however, failed to improve the symptoms [3]. Bone marrow transplantation (BMT) and mesenchymal cell transplantation have also been attempted. Those trials showed a slight improvement but an insufficient effect [65]. Successful ERT was reported in 2012, in which bioengineered TNAP was administered [7]. The C-terminal membrane-bound region of human TNAP was eliminated and replaced with the Fc region of human IgG and deca-aspartate sequences [66]. This bioengineered TNAP is, therefore, soluble, can be easily purified using the Fc region, and has high affinity for hydroxyapatite through acidic peptides such as deca-aspartate [66]. Before the trial, an animal experiment using the bioengineered

TNAP in a knockout mouse (*Akp2*$^{-/-}$; *AKP2* is the mouse homolog of the *ALPL*) that is a good mimic of the perinatal form of HPP, showed elongation of life and improvements in bone and dental defects without respiratory failure [66, 67]. The clinical trial with the bioengineered TNAP (ENB-0040; asfotase alfa) was conducted with five perinatal and six infantile patients [7]. It was administered first as a single intravenous infusion of 2 mg/kg, which was then followed by subcutaneous injections three times per week at a dose of 1 mg/kg for 48 weeks. With the exception of one case who died of respiratory failure that was unrelated with asfotase alfa, the recruited patients showed improvements in rickets and respiratory failure [7]. Asfotase alfa (StrensiqST; Alexion Pharmaceuticals, Inc.) was approved in Japan, the EU, Canada, and the USA in that order in 2015 [2]. Asfotase alfa has dramatically changed the treatment of HPP [68]. Asfotase alfa is indicated for the treatment of patients with perinatal-, infantile- and juvenile-onset HPP [69], in which juvenile-onset HPP means almost the same as the childhood form. The current protocol of the recommended administration is subcutaneous injection six times a week at a dose of 1 mg/kg or three times a week at 2 mg/kg, and the maximal volume of injection is 1 ml [69]. The half-life of asfotase alfa is 5 days in the case of subcutaneous administration. The most common adverse reactions (≥ 10%) are injection site reactions, lipodystrophy, ectopic calcifications, and hypersensitivity reactions. Patients with HPP are at increased risk for developing ectopic calcifications, especially of the eye including the cornea and conjunctiva, and the kidneys (nephrocalcinosis). Although ectopic calcification of the blood vessels has not been reported, it is conceivable that long -term administration may cause medial artery calcification. Medial artery calcification or Mönckeberg-type calcification is often shown as a lethal complication in chronic kidney disease (CKD) patients [70]. In CKD patients, hyperphosphatemia triggers transformation of smooth muscle cells in the media into osteoblastic cells that express elevated TNAP, which then stimulates calcification in the medial artery by a mechanism similar to that of bone mineralization [71, 72]. Asfotase alfa is still not indicated for milder form HPP patients. In this regards, the natural history of the adult form has not been well elucidated [44], and more study is needed. Similarly, odontohypophosphatasia may be still underdiagnosed, because dentists usually do not evaluate the serum ALP value. There should be more investigation into the feasibility of using asfotase alfa for those milder forms.

9. Future perspective

Although current ERT has drastically changed the treatment of HPP, many problems are indicated regarding asfotase alfa administration. First of all, two or three injections per week are needed for this ERT treatment, which burdens patients with injections and parents with administration fees. The interval between injections can be elongated by introducing some modifications into the enzyme preparation. Other possible therapies are bone marrow stem-cell transplantation and/or combination therapy of such transplantation with ERT. Another possible trial is a trial of gene therapy. Using viral vectors, gene therapy was successfully used to treat knockout mice (*AKP2*$^{-/-}$) [73, 74]. Since a viral vector containing *ALPL* cDNA that is injected into blood cannot maintain an effective concentration, gene therapy in combination with stem cell transplantation (*ex vivo* gene therapy) may be more effective [75].

Once gene-transferred stem cells are transplanted, no other injection may be necessary [2]. Although gene therapy seems to be a promising procedure, results have so far only been obtained for mouse models, and its feasibility and safety in humans must be investigated.

10. Conclusions

HPP is a systemic skeletal disorder that is caused by TNAP deficiency. Human TNAP is one of the four isoenzymes of alkaline phosphatase and is expressed ubiquitously. The TNAP protein is linked to the outer membrane of cells via a GPI anchor and works as an enzyme in a homodimer state. TNAP is essential for biomineralization; it is located on the MV membrane and plays a role in the elongation of hydroxyapatite crystals into the extracellular space.

HPP is classified into six forms and clinical severity varies among the forms. Hypomineralization of hard tissues is a common feature of HPP. In the severe forms, patients show rickets and respiratory failure that cause death. Milder forms exhibit musculoskeletal disorder or teeth problems. Although low serum ALP activity and an elevated urine PEA value are characteristic of HPP, genetic diagnosis is the definitive diagnosis. ERT using a genetically modified enzyme (asfotase alfa) opens up a new vista in the therapy of HPP, especially for severe forms of HPP. Although asfotase alfa has drastically changed the treatment of HPP, there remain still several problems with its use that need to be resolved.

Conflict of interest

The author has received honoraria from Alexion Pharmaceuticals, Inc. The author reports no other conflict of interest in this work.

Author details

Hideo Orimo

Address all correspondence to: orimohd@nms.ac.jp

Division of Metabolism and Nutrition, Department of Biochemistry and Molecular Biology, Nippon Medical School, Tokyo, Japan

References

[1] Whyte MP. Hypophosphatasia: Nature's Window on alkaline phosphatase function in man. In: Bilezikian JP, Raisz LG, Rodan GA, editors. Principles of Bone Biology. 2nd ed. San Diego, CA: Academic Press; 2002. p. 1229-1248

[2] Orimo H. Pathophysiology of hypophosphatasia and the potential role of asfotase alpha. Therapeutics and Clinical Risk Management. 2016;**12**:777-786

[3] Whyte MP. Hypophosphatasia: An overview for 2017. Bone. 2017;**102**:15-25. DOI: 10.1016/j.bone.2017.02.011

[4] Rathbun JC. "Hypophosphatasia": A new developmental anomaly. American Journal of Diseases of Children. 1948;**75**:822-831

[5] Mumm S, Jones J, Finnegan P, Whyte MP. Hypophosphatasia: Molecular diagnosis of Rathbun's original case. Journal of Bone and Mineral Research. 2001;**16**:1724-1727

[6] The Tissue-Nonspecific Alkaline Phosphatase Gene Mutations Database [Internet]. Available from: http://www.sesep.uvsq.fr/03_hypo_mutations.php [Accessed: 31 May 2017]

[7] Whyte MP, Greenberg CR, Salman NJ, Bober MB, McAlister WH, Wenkert D, Van Sickle BJ, Simmons JH, Edgar TS, Bauer ML, Hamdan MA, Bishop N, Lutz RE, McGinn M, Craig S, Moore JN, Taylor JW, Cleveland RH, Cranley WR, Lim R, Thacher TD, Mayhew JE, Downs M, Millán JL, Skinar AM, Crine P, Landy H. Enzyme-replacement therapy in life-threatening hypophosphatasia. New England Journal of Medicine. 2012;**366**:904-913

[8] Orimo H. The mechanism of mineralization and the role of alkaline phosphatase in health and disease. Journal of Nippon Medical School. 2010;**77**:4-12

[9] Millán JL. Mammalian Alkaline Phosphatases: From Biology to Applications in Medicine and Biotechnology. Weinheim, Germany: Wiley-VCH Verlag GmbH & Co.; 2006

[10] Harris H. The human alkaline phosphatases: What we know and what we don't know. Clinica Chimica Acta. 1989;**186**:133-150

[11] Smith M, Weiss MJ, Griffin CA, Murray JC, Buetow KH, Emanuel BS, Henthorn PS, Harris H. Regional assignment of the gene for human liver/bone/kidney alkaline phosphatase to chromosome 1p36.1-34. Genomics. 1988;**2**:139-143

[12] Weiss MJ, Ray K, Henthorn PS, Lamb B, Kadesch T, Harris H. Structure of the human liver/bone/kidney alkaline phosphatase gene. Journal of Biological Chemistry. 1988; **263**:12002-12010

[13] Matsuura S, Kishi F, Kajii T. Characterization of a 5′-flanking region of the human liver/bone/kidney alkaline phosphatase gene: Two kinds of mRNA from a single gene. Biochemical and Biophysical Research Communications. 1990;**168**:993-1000

[14] Kiledjian M, Kadesch T. Analysis of the human liver/bone/kidney alkaline phosphatase promoter *in vivo* and *in vitro*. Nucleic Acids Research. 1990;**18**:957-961

[15] Orimo H, Shimada T. Regulation of the human tissue-nonspecific alkaline phosphatase gene expression by all-*trans*-retinoic acid in SaOS-2 osteosarcoma cell line. Bone. 2005;**36**:866-876

[16] Orimo H, Shimada T. Posttranscriptional modulation of the human tissue-nonspecific alkaline phosphatase gene expression by 1,25-dihydroxyvitamin D3 in MG-63 osteoblastic osteosarcoma cells. Nutrition Research. 2006;**26**:227-234

[17] Orimo H, Shimada T. The role of tissue-nonspecific alkaline phosphatase in phosphate-induced activation of alkaline phosphatase and mineralization in SaOS-2 human osteoblast-like cells. Molecular and Cellular Biochemistry. 2008;**315**:51-60

[18] Delgado-Calle J, Sañudo C, Sánchez-Verde L, García-Renedo RJ, Arozamena J, Riancho JA. Epigenetic regulation of alkaline phosphatase in human cells of the osteoblastic lineage. Bone. 2011;**49**:830-838

[19] Henthorn PS, Raducha M, Kadesch T, Weiss MJ, Harris H. Sequence and characterization of the human intestinal alkaline phosphatase gene. Journal of Biological Chemistry. 1988;**263**:12011-12019

[20] Knoll BJ, Rothblum KN, Longley M. Nucleotide sequence of the human placental alkaline phosphatase gene: Evolution of the 5′ flanking region by deletion/substitution. Journal of Biological Chemistry. 1988;**263**:12020-12027

[21] Millán JL, Manes T. Seminoma-derived Nagao isozyme is encoded by a germ-cell alkaline phosphatase gene. Proceedings of the National Academy of Sciences of the United States of America. 1988;**85**:3124-3028

[22] Griffin CA, Smith M, Henthorn PS, Harris H, Weiss MJ, Raducha M, Emanuel BS. Human placental and intestinal alkaline phosphatase genes map to 2q34-q37. American Journal of Human Genetics. 1987;**41**:1025-1034

[23] Shibata H, Fukushi M, Igarashi A, Misumi Y, Ikehara Y, Ohashi Y, Oda K. Defective intracellular transport of tissue-nonspecific alkaline phosphatase with an Ala162→Thr mutation associated with lethal hypophosphatasia. Journal of Biochemistry. 1998;**123**:968-977

[24] Micanovic R, Bailey CA, Brink L, Gerber L, Pan Y-CE, Hulmes JD, Udenfriend S. Aspartic acid-484 of nascent placental alkaline phosphatase condenses with a phosphatidylinositol glycan to become the carboxyl terminus of the mature enzyme. Proceedings of the National Academy of Sciences of the United States of America. 1988;**85**:1398-1402

[25] Micanovic R, Gerber LD, Berger J, Kodukula K, Udenfriend S. Selectivity of the cleavage/attachment site of phosphatidylinositol-glycan-anchored membrane proteins determined by site-specific mutagenesis at Asp-484 of placental alkaline phosphatase. Proceedings of the National Academy of Sciences of the United States of America. 1990;**87**:157-161

[26] Silvent J, Gasse B, Mornet E, Sire JY. Molecular evolution of the tissue-nonspecific alkaline phosphatase allows prediction and validation of missense mutations responsible for hypophosphatasia. Journal of Biological Chemistry. 2014;**289**:24168-24179

[27] Le Du MH, Stigbrand T, Taussig MJ, Ménez A, Stura EA. Crystal structure of alkaline phosphatase from human placenta at 1.8Å Resolution. Journal of Biological Chemistry. 2001;**276**:9158-9165

[28] Ghosh K, Tagore DM, Anumula R, Lakshmaiah B, Kumar PPBS, Singaram S, Matan T, Kallipatti S, Selvam S, Krishnamurthy P, Ramarao M. Crystal structure of rat intestinal alkaline phosphatase – Role of crown domain in mammalian alkaline phosphatases. Journal of Structural Biology. 2013;**184**:182-192

[29] Le Du MH, Millán JL. Structural evidence of functional divergence in human alkaline phosphatases. Journal of Biological Chemistry. 2002;**277**:49808-49814

[30] Mornet E, Stura E, Lia-Baldini A-S, Stigbrand T, Ménez A, Le Du M-H. Structural evidence for a functional role of human tissue nonspecific alkaline phosphatase in bone mineralization. Journal of Biological Chemistry. 2001;**276**:31171-31178

[31] Nosjean O, Koyama I, Goseki M, Roux B, Komoda T. Human tissue-nonspecific alkaline phosphatases: Sugar-moiety-induced enzymic and antigenic modulation and genetic aspects. Biochemical Journal. 1997;**321**:297-303

[32] Fedde KN, Whyte MP. Alkaline phosphatase (tissue-nonspecific isoenzyme) is a phosphoethanolamine and pyridoxal-5′-phosphate ectophosphatase: Normal and hypophosphatasia fibroblast study. American Journal of Human Genetics. 1990;**47**:767-775

[33] Guilarte TR. Regional changes in the concentrations of glutamate, glycine, taurine, and GABA in the vitamin B-6 deficient developing rat brain: Association with neonatal seizures. Neurochemical Research. 1989;**14**:889-897

[34] Anderson HC. The role of matrix vesicles in physiological and pathological calcification. Current Opinion in Orthopaedics. 2007;**18**:428-433

[35] Cui L, Houston DA, Farquharson C, MacRae VE. Characterisation of matrix vesicles in skeletal and soft tissue mineralisation. Bone. 2016;**87**:147-158

[36] Shapiro IM, Landis WJ, Risbud MV. Matrix vesicles: Are they anchored exosomes? Bone. 2015;**79**:29-36

[37] Mebarek S, Abousalham A, Magne D, De LD, Bandorowicz-Pikula J, Pikula S, Buchet R. Phospholipases of mineralization competent cells and matrix vesicles: Roles in physiological and pathological mineralizations. International Journal of Molecular Sciences. 2013;**14**:5036-5129

[38] Roberts S, Narisawa S, Harmey D, Millán JL, Farquharson C. Functional involvement of PHOSPHO1 in matrix vesicle-mediated skeletal mineralization. Journal of Bone and Mineral Research. 2007;**22**:617-627

[39] Hessle L, Johnson KA, Anderson HC, Narisawa S, Goding JW, Terkeltaub R, Millán JL. Tissue-nonspecific alkaline phosphatase and plasma cell membrane glycoprotein-1 are central antagonistic regulators of bone mineralization. Proceedings of the National Academy of Sciences of the United States of America. 2002;**99**:9445-9449

[40] Yadav MC, Sper Simão AM, Narisawa S, Huesa C, McKee MD, Farquharson C, Millán JL. Loss of skeletal mineralization by the simultaneous ablation of PHOSPHO1 and alkaline phosphatase function: A unified model of the mechanisms of initiation of skeletal calcification. Journal of Bone and Mineral Research. 2011;**26**:286-297

[41] Harmey D, Hessle L, Narisawa S, Johnson KA, Terkeltaub R, Millán JL. Concerted regulation of inorganic pyrophosphate and osteopontin by *Akp2*, *Enpp1*, and *Ank*. American Journal of Pathology. 2004;**164**:1199-1209

[42] Wenkert D, McAlister WH, Coburn SP, Zerega JA, Ryan LM, Ericson KL, Hersh JH, Mumm S, Whyte MP. Hypophosphatasia: Nonlethal disease despite skeletal presentation in utero (17 new cases and literature review). Journal of Bone and Mineral Research. 2011;**26**:2389-2398

[43] van den Bos T, Handoko G, Niehof A, Ryan LM, Coburn SP, Whyte MP, Beertsen W. Cementum and dentin in hypophosphatasia. Journal of Dental Research. 2005;**84**: 1021-1025

[44] Berkseth KE, Tebben PJ, Drake MT, Hefferran TE, Jewison DE, Wermers RA. Clinical spectrum of hypophosphatasia diagnosed in adults. Bone. 2013;**54**:21-27

[45] Anderson HC, Hsu HH, Morris DC, Fedde KN, Whyte MP. Matrix vesicles in osteomalacic hypophosphatasia bone contain apatite-like mineral crystals. American Journal of Pathology. 1997;**151**:1555-1561

[46] Watanabe A, Karasugi T, Sawai H, Naing BT, Ikegawa S, Orimo H, Shimada T. Prevalence of c.1559delT in ALPL, a common mutation resulting in the perinatal (lethal) form of hypophosphatasia in Japanese and effects of the mutation on heterozygous carriers. Journal of Human Genetics. 2011;**56**:166-168

[47] Silverman JL. Apparent dominant inheritance of hypophosphatasia. Archives of Internal Medicine. 1962;**110**:191-198

[48] Fauvert D, Brun-Heath I, Lia-Baldini AS, Bellazi L, Taillandier A, Serre J-L, de Mazancourt P, Mornet E. Mild forms of hypophosphatasia mostly result from dominant negative effect of severe alleles or from compound heterozygosity for severe and moderate alleles. BMC Medical Genetics. 2009;**10**:51

[49] Macfarlane JD, Kroon HM, van den Harten JJ. Phenotypically dissimilar hypophosphatasia in two sibships. American Journal of Medical Genetics Part A. 1992;**42**:117-121

[50] Peach CA, Zhang Y, Wordsworth BP. Mutations of the tissue-nonspecific alkaline phos phatase gene (TNAP) causing a non-lethal case of perinatal hypophosphatasia. Rheumatology. 2007;**46**:1037-1040

[51] Fraser D. Hypophosphatasia. American Journal of Medicine. 1957;**22**:730-746

[52] Greenberg CR, Taylor CL, Haworth JC, Seargeant LE, Philipps S, Triggs-Raine B, Chodirker BN. A homoallelic $Gly^{317}\rightarrow$Asp mutation in ALPL causes the perinatal (lethal) form of hypophosphatasia in Canadian mennonites. Genomics. 1993;**17**:215-217

[53] Mornet E, Yvard A, Taillandier A, Fauvert D, Simon-Bouy B. A molecular-based estimation of the prevalence of hypophosphatasia in the European population. Annals of Human Genetics. 2011;**75**:439-445

[54] Watanabe A, Orimo H, Takeshita T, Shimada T. Prenatal diagnosis of severe perinatal (lethal) hypophosphatasia. In: Choy RKW, Leung TY, editors. Prenatal Diagnosis – Morphology Scan and Invasive Methods. Rijeka, Croatia: InTech; 2012. p. 27-32

[55] Mornet E. Hypophosphatasia. Orphanet Journal of Rare Diseases. 2007;**2**:40

[56] Watanabe A, Satoh S, Fujita A, Naing BT, Orimo H, Shimada T. Perinatal hypophosphatasia caused by uniparental isodisomy. Bone. 2014;**60**:93-99

[57] Orimo H, Goseki-Sone M, Hosoi T, Shimada T. Functional assay of the mutant tissue-nonspecific alkaline phosphatase gene using U_2OS osteoblast-like cells. Molecular Genetics and Metabolism. 2008;**94**:375-381

[58] Orimo H, Nakajima E, Hayashi Z, Kijima K, Watanabe A, Tenjin H, Araki T, Shimada T. First-trimester prenatal molecular diagnosis if infantile hypophosphatasia in a Japanese family. Prenatal Diagnosis. 1996;**16**:559-563

[59] Taillandier A, Cozien E, Muller F, Merrien Y, Bonnin E, Fribourg C, Simon-Bouy B, Serre JL, Bieth E, Brenner R, Cordier MP, De Bie S, Fellmann F, Freisinger P, Hesse V, Hennekam RC, Josifova D, Kerein-Storrar L, Leporrier N, Zobot MT, Mornet E. Fifteen new mutations (−195C>T, L-12X, 298-2A>G, T117N, A159T, R229S, 997+2T>a, E274X, A331T, H364R, D389G, 1256delC, R433H, N461I, C472S) in the tissue-nonspecific alkaline phosphatase (TNSALP) gene in patients with hypophosphatasia. Human Mutation. 2000;**15**:293

[60] Hérasse M, Spentchian M, Taillandier A, Mornet E. Evidence of a founder effect for the tissue-nonspecific alkaline phosphatase (TNSALP) gene E174K mutation in hypophosphatasia patients. European Journal of Human Genetics. 2002;**10**:666-668

[61] Whyte MP, Mumm S, Deal C. Adult hypophosphatasia treated with teriparatide. Journal of Clinical Endocrinology & Metabolism. 2007;**92**:1203-1208

[62] Orimo H, Goseki-Sone M, Inoue M, Tsubakio Y, Sakiyama T, Shimada T. Importance of deletion of T at nucleotide 1559 in the tissue-nonspecific alkaline phosphatase gene in Japanese patients with hypophosphatasia. Journal of Bone and Mineral Metabolism. 2002;**20**:28-33

[63] Michigami T, Uchihashi T, Suzuki A, Tachikwa K, Nakajima S, Ozono K. Common mutation F310L and T1559del in the tissue-nonspecific alkaline phosphatase gene are related to distinct phenotypes in Japanese patients with hypophosphatasia. European Journal of Pediatrics. 2005;**164**:277-282

[64] Whyte MP, McAlister WH, Patton LS, Magill HL, Fallon MD, Lorentz WB, Herrod MD. Enzyme replacement therapy for infantile hypophosphatasia attempted by intravenous infusions of alkaline phosphatase-rich Paget plasma: Results in three additional patients. The Journal of Pediatrics. 1984;**105**:926-933

[65] Taketani T, Oyama C, Mihara A, Tanabe Y, Abe M, Hirade T, Yamamoto S, Bo R, Kanai T, Tadenuma T, Michibata Y, Yamamoto S, Hattori M, Katsube Y, Ohnishi H, Sasao M, Oda Y,

Hattori K, Yuba S, Ohgushi H, Yamaguchi S. Ex vivo expanded allogeneic mesenchymal stem cells with bone marrow transplantation improved osteogenesis in infants with severe hypophosphatasia. Cell Transplantation. 2015;**24**:1931-1943

[66] Millán JL, Narisawa S, Lemire I, Loisel TP, Boileau G, Leonard P, Gramatikova S, Terkeltaub R, Camacho NP, McKee MD, Crine P, Whyte MP. Enzyme replacement therapy for murine hypophosphatasia. Journal of Bone and Mineral Research. 2008;**23**:777-787

[67] McKee MD, Nakano Y, Masica DL, Gray JJ, Lemire I, Heft R, Whyte MP, Crine P, Millán JL. Enzyme replacement therapy prevents dental defects in a model of hypophosphatasia. Journal of Dental Research. 2011;**90**:470-476

[68] Whyte MP, Rockman-Greenberg C, Ozono K, Riese R, Moseley S, Melian A, Thompson DD, Bishop N, Hofmann C. Asfotase alpha treatment improves survival for perinatal and infantile hypophosphatasia. Journal of Clinical Endocrinology & Metabolism. 2016;**101**:334-342

[69] STRENSIQ™ (Asfotase Alfa) for Strensiq [Prescribing Information]. Cheshire, CT: Alexion Pharmaceuticals, Inc. [Internet]; 2015. Available from: http://strensiq.com/images/pi.pdf [Accessed: 15 May 2017]

[70] Massy ZA, Drüeke TB. Vascular calcification. Current Opinion in Nephrology and Hypertension. 2013;**22**:405-412

[71] Shioi A, Katagi M, Okuno Y, Mori K, Jono S, Koyama H, Nishizawa Y. Induction of bone-type alkaline phosphatase in human vascular smooth muscle cells: Roles of tumor necrosis factor-α and oncostatin M derived from macrophages. Circulation Research. 2002;**91**:9-16

[72] Tani T, Orimo H, Shimizu A, Tsuruoka S. Development of a novel chronic kidney disease mouse model to evaluate the progression of hyperphosphatemia and associated mineral bone disease. Scientific Reports. 2017;**7**:2233. DOI: 10.1038/s41598-017-02351-6

[73] Yamamoto S, Orimo H, Matsumoto T, Iijima O, Narizawa S, Maeda T, Millán JL, Shimada T. Prolonged survival and phenotypic correction of *Akp2*$^{-/-}$ hypophosphatasia mice by lentiviral gene therapy. Journal of Bone and Mineral Research. 2011;**26**:135-142

[74] Matsumoto T, Miyake K, Yamamoto S, Orimo H, Miyake N, Odagaki Y, Adachi K, Iijima O, Narisawa S, Millán JL, Fukunaga Y, Shimada T. Rescue of severe infantile hypophosphatasia mice by AAV-mediated sustained expression of soluble alkaline phosphatase. Human Gene Therapy. 2011;**22**:1355-1364

[75] Iijima O, Miyake K, Watanabe A, Miyake N, Igarashi T, Kanokoda C, Nakamura-Takahashi A, Kinoshita H, Noguchi T, Abe S, Narisawa S, Millán JL, Okada T, Shimada T. Prevention of lethal murine hypophosphatasia by neonatal ex vivo gene therapy using lentivirally transduced bone marrow cells. Human Gene Therapy. 2015;**26**:801-881

Chapter 7

Dynamic Properties of Skeletal Muscle Contraction in Rats with Diabetes

Tetyana Volodymyrivna Beregova,
Dmytro Nozdrenko, Sergii Berehovyi, Natali Nikitina,
Tetyana Falalyeyeva and
Liudmyla Ivanivna Ostapchenko

Additional information is available at the end of the chapter

http://dx.doi.org/10.5772/intechopen.70600

Abstract

The study was conducted on 20 white nonlinear male rats, which were divided into 2 groups of 10 animals each. Rats in the first group were used as control. Rats in the second group were induced type I diabetes by intraperitoneal (i.p.) administration of streptozotocin (65 mg/kg). Diabetes in rats was confirmed by the presence of hyperglycemia. For the establishment of nociceptive pain sensation, mechanical nociceptive test and tail-flick test were conducted in rats. Further animals were anesthetized by i.p. administration of Nembutal (40 mg/kg). The study of dynamic properties of muscle contraction was performed under conditions of the tibia muscle activation by using the modulated stimulation of efferent n. tibialis. Streptozotocin (STZ) was injected in rats; as a result, the blood glucose level was increased by 4.4 times ($p \leq 0.001$). Pain sensitivity in diabetic rats was suppressed, indicating the development of peripheral neuropathy. In rats with diabetes, biomechanical parameters of tibia muscle contraction such as the maximum force of contraction, the speed of maximum force of contraction, the retention time of maximum force of contraction and integrated power of muscle contraction (it is calculated on the total area of the received force curves) were violated. This prevents adequate implementation motor neuron pools muscular system, which will have significant consequences in accurate positional movements.

Keywords: skeletal muscle, contraction, diabetes, neuropathy

1. Introduction

The damages of the peripheral nervous system in patients with diabetes mellitus are recorded in 40–60% of cases and manifests itself in the form of diabetic polyneuropathy. The incidence of diabetic polyneuropathy increases with age and duration of diabetes mellitus [1]. According to recent data, in the last 10 years, in young patients with type 1 diabetes, an increase in the incidence of diabetic polyneuropathy from 24.2% to 62.9% has been observed [2]. Diabetic neuropathy correlates with a high risk of cardiovascular complications [3, 4]. Patients with diabetic polyneuropathy are also at risk for the formation of trophic ulcers that do not heal for a long time and often lead to amputating a limb [5–7]. In the USA, 15% of all patients with diabetes will develop foot ulcers [8].

Mortality due to diabetes mellitus, complicated by diabetic polyneuropathy, remains high in all countries of the world, regardless of their socioeconomic status [3]. Patients with diabetic polyneuropathy often require outside help, which, of course, is reflected on the quality of their life [9, 10].

Metabolic, vascular and immune theories were proposed to explain the pathogenesis of diabetic polyneuropathy [11]. Independent causes of the risk of this serious complication of diabetes mellitus are age, male gender, unsatisfactory control of the level of glycaemia, elevated lipid levels in the blood, height, overweight and obesity, and insulin treatment [12–16]. Thus, the pathogenesis of diabetic polyneuropathy is multifactorial. It includes the increase of mitochondrial production of free radicals due to hyperglycemia-induced oxidative stress [1]. A number of other factors affect the activity of neurons, mitochondrial function, permeability of membranes and endothelial function. These include the activation of polyol aldose reductase pathway [17], activation of poly(ADP ribose) polymerase [18], and modified Na+/K+-ATPase pump function [19].

In diabetic polyneuropathy, autonomic, motor, large fiber and small fiber nerve functions are attacked [20]. The most frequent variant of defeat of peripheral nervous system at a diabetes is distal symmetric sensorimotor neuropathy [21]. As a rule, this complication occurs in a few years from the onset of the underlying disease [22]. This form of diabetic polyneuropathy develops slowly (chronically), the first symptoms (numbness and paresthesia) occur in the lower extremities, sometimes unilateral [23]. Distal symmetric sensorimotor neuropathy is the cause of the development of chronic neuropathic pain syndrome. Pain is the reason for 40% of patient visits in a primary care setting, and about 20% of these have had pain for more than 6 months [24]. In this form of neuropathy, poorly myelinated and thin nonmyelinated fibers are affected in various combinations. In most cases, at the onset of the disease, the neurological deficit is caused by the damages to fine fibers. Symptoms of their damages are manifested by burning or shooting pain, hyperalgesia, paresthesia, disturbances of pain and temperature sensitivity, ulceration of the feet and a decrease in pain sensitivity from the internal organs. With the defeat of myelinated (thick) fibers, there is a violation of deep and vibrational sensitivity, and a decrease or loss of tendon reflexes.

Diabetic polyneuropathy affects both type 1 and type 2 diabetes patients, although specific differences exist in the underlying pathobiology, pathology and clinical expression of the disease [25]. In type 1 diabetes patients, diabetic polyneuropathy is more rapid and severe.

The nerve conduction study is a reliable and objective diagnostic method to evaluate the diabetic polyneuropathy treatment response [26]. Although a nerve conduction study is regarded as the gold standard in clinical research, it is not useful in clinical practice because it is time-consuming, requires special devices and trained examiners, and has no general consensus regarding its criteria, even after multiple investigations [27]. That is why the experiments on the rats give us possibility to investigate the mechanisms of diabetic polyneuropathy development, to evaluate the quality of treatment, and to propose the new approaches to diagnostic and treatment of diabetic polyneuropathy.

In isometric conditions, analysis of registered effort developed by the muscle due to frequency-modulated stimulation of its nerve is the qualitative indicator of the level of neuro and myopathy pathological processes.

Phenomenological approach in the analysis of pathological processes that influence the mechanical properties of the muscle makes it possible to establish important relationships between the real macroscopic parameters of the muscle state, such as the strength, length and level of efferent activity. Frequently, the analysis of pathological changes in muscle dynamics is sufficient for the analysis of central regulatory processes, both motor activity and pathological state of the organism as a whole.

The dynamics of contractile component is determined by the delicate interaction of motor neuron pools that appeared in the muscle through the activated motor neuron and the activation of actin and myosin myofilaments interactions. Dependence of muscle force response on value, duration of applied stimulation (force-velocity for the initial site) and on time of achievement and retention of the stationary state of the contractile process makes possible to track the level of pathological processes development that affect the mechanisms of positioning in muscle dynamics. These processes play a huge role in the accurate positional movements of hands and fingers, even minor violations in the control system of these movements lead to serious domestic and physiological problems.

The rapid excitement of contractile apparatus, in the process of prolonged activation of muscle fibers, usually undergoes a slow and stable modification, which can partly be due to the phosphorylation of the so-called light chains of myosin located in the neck of the bridge. A slower dephosphorylation process under conditions of prolonged uninterrupted activation of the muscle fiber causes stable phosphorylation of myosin, which, apparently, increases the mobility of the bridges or changes their orientation. Analysis of amplitude-velocity changes of activated muscle's force response makes it possible to assess the influence of developing pathology on these processes. One of the most effective and widely used methods to identify the dynamic systems' levels pathologies is to determine the reaction in responses to the harmonic input effects of different velocity ranges of increase stimulating irritations.

2. Dynamic properties of skeletal muscle contraction in rats with diabetes

2.1. Methods of experiment conduction

The study was conducted on 20 white nonlinear laboratory male rats, which were divided into two groups of 10 animals each. The rats in the first group were used as control. Rats in the second group were induced type I diabetes by administration of streptozotocin (STZ) (65 mg/kg, i/p). Diabetes in rats was confirmed by the presence of hyperglycemia. On the 28th day of experiment, glucose loading test was conducted for the confirmation of diabetes presence. For the establishment of pain sensation, mechanical nociceptive test was conducted in rats (Randall-Selitto analgesiometer test) [28]. Also heat-induced rat tail-flick latency was determined as a measure for nociceptive pain [29].

Animals were anesthetized (Ketamine (100 mg/kg "Pfizer", USA), and tracheotomy and connection to lung ventilator were performed. In the area of the popliteal fossa, musculus gastrocnemius was isolated and cut down to be attached to the force sensors. Further, the animal was fixed in a stereotaxic machine with the head, pelvis and extremities rigid fixation system. Nerve that innervate musculus gastrocnemius was fixed on a bipolar platinum wire electrode for further electrical stimulation. The parameters of stimulation signals were programmed. The skin edges (hind legs) around the incision were sutured to the machine tool and formed trays with the muscle and nerve and were filled with liquid paraffin. Heart rate and ECG amplitudes were monitored during surgery and experiments [30].

Before stimulation of the spinal cord, the ventral root muscle was connected to a load that did not stretch it because of unilateral mechanical limiter, and only shortening of the muscle was possible. After activation, the isometric growth of the force began until the muscular effort reached the external load, after that the isotonic shortening of the muscle started.

In the initial stage of the shortening, it was possible to distinguish a near-linear part of motion due to velocity measurement at which it was possible to establish the empirical dependence of the contraction rate on the level of isotonic loads. The pathological processes that occurred during the development of diabetic polyneuropathy modulated the muscular response registered by us. The level of this modulation was a qualitative characteristic of residual physiological disorders both at the neuropathic and at the myopathy level of pathology development. The statistical analysis of the data was conducted in the program Statistica 8.0. To approximate this empirical dependence, several analytic approaches were selected.

As a modulating component, a stimulating signal of different amplitudes and times characteristics was used and regarded as an input effect, and the output signal was the first harmonic of the muscle-developed effort and the subsequent realization of the modulated stimulation pool.

2.2. The analysis of electro-physiological parameters used in work as indicators of pathological processes development during diabetic polyneuropathy

2.2.1. The changes in time of muscle force response beginning caused by a single stimulation pool

Time between first and second mitotic response that was caused by successive stimulation with fixed meaning between them (2000 ms). This indicator makes it possible to assess the presence or absence of pathologies (neuropathy or myopathy) during the initial stages of the study, and to correct the algorithm of further investigation whether pathological changes are present.

2.2.2. The changes in time of muscle force response beginning caused by 10 consecutive stimulation pools with 10 s relaxation time between them

When the intensity of stimulation changes, the temporal parameters of the stimulation pools conduction in axon do not remain constant. The investigation of changes of time delays of impulses conduction with an increase number of stimuli makes it possible to assess the level of pathological changes in the neuromuscular preparation with prolonged, static reactions of the muscular system. High-frequency stimulation of peripheral afferents that form monosynaptic contacts with motor neuron causes an effective summation of successive action potentials and stable depolarization of the cell membrane. In this case, the pulse frequency is determined by the average level of membrane depolarization and increases with rise of frequency stimulation. During the development of pathological processes associated with diabetic polyneuropathy, the use of stimulation without relaxation of the corresponding long transsynaptic activation of motor neurons causes adaptive time decrease of stimuli conduction. Change in this parameter is the marker of pathological processes presence in the neuromuscular preparation while applying stimulation signals close to physiological parameters.

We analyzed several basic biomechanical parameters during studying the myotonic response of the muscle. These parameters are universal markers that show the presence of biomechanical disturbances caused by factors of different nature.

Changes in each of described biomechanical parameters is an indicative marker of the dysfunction presence in the excitation-response chain of both the neuromuscular preparation and the state of the organism as a whole.

We have designated the investigated segments of biomechanical responses for more favorable description of the changes in the obtained curves (**Figure 1**).

2.2.3. The changes in time to reach maximum force response

The maximum force generation on which the active muscle is capable is an important indicator for fast, ballistic, nontargeted movements (**Figure 1**—Δt_1) The changes of this indicator show the level of physiological dysfunction of neuromuscular preparation when it implements the maximum power tasks.

2.2.4. The changes in time of achievement of stationary state of contraction, with the use of modulated stimulation signal

The stationary state of the active muscle is a temporal area of the contractile activity of the muscle tissue without the presence of a significant trend in one or the other direction, during the activation of the muscle (**Figure 1**—Δt_2). Physiologically, the stationary state of the active muscle is the level of muscle force production that corresponds to the physiological state of the

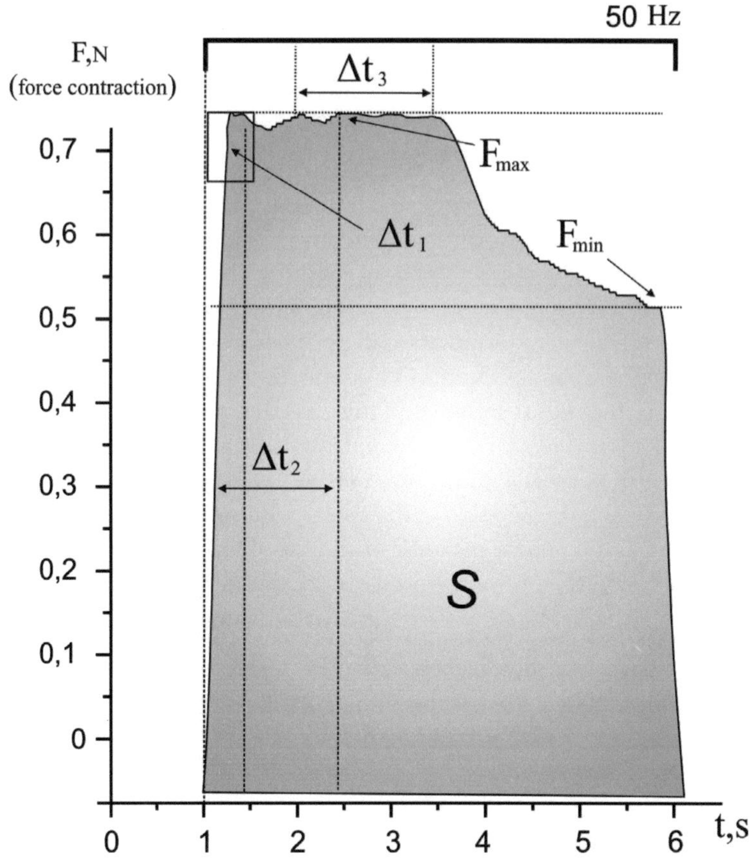

Figure 1. Schematic representation of analyzed biomechanical parameters of muscles gastrocnemius contraction using a modulated stimulation signal.

neuromuscular preparation at this moment. The time of its establishment is a time of adaptation processes passage in the muscle during its activation by stimulating pools, to select the optimal amplitude-strength characteristics of the contracting muscle in order to realize the incoming stimulations with the least deviations from the CNS tasks.

2.2.5. The changes in time of stationary state retention, with the use of modulated stimulation signal

The retention of stationary state is an indicator of adaptability of the muscular system to a new state of the neuromuscular system, altered by a pathological action (**Figure 1**—Δt_3). In some cases, we could record relatively stable periodic changes in the level of stationary state at the applied pulse activity frequency, but without significant dependencies of these fluctuations to the level of pathology development or methods of drug administration. We consider the presence of oscillations at the phases of stationary state retention is a consequence of individual differences in the muscular system of experimental laboratory animals.

2.2.6. The changes in time of maximum contraction force generation

This marker is an indicator of the general dysfunction of the muscular system, index of decrease (with pathologies development) of the maximum possible force response (**Figure 1**—F_{max}). The change in this parameter can be related either to a violation in the neuronal component or to the miotic components of the studied pathology. The dysfunction of this parameter can also be associated with a violation of the integrity of the signals that generate motor neurons in the synaptic current, and as a result, the violation of the summation of the transmembrane currents occurred in accordance with the internal membrane properties. That influences the pathological transformation of the sequence of action potentials that trigger a muscle contraction that causes the maximum force response.

2.2.7. The changes in minimum contraction force generation

This data show the maximum pathological changes caused by the pathological process during analyzing changes in contraction of each successive contractile act (**Figure 1**—F_{min}). This marker is the main indicator of muscle dysfunction while performing simple one-joint movements. The phenomenological analysis of it makes possible to establish the presence of cause-effect relationships between the level of decrease in biomechanical activity of muscles, the basic mechanical parameters of movements and the level of development of the pathological process. The accuracy of such conclusions is enhanced due to multiple repetitions of these stimuli and stimulation time increase.

2.2.8. The changes in integrated power of muscle contraction

The integrated power is subtracted from the total area of force curves (**Figure 1**—S) and is an indicator of the overall capacity of the muscle with the use of applied stimulation pools. Analysis of this value makes it possible to evaluate the mechanisms of the formation of muscular activity in the equilibrium system, in the force-external load system, that is, a physiological analogue of the working capacity of the muscular system as a whole.

2.2.9. The changes in fatigue processes of the neuromuscular preparation accompanied by diabetic polyneuropathy

In condition of 1 and 2 Hz, unrelaxed stimulation of the analysis of fatigue processes development was made, which makes it possible to evaluate the development of fatigue in different time ranges. Fatigue evaluation was calculated by time intervals with achievements of 50 and 30% force responses, with stimulation irritations. It should be noted that in control, the change of this data had a long time frame, which complicated the description of fatigue processes development during pathology. Therefore, for more precise description of results, the change in control values was considered 100%, and while analyzing the data, the percentage difference was described.

2.2.10. Analysis of fusion index

To analyze the dynamics of real movements, we considered the peculiarities of the transformation of segmental and descending activity during the development of polyneuropathy. An important role in the realization of the motor function belongs dedicated to asymmetric nature of the muscle reactions as a result of increase in the level of incoming efferent activity. In our work, almost all movements are relatively simple and are provided with straight pattern of motor neuron populations. Since motor neurons directly control muscle contraction, the nature of the transformation of activity coming to them from multiple sources is largely predetermined by the peculiarities of muscle dynamics. The significant inertia of muscle contraction during the development of the pathological process requires motor neurons to have such dynamic properties that could compensate for the insufficiently high-speed parameters of muscle contraction. Thus, the slowdown of smooth tetanus appearance can be used as another parameter to describe the dynamics of pathologies development. We investigated the transition of active muscle force response from the state of the unfused tetanus to the fused one. We had also analyzed the time variation between the peaks of the force response and their maximum force. Two above-described parameters are important for the transition of the active muscle from the state of unfused tetanus to the fused one. The analysis of their changes shows us the peculiarities of dysfunction generation by individual motor units, and the consistent nature of their activation provides the possibility of smooth regulation of the force developed by the whole muscle.

3. Electrophysiology

STZ was injected in rats on 28th day of experiment; as a result, blood glucose level was increased by 4.4 times ($p \leq 0.001$). On the 14th and 28th day of development of diabetes, the threshold of pain sensitivity increased by 26.4% ($p < 0.05$) and 95.86% ($p < 0.01$), accordingly, by comparison to an initial level (before STZ injection). Therefore, pain sensitivity in diabetic rats was suppressed, indicating the development of peripheral neuropathy.

Force response of musculus gastrocnemius in rats with diabetic polyneuropathy caused by single stimulation pool with frequency of 50 Hz showed that time of the force response beginning increased by 119.34% with stimulation through the nerve (**Figures 2** and **3**). It should be noted that time of force response in the condition of direct stimulation though the muscle did not change.

The time of force response beginning increased from 121.25% at the first run till 142.27% at the tenth run in case of 10 consecutive stimulation pools usage (**Figures 1** and **3**). It was concluded the presence of neuropathic changes associated with the impossibility of generation of 10 consecutive stimulation pulses without significant physiological disturbances of myopathy origin.

http://dx.doi.org/10.5772/intechopen.70600

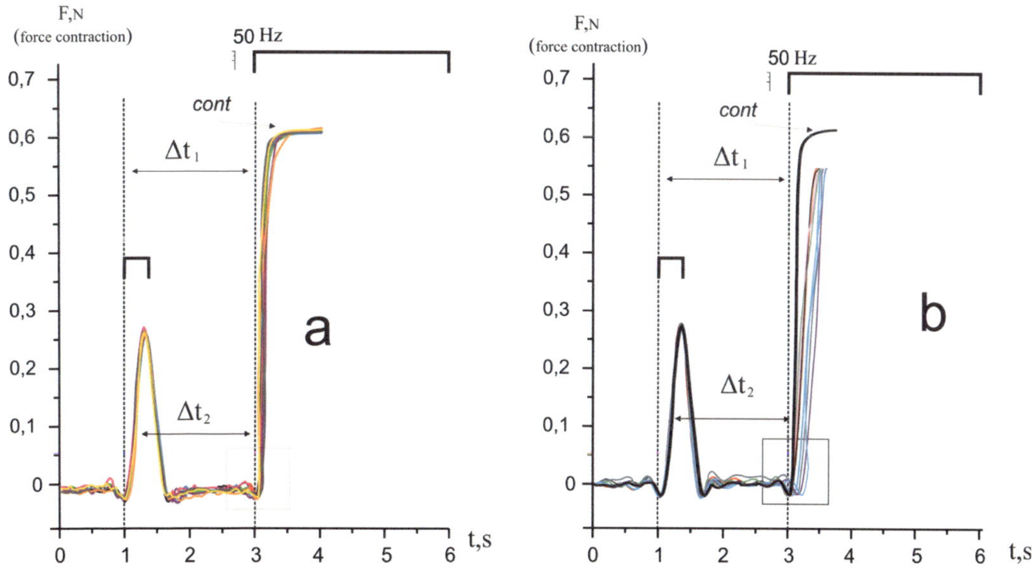

Figure 2. The change in time of muscle force response in rats with diabetic neuropathy caused by 10 consecutive irritation pools by modulated electrostimulation with 50 Hz frequency. The relaxation time is 10 s. Cont—control; Δt_1—time between two consecutive stimulation pools; Δt_2—time of muscle force response beginning; a—direct stimulation of the muscle, rat with diabetic neuropathy; b—stimulation through the nerve, rat with diabetic neuropathy.

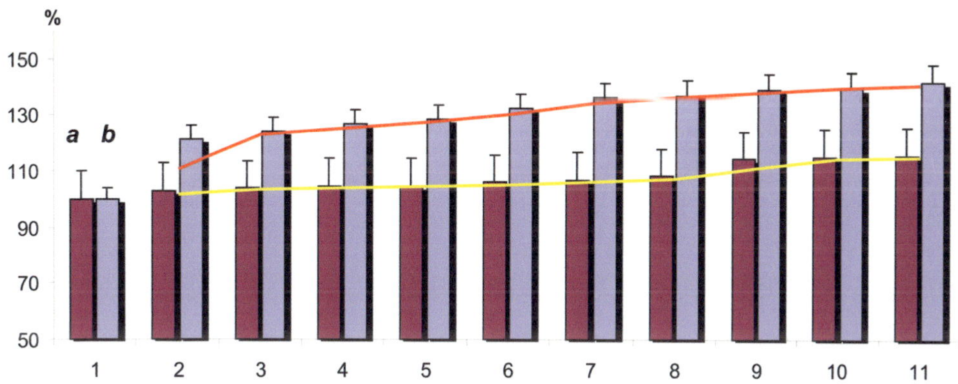

Figure 3. The change in time of muscle force response in rats with diabetic neuropathy caused by 10 consecutive irritation pools by modulated electrostimulation with 50 Hz frequency. The relaxation time is 10 s. The meanings are represented as percentages from control values considered as 100%. 1—control values; 2–11—consecutive irritation pools; a—direct stimulation of the muscle; b—stimulation through the nerve.

It was shown that the diabetic polyneuropathy leads to significant dysfunctions during stimulation signal transfer to effector. When the parameters of stimulation signal approach to the physiological level, the dysfunction of neuromuscular activity increases till the level that is capable to disturb the overall dynamics of the contractile process.

Thus, the use of streptozotocin increases time of force response, which is an adequate criterion for the presence of neuropathy in rats with diabetic neuropathy.

As a result, amplitude-force changes in the muscle response were revealed (**Figure 4**), both compared to control or to direct muscle stimulation. It should be noted that the presence of clearly expressed fluctuation changes in the phase of stationary state retention in rats with diabetic polyneuropathy with stimulation through the nerve.

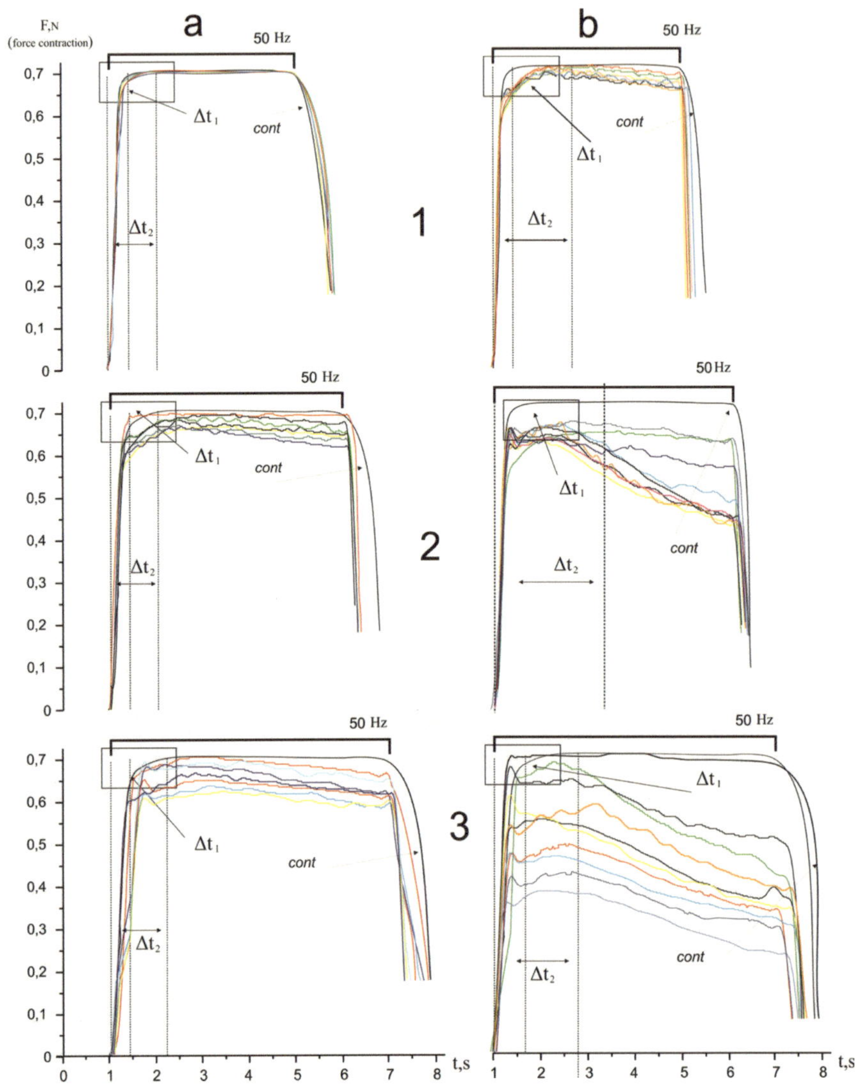

Figure 4. The changes in the dynamic parameters of musculus gastrocnemius contraction in rats with diabetic polyneuropathy, stimulated by modulated electrostimulation with 50 Hz frequency and duration of 2, 4 and 6 s. The relaxation time is 10 s. a—direct stimulation of the muscle; b—stimulation through the nerve; 1, 2, 3—stimulation time 2, 4 and 6 s, respectively; Cont—control, Δt_1—phase of the maximum force response, Δt_2—phase of stationary state of contraction.

The change in time of maximum force reach (**Figure 5**) caused by 10 consecutive stimulation pools modulated by electrostimulation with 50 Hz frequency and duration of 2 s was 183.41% at the first and 213.27% at the tenth run, respectively. When stimulation time was increased till 4 and 6 s, the data were 188.49% (1), 243.47% (10), 188.49% (1) and 243.47% (10), respectively.

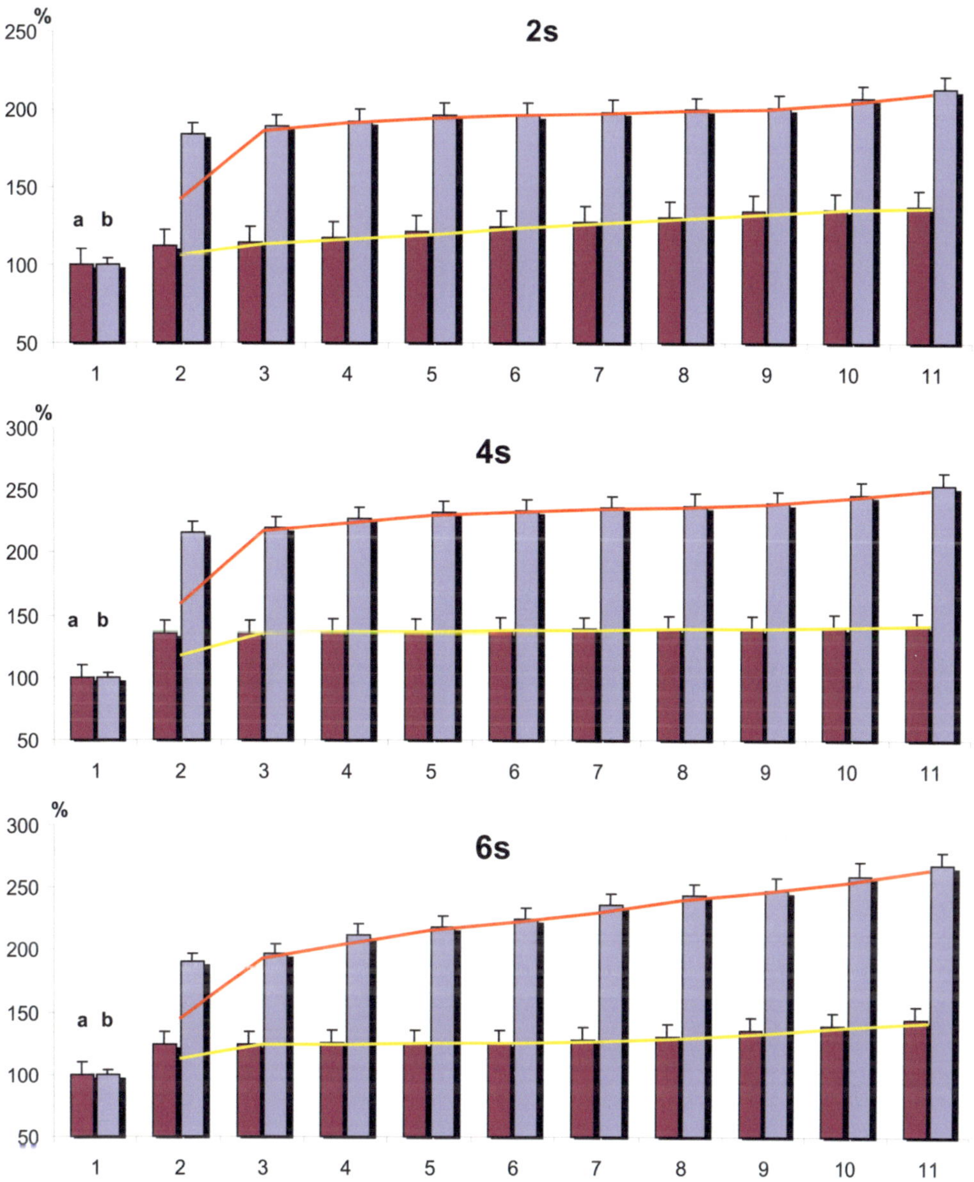

Figure 5. The change in time of maximum force reach by musculus gastrocnemius in rats with diabetic polyneuropathy caused by 10 consecutive stimulation pools with electrostimulation with 50 Hz frequency and duration 2, 3 and 4 s. The relaxation time is 10 s. The meanings are represented as percentages from control values considered as 100%. 1—control values; 2–11—consecutive irritation pools; a—direct stimulation of the muscle; b—stimulation through the nerve.

The time of stationary state reach by musculus gastrocnemius in rats with diabetic neuropathy by stimuli for 2 s showed that the time increased from 211.34% at the first till 249.14% at the tenth run corresponding (**Figure 6**). When stimulation time was increased till 4 and 6 s—215.64% (1), 253.78% (10) and 234.12% (1) 297.66% (10), respectively. At the same time, the time of stationary state retention also decreased linearly as with the increase in the number of stimulating pools and with an increase in the stimulation longevity (**Figure 7**).

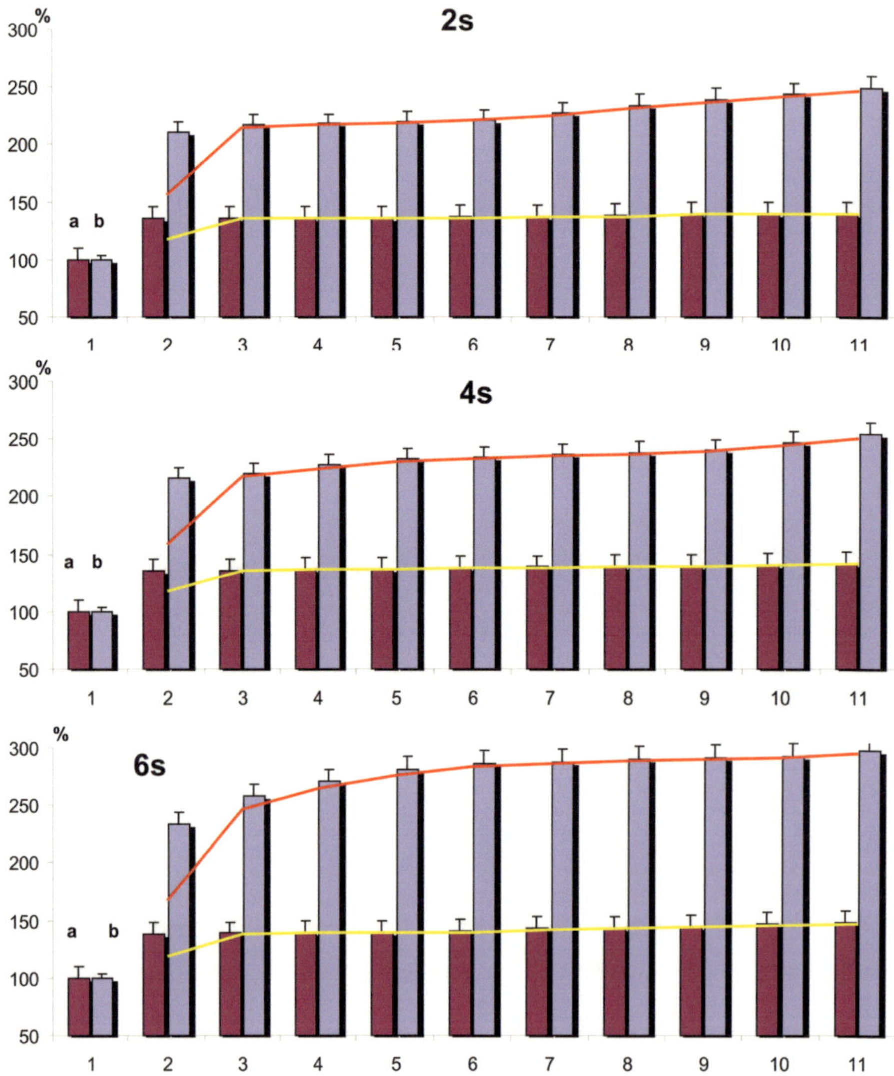

Figure 6. The change in time of stationary state reach by musculus gastrocnemius in rats with diabetic polyneuropathy caused by 10 consecutive stimulation pools with electrostimulation with 50 Hz frequency and duration 2, 4 and 6 s. The relaxation time is 10 s. The meanings are represented as percentages from control values considered as 100%. 1—control values; 2–11—consecutive irritation pools; a—direct stimulation of the muscle; b—stimulation through the nerve.

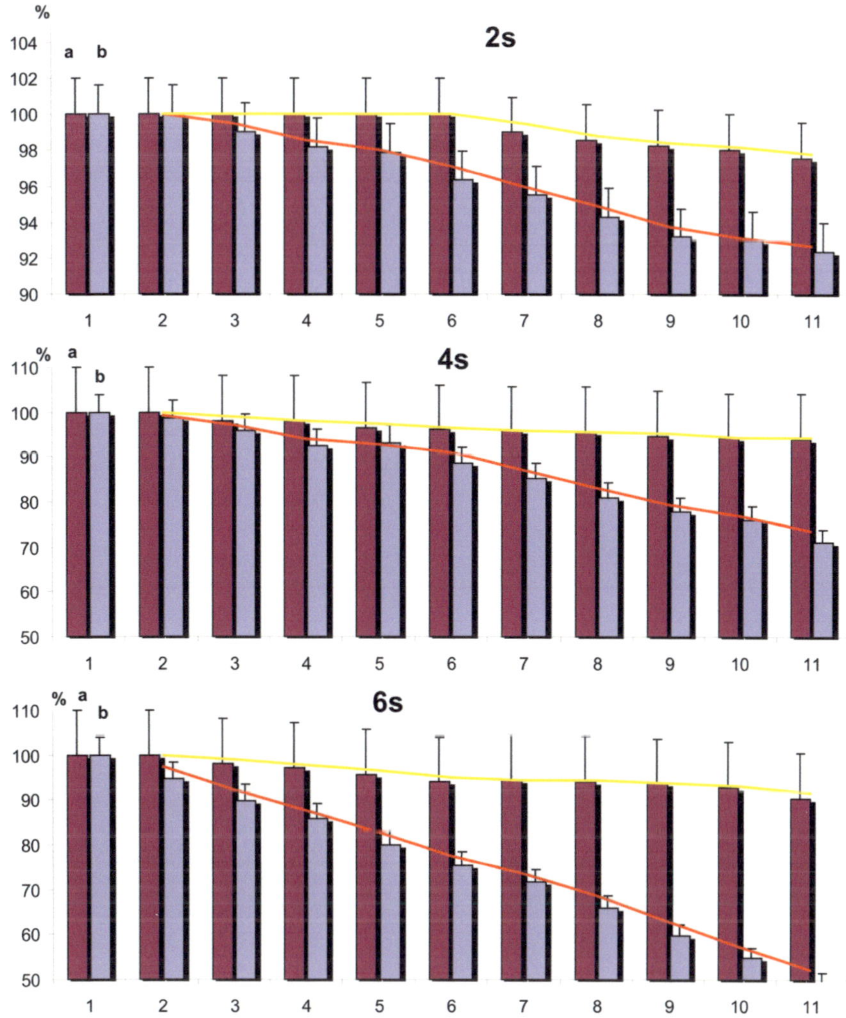

Figure 7. The change of integrated power of musculus gastrocnemius in rats with diabetic polyneuropathy caused by 10 consecutive stimulation pools with electrostimulation with 50 Hz frequency and duration 2, 3 and 4 s. The relaxation time is 10 s. The meanings are represented as percentages from control values considered as 100%. 1—control values; 2–11—consecutive irritation pools; a—direct stimulation of the muscle; b—stimulation through the nerve.

The changes in the maximum and minimum force of muscle contraction in rats with diabetic neuropathy caused by 10 consecutive stimulation pools with modulated electrostimulation with 50 Hz frequency and duration 2, 4 and 6 s were analyzed. The decrease in the maximum force was found from 99.34% at first run till 91% at tenth run, as well as decrease in the minimum force response was found from 99% (1) till 90.78% (10). The changes in these indicators with increasing stimulation duration up to 4 s were as follows: 98.71% (1) to 78.58% (10) and 97% (1) to 51.8% (10) for the maximum and minimum force, respectively. Increase in stimulation up to 6 s: 97% (1) to 51.8% (10) and 91.18% (1) to 65.34% (1) for the maximum and minimum force, respectively.

Integrated power in rats with diabetic polyneuropathy showed a slight decrease from 100% at the first run to 92.37% at the tenth run with stimulation duration of 2 s. More significant changes were recorded at 4 and 6 s stimulation from 98.7% (1) to 71.16% (10) and from 94.71% (1) to 49.6% (10), respectively.

Based on the obtained data, it could be concluded that with the development of diabetic neuropathy for all 10 consecutive stimulation pools, the formation of a stable muscle response in the phases of the maximum force retention (and stationary state) does not occur. The dynamics of amplitude-force formation had a clear tendency to reduce the stabilization time of the constant power characteristics.

Biomechanical curves showed that prolonged stimulation with 1 and 2 Hz frequency (**Figure 8**) decreased the maximum force response of the muscle throughout the period of stimulation. Stimulation of 2 Hz caused the development of rapid fatigue processes, and the maximum change in muscle power productivity occurs on 1 min of force parameters registration (**Figures 8** and **9**). If we continue stimulation in the same way, after 150 s, the muscle passes into a state of complete nonexcitability (**Figure 10**).

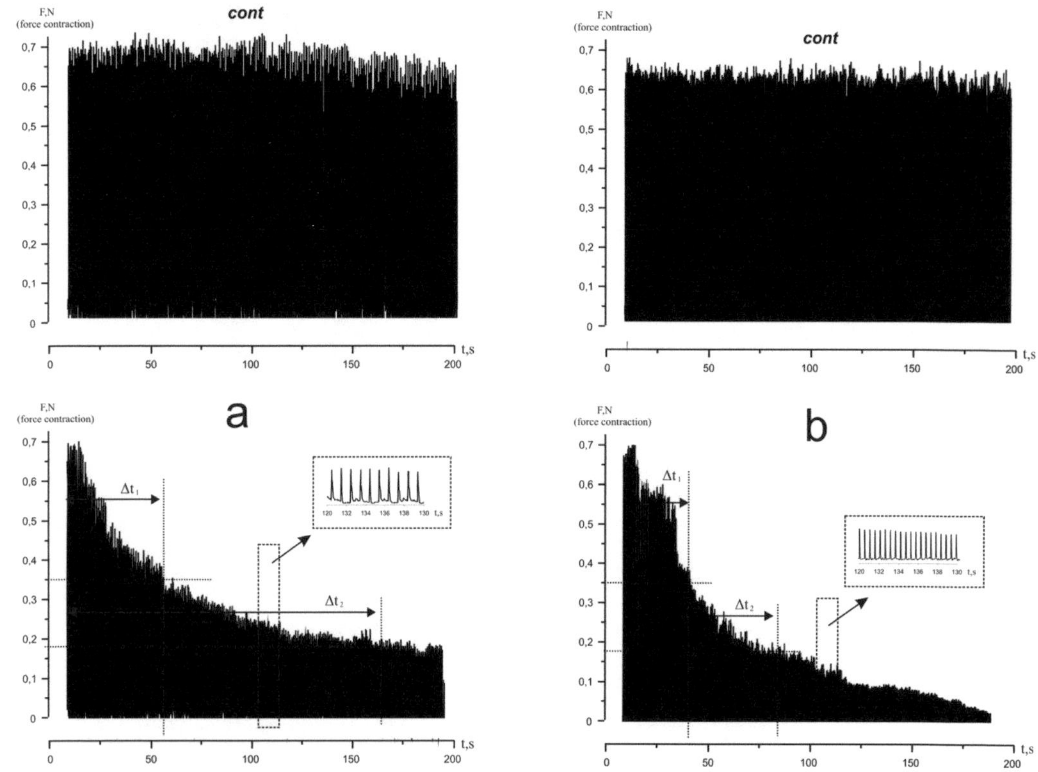

Figure 8. Curves of musculus gastrocnemius force generation caused by unrelaxed stimulation by electrostimulation with 1 Hz (a) and 2 Hz (b) frequency. Δt_1—time of force reduction by 50% compared to the initial level; Δt_2—time of force reduction by 30% compared to the initial level.

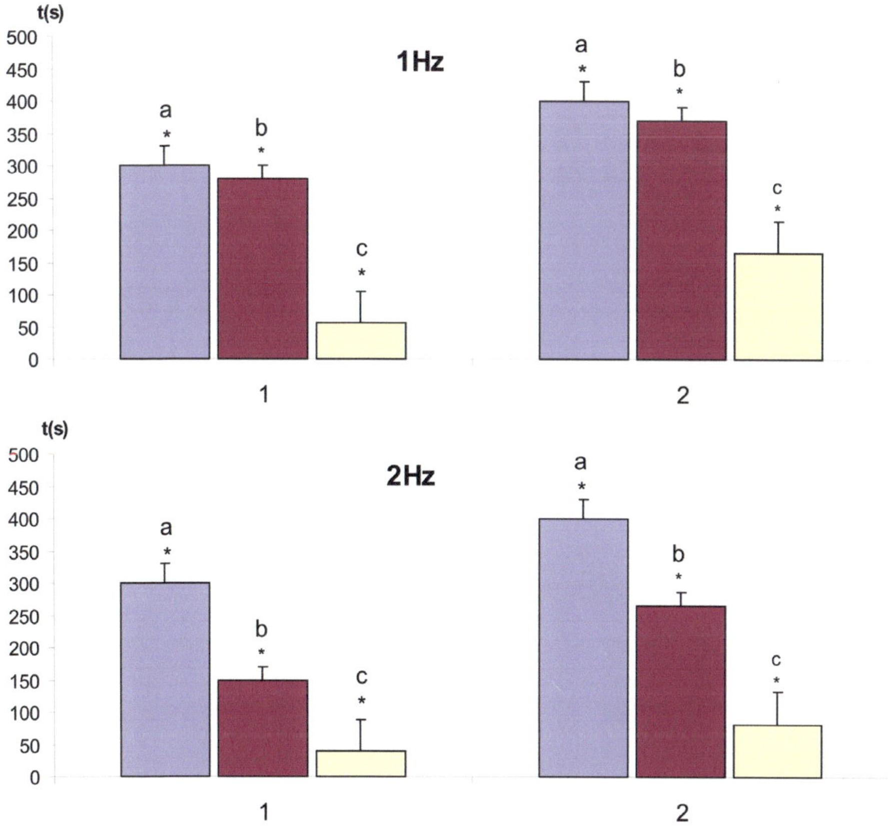

Figure 9. Time of musculus gastrocnemius force reduction in rats with diabetic neuropathy by 50% (1) and 30% (2) compare to initial level caused by unrelaxed stimulation by electrostimulation with frequency 1 Hz and 2 Hz. a—control; b—direct stimulation of the muscle; c—stimulation of the muscle through the nerve; 1—time of force reduction by 50% compared to the initial level; 2—time of force reduction by 30% compared to the initial level.

The time of muscle contraction force reduction during diabetic polyneuropathy by 50% was 55 and 39 s, respectively. The time of muscle contraction force reduction by 30% was 165 s at 1 Hz and 82 s at 2 Hz (**Figure 9**).

Thus, it can be assumed that the conversion of the depolarization current to the impulse frequency of the outgoing motor neuron during the development of these pathological processes is a linear process of the development of fatigue with the absence of rapid adaptation by a constant frequency stimulus. The registered parameters during fatigue process development were similar to the processes of motor neuron impulse frequency changing caused by severe pathological disorders of the neuromuscular preparation. The transformation of depolarization current into the pulse frequency in this case is a nonlinear process, most likely connected with numerous pathological processes in organism. The absence of both initial and subsequent adaptation of the induced fatigue process can be associated with processes of inactivation of Ca channels located in the initial axon segments.

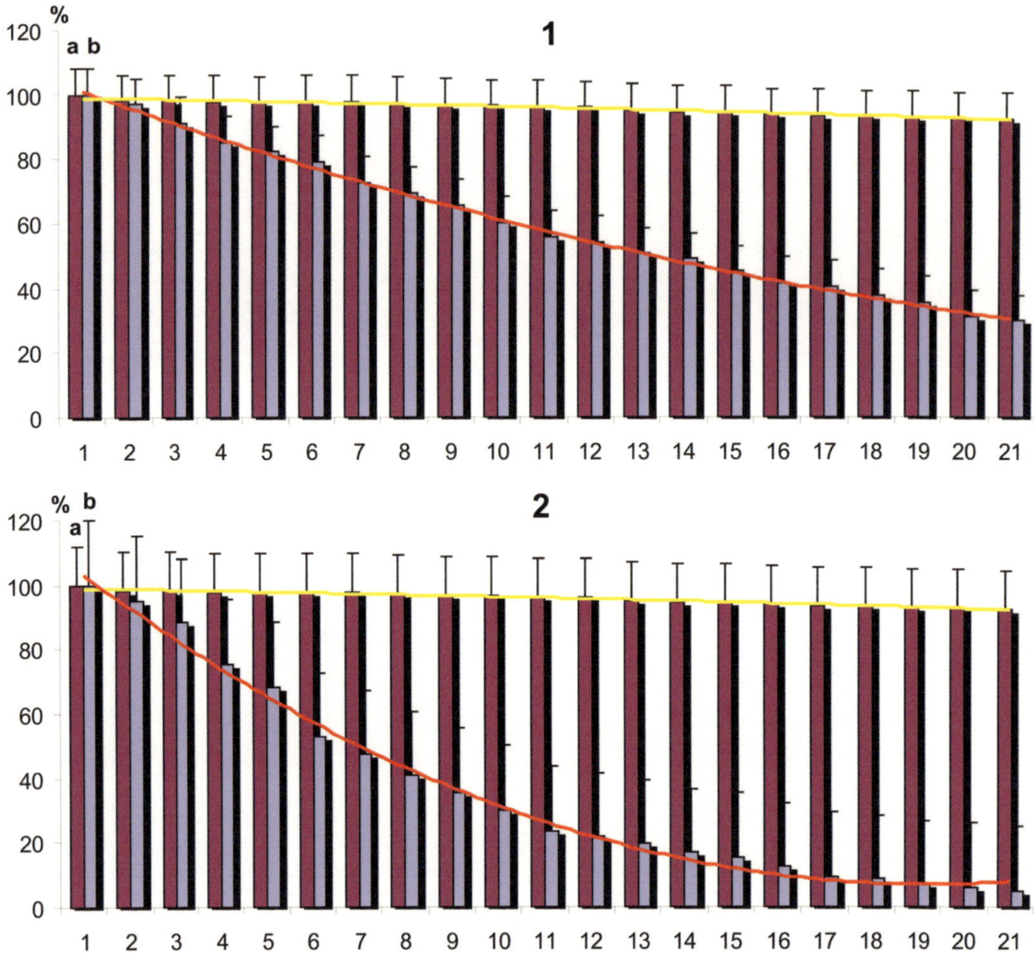

Figure 10. Musculus gastrocnemius maximum force reduction in rats with diabetic neuropathy compared to the initial level caused by unrelaxed stimulation by electrostimulation with 1 Hz and 2 Hz frequency and duration of 200 s. The meanings are represented as percentages from control values considered as 100%. a—control; b—rat with diabetic neuropathy; 1–21—consecutive irritation pools.

Maximum force contraction during diabetic neuropathy decreased from 97% till 30% with stimulation of 1 Hz and duration of 200 s (**Figure 11**).

With stimulation of 2 Hz and duration of 200 s, the maximum force contraction of musculus gastrocnemius in rats with diabetic neuropathy decreased significantly from 95 to 5%, respectively (**Figure 10**).

Time between the development of the maximum force response decreased by 65 min during first unfused tetanus till 53 min during the fifth contraction (**Figures 10**). The change in peaks force is 311 mN at the first contraction and 331 mN at the fifth contraction of the unfused tetanus. The time for establishing of fused tetanus caused with stimulation of 20 Hz and 6 s duration was 4789 ms. In control this time was 3456 ms (**Figure 12**).

http://dx.doi.org/10.5772/intechopen.70600

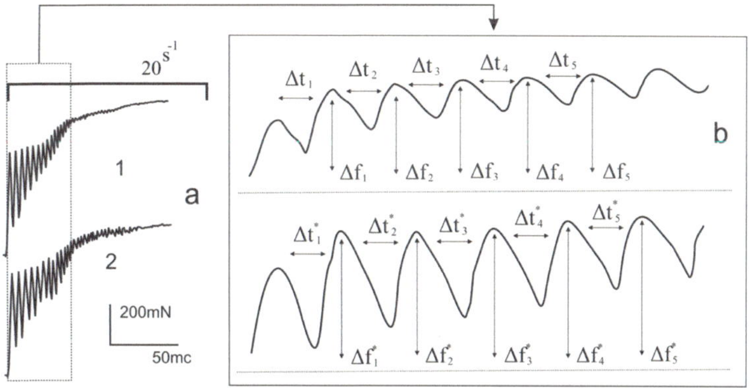

Figure 11. The changes in musculus gastrocnemius maximum force response development at five first peaks of the unfused tetanus caused by stimulation with 20 Hz frequency in rats with diabetic neuropathy. a—it is the general view of the muscle force response caused by stimulation with 20 Hz frequency, for 6 s control (1), rats with diabetic neuropathy (2); b—five consecutive peaks of the tetanus; *—indicated parameters of the investigated rats; Δt_1–Δt_5—time of force response development 1–5 consecutive reductions; Δf_1–Δf_5—the force of consecutive peaks of the first contractions of musculus gastrocnemius.

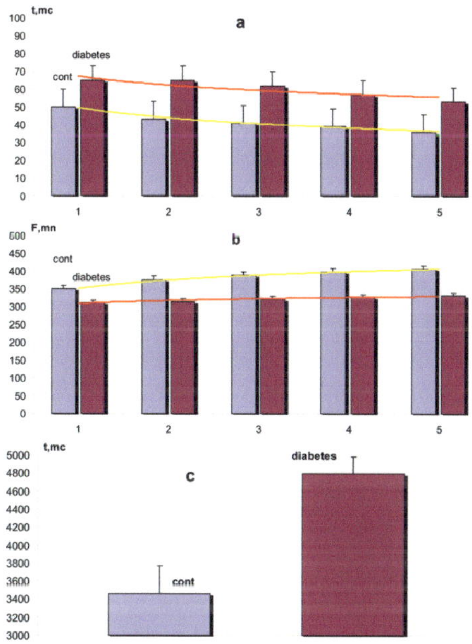

Figure 12. The changes in time between the development of the maximum force response (a), force (b), during the first five contractions of unfused tetanus and the time of its establishment (c), stimulation with 20 Hz frequency of the control (cont) and diabetic (diabete) rats. 1–5—consecutive irritation pools.

4. Conclusions

To form macroindicators of neuromuscular activity during the development of diabetic polyneuropathy numerous complex, nonlinear nonstationary processes occur. The influence of pathological factors on these processes leads to either complete dysfunction of these parameters or their desynchronization. As a result, the whole muscle as a dynamic system is not able to adequately implement the pool of neural activity getting from the central nervous system. The nature and level of these dysfunctions is linearly related to the level of pathological processes development, the analysis of which at present can be carried out exclusively at the phenomenological level. Despite new experimental approaches in studying microlevel of neuromuscular regulation, traditional electro-physiological models with usage of neuromuscular preparation in vivo are still important. Such studies should be conducted not only to obtain accurate quantitative analysis of the pathologies of muscle dynamics but also to study the totality of the central processes involved in the regulation of muscle contraction.

In condition of diabetic polyneuropathy development, differences in the response of the muscle to frequency changes indicate that to determine the contractile properties of the muscle, it is important to know not only the current values of the force response and activation intensity but also the history of changes in these parameters. The consequence of above-described dysfunction of the neuromuscular complex is the need of motor neurons to generate powerful dynamic discharge components to resume the error-free operation of the muscular system. Thus, at the same levels of the stationary state of the efferent command, an increase in the duration of the preceding dynamic component not only slows down the transition to a new equilibrium force but also leads to decrease in the maximum force response. The mechanokinetic curves showed the changes in the implementation of complex stimulation programs during the development of polyneuropathy. The analysis of dynamic properties of various parts of the motor system gives an idea of the presence of changes in the dynamics of complex movements associated with the precision positioning of joints and the ability of the system to correct the descending motor commands by adaptation processes in the central neurons.

Usage of static characteristics "stimulation signal-reduction force" to analyze the pathological processes during diabetic polyneuropathy development will lead to incomplete picture of pathology development. For an adequate understanding and analysis of these changes, a multifaceted experimental approach is needed with the possibility of simultaneous monitoring of various biomechanical parameters with different amplitude-time intervals and a labile system of external stimulation. Only in this case it becomes possible to trace the changes in the reaction of neuromuscular preparation to stimulation that are responsible for the development of ballistic precision positional movements, the analysis of which will be a critical factor in concluding the level of development of pathologies in diabetic polyneuropathy.

Author details

Tetyana Volodymyrivna Beregova*, Dmytro Nozdrenko, Sergii Berehovyi, Natali Nikitina, Tetyana Falalyeyeva and Liudmyla Ivanivna Ostapchenko

*Address all correspondence to: tetyana_beregova@ukr.net

Taras Shevchenko National University of Kyiv, Kyiv, Ukraine

References

[1] Albers JW, Rodica Pop-Busui R. Diabetic neuropathy: Mechanisms, emerging treatments, and subtypes. Current Neurology and Neuroscience Reports. 2014;**14**(8):473-491

[2] Hajas G, Kissova V, Tirpakova A. A 10-yr follow-up study for the detection of peripheral neuropathy in young patients with type 1 diabetes. Pediatric Diabetes. 2016;**17**(8):632-641

[3] Khandoker AH, Jelinek HF, Moritani T, Palaniswami M. Association of cardiac autonomic neuropathy with alteration of sympatho-vagal balance through heart rate variability analysis. Medical Engineering & Physics. 2010;**32**(2):161-167

[4] Spallone V, Ziegler D, Freeman R, Bernardi L, Frontoni S, Pop-Busui R, et al. Cardiovascular autonomic neuropathy in diabetes: Clinical impact, assessment, diagnosis, and management. Diabetes/Metabolism Research and Reviews. 2011;**27**(7):639-653

[5] Callaghan BC, Price RS, Feldman EL. Distal symmetric polyneuropathy: A review. Journal of the American Medical Association. 2015;**314**(20):2172-2181

[6] Thomas PK. Diabetic peripheral neuropathies: Their cost to patient and society and the value of knowledge of risk factors for development of interventions. European Neurology. 1999;**41**(Suppl 1):35-43

[7] The Look AHEAD Research Group. Effects of a long-term lifestyle modification programme on peripheral neuropathy in overweight or obese adults with type 2 diabetes: The look AHEAD study. Diabetologia. 2017;**60**(6):980-988

[8] Gordois A, Scuffham P, Shearer A, Oglesby A, Tobian JA. The health care costs of diabetic peripheral neuropathy in the US. Diabetes Care. 2003;**26**(6):1790-1795

[9] Rijken PM, Dekker J, Dekker E, et al. Clinical and functional correlates of foot pain in diabetic patients. Disability and Rehabilitation. 1998;**20**(9):330-336

[10] Type 1 Diabetes in Adults: Diagnosis and Management. NICE Guideline—National Clinical Guideline Centre (UK): 2015;(17)

[11] Pasnoor M, Dimachkie MM, Kluding P, Barohn RJ. Diabetic neuropathy part 1: Overview and symmetric phenotypes. Neurologic Clinics. 2013;**31**(2):425-445

[12] Pittenger GL, Ray M, Burcus NI, McNulty P, Basta B, Vinik AI. Intraepidermal nerve fibers are indicators of small-fiber neuropathy in both diabetic and nondiabetic patients. Diabetes Care. 2004;**27**:1974-1979

[13] Grandinetti A, Chow DC, Sletten DM, et al. Impaired glucose tolerance is associated with postganglionic sudomotor impairment. Clinical Autonomic Research. 2007;**17**:231-233

[14] Callaghan BC, Little AA, Feldman EL, Hughes RA. Enhanced glucose control for preventing and treating diabetic neuropathy. Cochrane Database of Systematic Reviews. 2012;**6**:CD007543

[15] Van Acker K, Bouhassira D, De Bacquer D, et al. Prevalence and impact on quality of life of peripheral neuropathy with or without neuropathic pain in type 1 and type 2 diabetic patients attending hospital outpatients clinics. Diabetes & Metabolism. 2009;**35**:206-213

[16] Román-Pintos LM, Villegas-Rivera G, Rodríguez-Carrizalez AD, Miranda-Díaz AG, Cardona-Muñoz EG. Diabetic polyneuropathy in type 2 diabetes mellitus: Inflammation, oxidative stress, and mitochondrial function. Journal of Diabetes Research. 2016;**2016**:3425617

[17] Shakher J, Stevens MJ. Update on the management of diabetic polyneuropathies. Diabetes, Metabolic Syndrome and Obesity: Targets and Therapy. 2011;**4**:289-305

[18] Curtin N, Szabo C. Therapeutic applications of PARP inhibitors: Anticancer therapy and beyond. Molecular Aspects of Medicine. 2013;**34**(6). DOI: 10.1016/j.mam.2013.01.006

[19] Pop-Busui R, Ang L, Holmes C, Gallagher K, Feldman EL. Inflammation as a therapeutic target for diabetic neuropathies. Current Diabetes Reports. 2016;**16**(3):29

[20] Tracy JA, Dyck PJB. The Spectrum of diabetic neuropathies. Physical Medicine and Rehabilitation Clinics of North America. 2008;**19**(1):1-v

[21] Callaghan BC, Hur J, Feldman EL. Diabetic neuropathy: One disease or two? Current Opinion in Neurology. 2012;**25**:536-541

[22] Timar B, Timar R, Schiller R, Oancea C, Roman D, Vlad M, Balinisteanu B, Mazilu O. Impact of neuropathy on the adherence to diabetes-related self-care activities: A cross-sectional study. Patient Preference and Adherence. 2016;**10**:1169-1175

[23] Tesfaye S, Boulton AJ, Dyck PJ, et al. Diabetic neuropathies: Update on definitions, diagnostic criteria, estimation of severity, and treatments. Diabetes Care. 2010;**33**:2285-2293

[24] Vinik AI, Casellini CM. Guidelines in the management of diabetic nerve pain: Clinical utility of pregabalin. Diabetes, Metabolic Syndrome and Obesity: Targets and Therapy. 2013;**6**:57-78

[25] Sima AA, Kamiya H. Diabetic neuropathy differs in type 1 and type 2 diabetes. Annals of the New York Academy of Sciences. 2006;**1084**:235-249

[26] Kanji JN, Anglin RE, Hunt DL, Panju A. Does this patient with diabetes have large-fiber peripheral neuropathy? Journal of the American Medical Association. 2010;**303**(15): 1526-1532

[27] England JD, Gronseth GS, Franklin G, Miller RG, Asbury AK, Carter GT, et al. Distal symmetric polyneuropathy: A definition for clinical research: Report of the American Acad-emy of Neurology, the American Association of Electrodi-Agnostic Medicine, and the American Academy of Physical Medicine and Rehabilitation. Neurology. 2005;**64**:199-207

[28] Sambasevam Y, Omar Farouk AA, Tengku Mohamad TA, Sulaiman MR, Bharatham BH, Perimal EK. Cardamonin attenuates hyperalgesia and allodynia in a mouse model of chronic constriction injury-induced neuropathic pain: Possible involvement of the opioid system. European Journal of Pharmacology. 2017;**796**:32-38

[29] D'Amour FE, Smith DLA. Method for determining loss of pain sensation. The Journal of Pharmacology and Experimental Therapeutics. 1941;**72**(1):74-78

[30] Nozdrenko DM, Zavodovskyi DO, Matvienko TY, Zay SY, Bogutska KI, Prylutskyy YI, Ritter U, Scharff P. C60 fullerene as promising therapeutic agent for the prevention and correction of skeletal muscle functioning at ischemic injury. Nanoscale Research Letters. 2017;**12**(1):115

Section 4

Renal Pathophysiology

Chapter 8

Immunopathology of Kidney Transplantation

Zesergio Melo, Juan A. Ruiz-Pacheco,
Claudia A. Mendoza-Cerpa and Raquel Echavarria

Additional information is available at the end of the chapter

http://dx.doi.org/10.5772/intechopen.70596

Abstract

Renal transplantation is currently the best alternative for patients with end-stage renal disease. Immune responses activated against the allograft are a decisive factor in transplantation outcomes and patient survival. Although short-term graft and patient survival have improved significantly as a result of better donor matching systems, novel immunosuppressive agents and enhanced care, long-term outcomes remain unfavorable and reflect sub-clinical injury caused by chronic rejection. The immune system lies at the intersection of immunogenic tolerance and graft failure; thus, it is a major determinant of pathology in the context of renal transplantation. During the early stages of transplantation increased expression of cytokines has been observed in addition to increased expression of adhesion proteins and immune cells. This early inflammatory response does not necessarily end in graft rejection, although this will depend on the severity of the inflammation. Activation of Toll-like Receptors (TLRs), damaging molecular patterns (DAMPs), and other components of innate immunity is key to the formation of atherosclerotic plaques and the development of autoimmune diseases. Initially the donor antigens are presented to the T lymphocytes of the recipient. This activation induces their proliferation, differentiation and cytokine production. Successful kidney transplant recipients need to develop immunologic tolerance against donor antigens. In this chapter, we address some of the innate and adaptive immune mechanisms associated with kidney transplantation; emphasizing their role in allograft rejection.

Keywords: kidney, transplantation, immunopathology, graft rejection, immunology

1. Introduction

According to statistics from the United States Renal Data System (UNOS) and the U.S. Department of Health & Human Services Organ Procurement and Transplantation Network

(OPTN), there are currently close to 100,000 people in the U.S. waiting for a lifesaving kidney transplant. Only between January and May 2017, 14,075 kidney transplants took place in the United States; of which 11,702 organs came from deceased donors and 2373 came from living donors. Renal transplantation has become the treatment of choice for patients with end-stage renal disease (ESRD); though its success and widespread use are still limited by the availability of suitable organs and allograft rejection [1]. In recent decades, short-term graft survival has improved significantly as consequence of better donor matching systems, novel immunosuppressive agents and enhanced care. Unfortunately, long-term outcomes remain unfavorable and reflect subclinical injury caused by antibody-mediated allograft rejection (ABMR) [2]. The immune system lies at the intersection between immunogenic tolerance and graft failure and as such, it is a major determinant of pathology in the context of renal transplantation [3]. The immune system is a complex network of lymphoid organs, cells, and molecules responsible for body homeostasis and host defense. Although the main function of the immune system is to protect against external pathogens and molecules, the presence of foreign antigens on the donor organ also triggers innate and adaptive immune responses in the recipient that will largely determine graft performance and patient survival.

2. Activation of innate immunity in kidney transplantation

Innate immune responses are required for the activation of cellular and molecular mechanisms behind the physiopathology of kidney transplantation [4]. During the early stages of transplantation, innate immunity is essential for the activation of the adaptive immune system, whereas at later stages, innate components promote an inflammatory microenvironment that enhances allograft damage.

2.1. Cells of the innate immune system

The cellular components of innate immunity are phagocytic leukocytes (neutrophils, monocytes, eosinophils, and basophils), natural killer (NK) cells, and dendritic cells (DCs). Ischemic injury that occurs during organ transplantation promotes alloimmune responses including innate cell recruitment [5]. Infiltrating neutrophils release proteases, free radicals, and proinflammatory molecules such as interleukin 6 (IL-6), interleukin 8 (IL-8), and tumor necrosis factor alpha (TNF-α) within the graft. It has been demonstrated that a high neutrophil-lymphocyte ratio amplifies the inflammatory process during acute renal failure [6]. Furthermore, neutrophil-depleted mice and intracellular adhesion molecule 1 (ICAM-1) knockouts are more resistant to renal ischemic injury; suggesting that neutralizing neutrophil activity could increase transplant success rates by reducing early graft damage [7]. Macrophages are also an important source of interleukin 1 (IL-1), IL-6, transforming growth factor beta (TFG-β), interferon γ-induced protein 10 (IP-10), monocyte chemoattractant protein 1 (MCP-1), and macrophage inflammatory protein 2 (MIP-2) during ischemia [8]. In the context of renal damage, monocytes are recruited within the first few days thanks to C–C chemokine receptor type 2 (CCR2) and CX3C chemokine receptor 1 (CX3CR1) ligand release. Subsequently, these monocytes are transformed into macrophages able to phagocyte damaged cells and present peptides to alloreactive T cells in peripheral lymph nodes [8, 9]. There is NK cell recruitment after ischemia and during the early stages of renal transplantation [10, 11]. NK cells keep other cells in check for major histocompatibility complex (MHC) surface expression through killer Ig-like receptors (KIR) [12]. In allotransplantation, lack of MHC Class I recognition triggers NK effector mechanisms, including perforin-dependent cell lysis and cytokine production [13]. NK cells seem to play an important role in the induction of acute renal damage and long-term graft survival as demonstrated in mice that exhibit abnormalities in recruitment of these cells and are more resistant to kidney damage [10, 11].

2.2. Role of pattern recognition receptors and damaging molecular patterns in renal transplantation

In the early 1990s, Janeway proposed that all innate immune cells had pattern recognition receptors (PRRs) that can discriminate between self-components and pathogens. Soon after, Polly Matzinger suggested that our immune system is designed to recognize signs of harm rather than to discriminate between self and nonself, which could explain how innate immune activation can occur under sterile conditions such as in allotransplantation [14]. Consequently, pathogen-associated molecular patterns (PAMPs) and DAMPs are designed to signal damage threats [15]. DAMPs and PAMPs arise in the allograft during pre- and post-transplant periods; and activation of vascular PRRs such as TLRs, C-type lectin receptors, Nod-like receptors, and retinoic acid-inducible gene-I-like receptors can trigger production of proinflammatory cytokines [4].

The surgical process as well as ischemic injury, precondition for a systemic inflammatory reaction by releasing high mobility group box 1 (HMGB1) and heat shock proteins; as well as by increasing Toll-like receptor 4 (TLR4) expression in endothelial and peripheral blood cells [16]. The immunosuppressant cyclosporin A also induces HMGB1 release and promotes immune cell infiltration into the renal graft [17]. Furthermore, blocking HMGB1 reduced cellular infiltrate, IL-6 and TNF-α production in kidneys subjected to ischemia, and decreased of MCP-1 which is reflected in reduced nephrotoxicity [18]. On the other hand, HMGB1 appears to play a protective role; the administration of recombinant HMGB1 prevents dysfunction, tissue damage, and inflammation in animals subjected to ischemia [19].

2.3. The complement system

The complement system is a set of membrane-anchored and serum proteins that work in a coordinated way to eliminate microorganisms or damaged cells. The functions of complement include opsonization, inflammation through secondary products that result from the degradation of anaphylatoxins and formation of the membrane attack complex (MAC). There are three known complement pathways: the classical pathway that depends on the previous binding of antibodies, the alternate pathway that depends on the spontaneous hydrolysis and binding of C3 and the pathway of lectins that depends on the binding of proteins to carbohydrates. Currently, there is evidence to suggest the participation of the three complement pathways during renal transplantation [20–22].

2.4. Innate-adaptive immunity interactions

Communication between innate and adaptive immunity largely depends on antigen presentation. T and B cells express antigen-specific receptors (TCR and BCR). The signals elicited by the TCR and BCR are insufficient to achieve the proper activation state, and costimulatory molecules and cytokines provided by innate immune cells are necessary [4]. Although DCs are the most efficient APCs, neutrophils, basophils, and eosinophils also influence the outcome of adaptive immunity. Neutrophils can recruit IL-17-producing Th17 lymphocytes by releasing CCL2 and CCL20. Interestingly, patients with a history of chronic renal dysfunction showed a significant increase in IL-17 producing cells [23]. Basophils are normally activated by IL-3 or immunoglobulin binding in different renal structures; and are an important source of cytokines, thymic stromal lymphopoietin, leukotrienes and histamines which may influence the outcome of adaptive immune responses [24, 25]. Basophils express MCH Class II and are considered important regulators of T and B cell activation. Moreover, an increase in eosinophils in renal transplant, recipients has been proposed as a predictor of allograft success [26].

3. Adaptive immune responses

3.1. Allorecognition, T-cell activation, T cell–mediated cytotoxicity, and B lymphocytes

The term allorecognition refers to recognition of diverse forms of genes between a member of the same species by T cells and involve Human major histocompatibility complex (MHC) glycoproteins. MHC is a family composed by the most studied antigens in transplantation field. These antigens are widely known as human leukocyte antigens (HLA). The genes encoding HLA antigens are highly polymorphic, this feature represents a big obstacle in the study of mechanisms of graft rejection. Class I HLA are present in membranes of the nucleated cell of humans and its function is to present small endogenous antigens to CD8 T lymphocytes. Class II are expressed on dendritic cells, macrophages, B cells, endothelial, and some types of epithelial cells. This T cell recognition event is the first step of graft rejection. There are two different ways in which T cells recognize alloantigens, i.e., direct and indirect. Direct recognition is when CD8+ and CD4+ T cells from the recipient recognize MHC class I and class II presented by APCs and donor peptides. Indirect recognition is mediated by specialized APCs form the recipient presenting to T cells [27]. Donor endothelial cells express molecules that stimulate T cells, these activated cells provide help to B cells resulting in the production of alloantibodies [28]. Although the most studied role of B cells is associated with alloantibodies and donor specific antibodies, there are controversial opinions about the deleterious role of these antibodies and its association with poor graft outcomes [29].

4. Immunotolerance in transplantation

The term immunotolerance implies the absence of recognition and renal graft attack by the immune cells of the recipient. One of the most important developments in the field of organ transplantation has been the use of immunosuppressive therapies that interfere with immune recognition and consequently delay graft rejection. Nonetheless, although immunosuppression is used, some immune adaptation may develop in the graft. To choose a clinically successful immunosuppressive therapy, several factors must be considered: they must be easily applicable in clinical practice, there should be enough evidence of their effectiveness, they must be stable over time even in conditions where the immune system is altered, and their mechanism of action should not have cross-reactions with other therapies. As a final point, it should be possible to measure and control its levels in the transplanted patient [30]. Induction of tolerance can occur through various mechanisms that include thymic deletional, central and peripheral deletional, and nondeletional mechanisms.

4.1. Mechanisms of -cell tolerance

T cell tolerance in transplantation is a regulated process that ensures the tolerance and permanence of antigens, similarly to tolerance required for the maintenance of self-antigens [31]. It consists of several stages: deletion, anergy, suppression, and ignorance. Tolerance is maintained by several mechanisms initiating in the thymus, where T cells are chosen by negative selection. The main mechanism of transplanted antigens tolerance is through intrathymic deletion of donor-reactive T cells [32]. Although there are additional mechanisms of peripheral tolerance, most T cells are eliminated by this mechanism. Peripheral deletion of T cells is an important mechanism of tolerance, in which CD4 T cells reactive to donor antigens show activation, as well as apoptotic cell death. Once the tolerance is given T cells cannot respond to antigens, a state known as anergy. A costimulatory block induces anergy and has been successfully applied for tolerance induction. The activation of the T cell requires at least two signals: an antigen-dependent T cell receptor-mediated signal 1 and an antigen-independent costimulatory signal 2 [33]. CD4 and CD25 T cell regulators are actively involved in the development of immunological tolerance toward the graft. Ignorance is another mechanism that occurs when donor antigens are not recognized by the lymphoid system of the recipient or when lymphocytes fail to invade the graft. However, this mechanism applies to nonvascularized grafts.

The aim of tolerance induction in renal transplantation is to block direct and indirect alloresponse pathways. In the first, it is necessary to establish the depletion of the recipient T cells and the activation of suppressor cells capable of regulating T cells. Some drugs can induce the death of alloreactive T cells. On the other hand, oral administration of allopeptides may also produce specific tolerance to corresponding alloantigens and generate specific production and activation of regulatory T cells.

4.2. Induction of immunologic tolerance

Tolerance induction requires alloreactive T-cell deletion in the thymus before these cells can be released to the periphery. Hematopoietic chimerism is a widespread method to induce tolerance. Animal models have improved our understanding of this mechanism that ranges from tolerance induction through the injection of allogeneic cells into newborn mice to the use of adult irradiated animals injected with allogeneic donor bone marrow [34]. Tolerance induction at the peripheral systemic level needs to target mature T cells by blocking T cell molecules located on its surface, which have important roles in the activation of signaling pathways that impact cell function directly. To this end, antibodies directed against CD4 or CD8 or costimulatory molecules have been used. CD28 receptor blockade prevents proinflammatory cytokine production, as well as T cell survival and proliferation. It is also possible to interfere with the signaling pathways involved in T cell survival and proliferation, which is the case of the mTOR pathway inhibitor rapamycin. Clinical studies in humans have focused on graft tolerance induction by pretransplanting donor hematopoietic cells in human leukocyte antigen (HLA)-matched and mismatched kidney transplant recipients [35, 36].

4.3. Immunosuppressive therapy in renal transplantation

The discovery of effective immunosuppressive drugs has had great impact in the field of transplantation. Currently available immunosuppressive therapies focus on three main objectives: induction, maintenance, and treatment of rejection. For induction therapy three types of antibodies are used, the lymphocytes depleting agents, antithymocyte globulin and alemtuzumab, and basiliximab (nondepleting) [37]. Basiliximab, an IL-2 receptor antagonist and it is used in combination with other immunosuppressants, significantly reduces acute rejection in large clinical studies [38]. The use of antithymocyte antibodies in diseased donor recipients also reduces early acute rejection incidence. Nevertheless, its use has been associated with reversible leukopenia, thrombocytopenia, and cytomegalovirus infection [39].

The use of calcineurin inhibitors cyclosporine and tacrolimus has been key in reducing the risk of rejection and has greatly improved short-term graft survival outcomes. Unfortunately, in the long run they also help develop histological changes typical of nephropathy that diminish kidney graft function and increase risk of graft loss [40, 41]. A T cell costimulatory inhibitor called belatacept was introduced to avoid the deleterious effects of calcineurin inhibitors. In several studies, belatacept prevents acute rejection in renal transplantation comparable to cyclosporine [42]. Since the 1980s, several options have been developed to reduce kidney transplant rejection. Monoclonal muromonab-CD3/OKT3, monoclonal interleukin-2 receptor (IL-2R) antibodies (daclizumab and zenapax), and antiproliferative agents (mycophenolate mofetil) are part of a large list of options currently available in renal transplantation [43]. Nevertheless, some transplant experts propose a reduction in the use of immunosuppressive drugs in order to reduce the nephrotoxicity that can also end in fibrosis and graft rejection. Additionally, some transplant recipients develop diabetes, cardiovascular disease, dyslipidemia associated to immunosuppressant therapies. For this reason, it is estimated that kidney grafts can function on average 10 years after the transplantation [44, 45].

5. Graft rejection

Current immunosuppressant therapies have drastically reduced acute rejection events in kidney transplant recipients [46, 47]. Unfortunately, there is still a high percentage of short- and long-term kidney graft loses secondary to ABMR [2]. Here, we will discuss the contribution of adaptive and innate immune cells; as well as antibodies, molecules from the complement system and chemokines to disease states that lead to kidney graft rejection (**Figure 1**).

5.1. T cell–mediated rejection

T cell mediated rejection (TCMR) is characterized by infiltration of the donor graft interstitium by host CD4 and CD8 T effector and memory cells, macrophages, and dendritic cells; followed by epithelial dedifferentiation and tubulitis [48, 49] (see histopathological findings in **Figure 2**). TCMR is the predominant phenotype found in kidney transplant recipients with early rejection and it is still an important cause of graft dysfunction that when left untreated causes fibrosis, tubular atrophy, and irreversible nephron loss [50]. Genes expressed by effector T cells, APCs, and macrophages stimulated with IFN-γ are abundant in the transcriptomic signature of TCMR. These transcripts are mostly related to T cell receptor signaling, T helper differentiation and communication between adaptive and innate immune cells; highlighting the importance of these pathways in TCMR [51]. Cytotoxic molecules like perforin, granulysin,

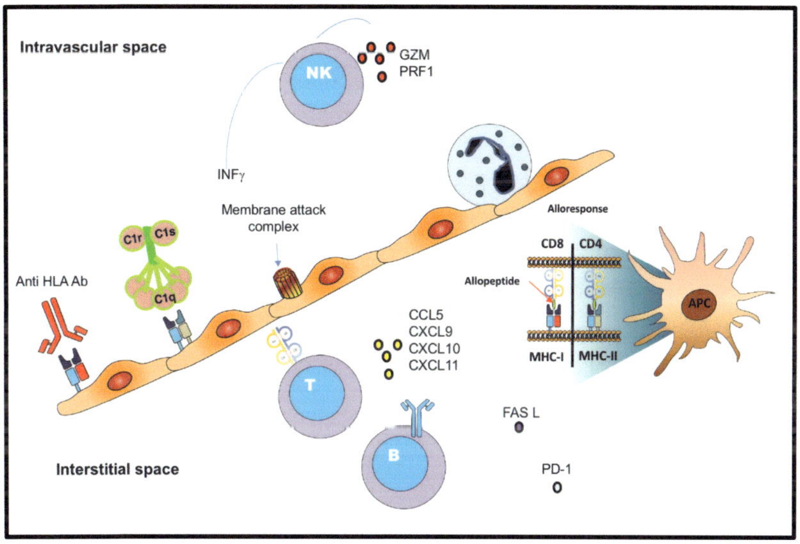

Figure 1. Mechanisms of ABMR and TCMR in kidney transplantation. Preformed and *de novo* DSAs, complement proteins, and antibody-dependent NK cell-mediated IFN-γ release and cytotoxicity have emerged as key immune players in the development of the microvascular damage characteristic of ABMR. Meanwhile, in TCMR the interaction of infiltrating T cells with intragraft APCs and macrophages triggers an inflammatory response dependent on TCR synapse and subsequent activation, and characterized by chemokine (CCL5) and cytokine (CXCL9, CXCL10, and CXCL11) release.

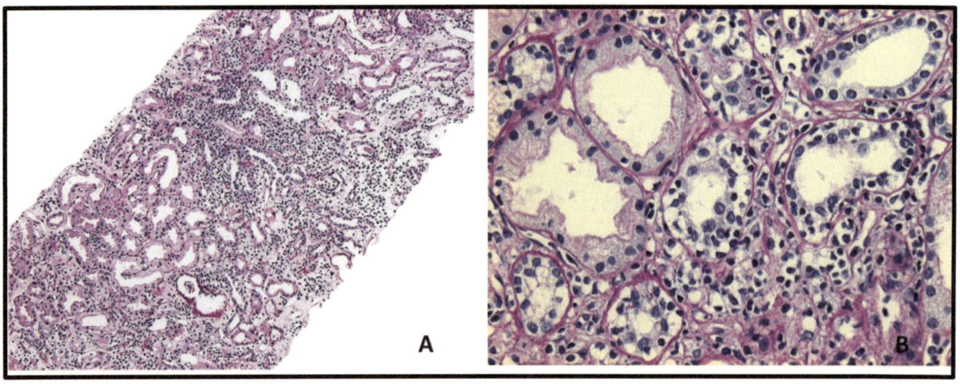

Figure 2. T cell-mediated rejection. The hallmark of TCMR is the infiltration of mononuclear cells to the interstitium and tubules. (A) Prominent intersticial inflamatory cell infiltrate. PAS 5×. (B) Higher magnification reveals infiltration of the tubular epithelium by mononuclear cells (tubulitis). PAS 40×. Courtesy of Dr. Claudia Mendoza-Cerpa, Laboratory of Pathology, IMSS-CMNO, Guadalajara; México.

Fas ligand, and granzyme A and B are also expressed in TCMR; though it has been demonstrated that they are not directly linked to the mechanism of injury [48, 52]. Instead, TCMR is considered an inflammatory reaction initiated by the engagement of TCR on cognate T cells with its antigen on APCs [53, 54]. It has been suggested that a very small proportion of infiltrating T cells are able to establish a TCR-mediated interaction with the allograft [55]. However, this interaction is important in the establishment of TCMR inflammatory phenotype since it activates the effector T cell and APC, induces INF-γ secretion and further promotes myeloid and T cell recruitment by inducing chemokines and adhesion molecules [56]. Interestingly, increased expression of immune checkpoints responsible for modulating T cell activation such as cytotoxic T-lymphocyte antigen 4, programmed death-ligand 1 and 2 have also been associated with TCMR; suggesting these molecules might be regulating some of the interactions between T cells and APCs within the graft microenvironment [51]. Moreover, evidence that the programmed cell death protein 1 (PD1) pathway may be critical in maintaining tolerance and preventing TCMR comes from a report case in which administration of an anti-PD1 antibody to a kidney transplant recipient with metastatic cutaneous squamous-cell carcinoma resulted in allograft rejection [57].

B cells are robust APCs that can readily capture, process and present antigen for T cell recognition. Still, the role of B cells in TCMR development was initially overlooked since studies in B cell-deficient mice reported similar rejection rates in skin and heart transplants, as well as efficient CD4 T cell priming [58, 59]. The first evidence of a possible role of B cells in TCMR came from a systematic study of gene expression patterns using DNA microarrays in biopsy samples from renal allografts that found a surprising association between dense CD20+ B cell infiltrates and both, steroid resistance and graft loss [60]. Although the prognostic significance of CD20+ B cell infiltrates in acute cellular rejection is a matter of debate, the presence of these B cell clusters in cases of pure TCMR and their close proximity to CD4+ T cells suggests they might have antibody-independent functions in allograft rejection by acting as APCs [61–64]. Interestingly, reversible rejection episodes with monocytic infiltrates and scant T cells have been described in severely T cell-depleted patients, emphasizing the central role of macrophages in allograft rejection [65].

Macrophages in TCMR exert dual functions by promoting initiation and progression of kidney injury through secretion of proinflammatory mediators and interaction with other cells in the graft; whilst also in charge of tissue remodeling and repair during the recovery phase [66, 67]. Interestingly, reversible rejection episodes with monocytic infiltrates and scant T cells have been described in severely T cell-depleted patients, emphasizing the central role of macrophages in allograft rejection [65].

An increase in IFN-γ induces CCL5, CXCL9, CXCL10, CXCL11, and MHC class I and II expression; and is an important feature of TCMR [68, 69]. In the context of TCMR, IFN-γ has protective and proinflammatory functions as evidenced by IFN-γ-deficient recipient animals or donors lacking IFN-γ receptors or IFN-γ-regulated factor 1 [68, 70].

5.2. Antibody-mediated rejection

Evidence form multiple studies supports the humoral theory of transplantation strongly advocated by Dr. Paul Terasaki, in which antibodies are not only responsible for immediate hyperacute allograft rejection but can produce chronic vascular damage, fibrosis, and graft rejection months or even years posttransplantation [71]. Hyperacute allograft rejection occurs soon after the graft is perfused with blood of the recipient due to preformed

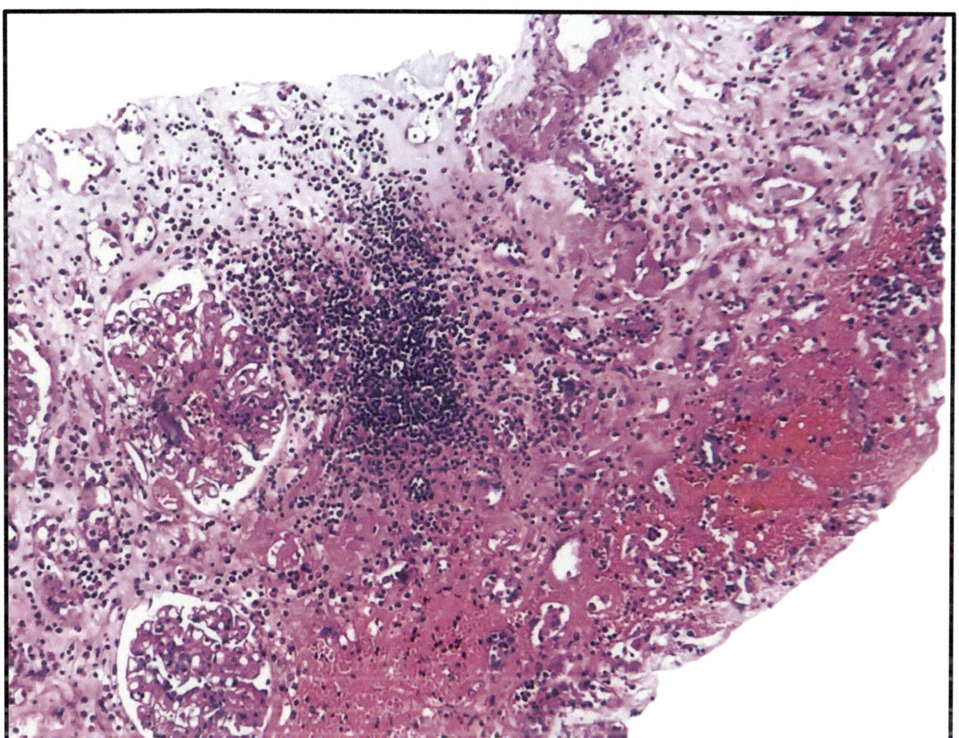

Figure 3. Interstitial hemorrhage in hyperacute allograft rejection. Microphotography shows severe capillary injury with subsequent peritubular capillary disruption. Hematoxylin & eosin 10×. Courtesy of Dr. Claudia Mendoza-Cerpa. Laboratory of Pathology, IMSS-CMNO, Guadalajara; México.

antibodies directed primarily at the vasculature of the donor organ [72]. These antibodies activate the complement cascade and induce neutrophil infiltration, endothelial damage, interstitial hemorrhage (**Figure 3**), edema, fibrin deposition, platelet aggregation, and thrombosis; causing the organ to fail within a few hours after transplantation. Hyperacute rejection used to be a frequent occurrence in transplantation before cross-match tests were designed to screen potential recipients for circulating anti-HLA antibodies to the prospective donor [73].

Antibody-mediated rejection (ABMR) pathogenesis involves mechanisms of graft injury caused by donor-specific anti-HLA antibodies (DSAs) and non-HLA antibodies; and has been associated with progressive decline in graft function and poor transplantation outcomes [74]. Molecular changes in the microvasculature characteristic of tissue remodeling and repair are common manifestations of ABMR, as well as neutrophilic infiltration and fibrosis (**Figure 4**) [50]. ABMR can be acute or chronic, and can also manifest in cases of mixed TCMR/AMBR rejection [2]. It is estimated that close to 20% of renal allograft recipients will develop *de novo* DSAs within 10 years posttransplant [75]. DSAs bind to allogenic HLA and non-HLA targets

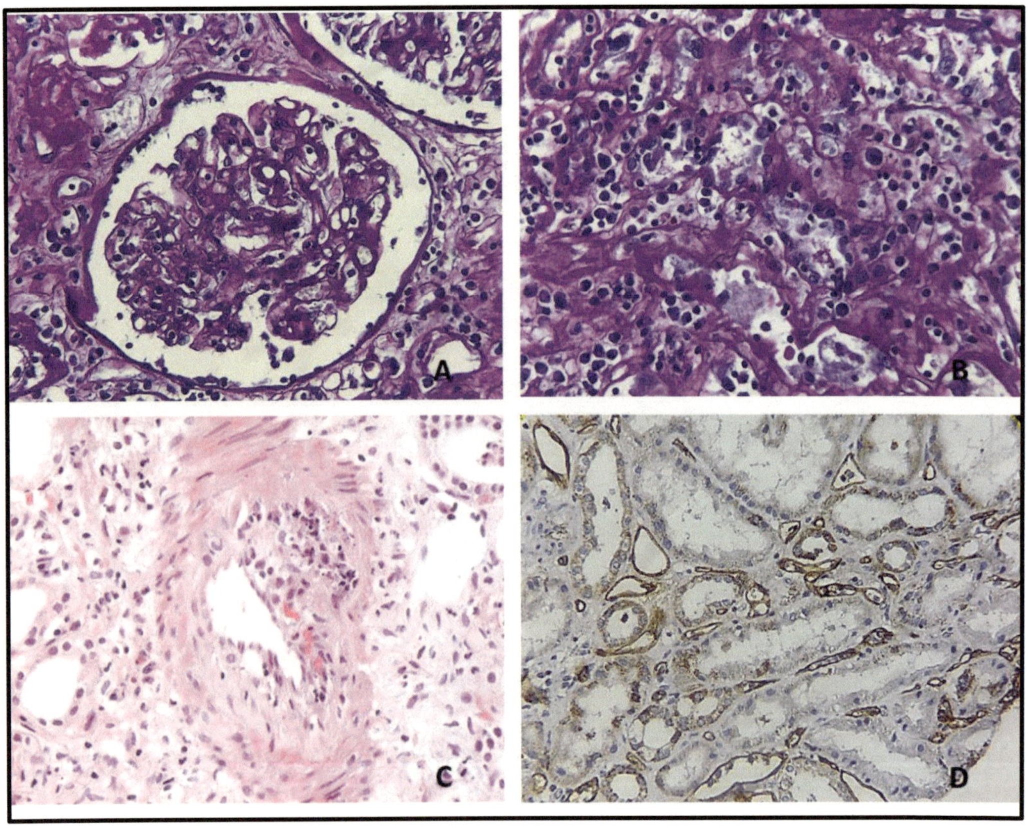

Figure 4. Antibody-mediated rejection. Two of the three criteria required for AMR. (A to C) Microvascular inflammation: glomerulitis, peritubular capilaritis, and intimal arteritis. PAS and H&E 40×. (D) Linear staining of C4d in peritubular capillaries IP 40×. Courtesy of Dr. Claudia Mendoza-Cerpa, Laboratory of Pathology, IMSS-CMNO, Guadalajara; México.

expressed by graft microvasculature and induce antibody-dependent cell cytotoxicity, complement activation and modulation of signaling pathways within vascular cells. These events promote the development of irreversible lesions that compromise graft function that eventually lead to rejection [76].

Complement activation is a well-established mechanism of ABMR [22, 77–79]. Although in some models, a causal relationship between antibody-mediated complement activation and graft damage has not been demonstrated [80]. DSAs bind to their targets on donor endothelial cells where they cause complement activation, and membrane attack complex formation. Interestingly, DSAs also activate an endothelial proinflammatory gene program to support allograft injury through noncanonical NF-κB signaling [81]. The graft microvasculature limits antibody injury by inducing the expression of the complement inhibitors CD55 and CD59 [82]. IgG subclasses exhibit variability in their hinge region that controls Fc region affinity for FcγRs and complement components [83]. Transcriptomic studies of ABMR biopsies have revealed an enrichment of endothelial, NK cells and IFN-γ-inducible transcripts. NK cells secrete IFN-γ upon FcγR crosslinking, a positive feedback mechanism that enhances HLA expression on endothelial cells and results in more DSA deposition and activation of local immunity [82].

6. Future directions

Improving kidney transplantation outcomes and patient survival is a challenging task. It is now clear that the cooperation between the innate and humoral arms of the immune system plays complex roles in graft tolerance and rejection. For this reason, understanding the immune mechanisms responsible for graft rejection in allotransplantation has becomes essential in our quest to develop better diagnostic tools and immunosuppressant therapies that can successfully be translated into the clinic.

Acknowledgements

This work was supported by the National Council of Science and Technology of Mexico (CONACYT project number 653).

Author details

Zesergio Melo[1,2]*, Juan A. Ruiz-Pacheco[1], Claudia A. Mendoza-Cerpa[2] and Raquel Echavarria[1]

*Address all correspondence to: zesergiomelo@gmail.com

1 CONACyT-Centro de Investigacion Biomedica de Occidente, IMSS-Guadalajara, Mexico

2 Laboratory of Pathology, IMSS-CMNO, Guadalajara, Mexico

References

[1] Levey AS, Coresh J. Chronic kidney disease. Lancet. 2012;**379**(9811):165-180

[2] Djamali A, Kaufman DB, Ellis TM, Zhong W, Matas A, Samaniego M. Diagnosis and management of antibody-mediated rejection: Current status and novel approaches. American Journal of Transplantation. 2014;**14**(2):255-271

[3] Gaber LW, Knight RJ, Patel SJ. A surgeons' guide to renal transplant immunopathology, immunology, and immunosuppression. Surgical Clinics of North America. 2013; **93**(6):1293-1307

[4] Cucchiari D, Podestà MA, Ponticelli C. The critical role of innate immunity in kidney transplantation. Nephron. 2016;**132**(3):227-237

[5] Salvadori M, Rosso G, Bertoni E. Update on ischemia-reperfusion injury in kidney transplantation: Pathogenesis and treatment. World Journal of Transplantation. 2015;**5**(2):52-67

[6] Erdem E. Neutrophil lymphocyte ratio in aute renal failure. Indian Journal of Nephrology. 2015;**25**(2):126-127

[7] Kelly KJ, Williams WW, Colvin RB, Meehan SM, Springer TA, Gutierrez-Ramos JC, et al. Intercellular adhesion molecule-1-deficient mice are protected against ischemic renal injury. Journal of Clinical Investigation. 1996;**97**(4):1056-1063

[8] Takada M, Nadeau KC, Shaw GD, Marquette KA, Tilney NL. The cytokine-adhesion molecule cascade in ischemia/reperfusion injury of the rat kidney. Inhibition by a soluble P-selectin ligand. Journal of Clinical Investigation. 1997;**99**(11):2682-2690

[9] Li L, Huang L, Sung SS, Vergis AL, Rosin DL, Rose CE, et al. The chemokine receptors CCR2 and CX3CR1 mediate monocyte/macrophage trafficking in kidney ischemia-reperfusion injury. Kidney International. 2008;**74**(12):1526-1537

[10] Zhang ZX, Wang S, Huang X, Min WP, Sun H, Liu W, et al. NK cells induce apoptosis in tubular epithelial cells and contribute to renal ischemia-reperfusion injury. Journal of Immunology. 2008;**181**(11):7489-7498

[11] Zhang ZX, Huang X, Jiang J, Lau A, Yin Z, Liu W, et al. Natural killer cells mediate long-term kidney allograft injury. Transplantation. 2015;**99**(5):916-924

[12] Ljunggren HG, Kärre K. In search of the 'missing self': MHC molecules and NK cell recognition. Immunology Today. 1990;**11**(7):237-244

[13] Moretta A, Pende D, Locatelli F, Moretta L. Activating and inhibitory killer immunoglobulin-like receptors (KIR) in haploidentical haemopoietic stem cell transplantation to cure high-risk leukaemias. Clinical and Experimental Immunology. 2009;**157**(3):325-331

[14] Matzinger P. Tolerance, danger, and the extended family. Annual Review of Immunology. 1994;**12**:991-1045

[15] Medzhitov R, Janeway CA. Decoding the patterns of self and nonself by the innate immune system. Science. 2002;**296**(5566):298-300

[16] Wu H, Chen G, Wyburn KR, Yin J, Bertolino P, Eris JM, et al. TLR4 activation mediates kidney ischemia/reperfusion injury. Journal of Clinical Investigation. 2007;**117**(10):2847-2859

[17] González-Guerrero C, Cannata-Ortiz P, Guerri C, Egido J, Ortiz A, Ramos AM. TLR4-mediated inflammation is a key pathogenic event leading to kidney damage and fibrosis in cyclosporine nephrotoxicity. Archives of Toxicology. 2017;**91**(4):1925-1939

[18] Wu H, Ma J, Wang P, Corpuz TM, Panchapakesan U, Wyburn KR, et al. HMGB1 contributes to kidney ischemia reperfusion injury. Journal of the American Society of Nephrology. 2010;**21**(11):1878-1890

[19] Wang C, Liu XX, Huang KB, Yin SB, Wei JJ, Hu YF, et al. Preconditioning with recombinant high-mobility group box 1 induces ischemic tolerance in a rat model of focal cerebral ischemia-reperfusion. Journal of Neurochemistry. 2016;**137**(4):576-588

[20] Frémeaux-Bacchi V, Legendre CM. The emerging role of complement inhibitors in transplantation. Kidney International. 2015;**88**(5):967-973

[21] Sacks SH, Zhou W. The role of complement in the early immune response to transplantation. Nature Reviews. Immunology. 2012;**12**(6):431-442

[22] Stegall MD, Chedid MF, Cornell LD. The role of complement in antibody-mediated rejection in kidney transplantation. Nature Reviews. Nephrology. 2012;**8**(11):670-678

[23] Chung BH, Kim KW, Kim BM, Doh KC, Cho ML, Yang CW. Increase of Th17 cell phenotype in kidney transplant recipients with chronic allograft dysfunction. PLoS One. 2015;**10**(12):e0145258

[24] Colvin RB, Dvorak HF. Letter: Basophils and mast cells in renal allograft rejection. Lancet. 1974;**1**(7850):212-224

[25] Stone KD, Prussin C, Metcalfe DD. IgE, mast cells, basophils, and eosinophils. The Journal of Allergy and Clinical Immunology. 2010;**125**(2 Suppl 2):S73-S80

[26] Weir MR, Hall-Craggs M, Shen SY, Posner JN, Alongi SV, Dagher FJ, et al. The prognostic value of the eosinophil in acute renal allograft rejection. Transplantation. 1986; **41**(6):709-712

[27] Game DS, Lechler RI. Pathways of allorecognition: Implications for transplantation tolerance. Transplant Immunology. 2002;**10**(2-3):101-108

[28] Vella JP, Vos L, Carpenter CB, Sayegh MH. Role of indirect allorecognition in experimental late acute rejection. Transplantation. 1997;**64**(12):1823-1828

[29] Coelho V, Saitovitch D, Kalil J, Silva HM. Rethinking the multiple roles of B cells in organ transplantation. Current Opinion in Organ Transplantation. 2013;**18**(1):13-21

[30] Auchincloss H Jr. In search of the elusive Holy Grail: The mechanisms and prospects for achieving clinical transplantation tolerance. American Journal of Transplantation. 2001;**1**(1):6-12

[31] Alpdogan O, van den Brink MR. Immune tolerance and transplantation. Seminars in Oncology 2012;**39**(6):629-642

[32] Manilay JO, Pearson DA, Sergio JJ, Swenson KG, Sykes M. Intrathymic deletion of alloreactive T cells in mixed bone marrow chimeras prepared with a nonmyeloablative conditioning regimen. Transplantation. 1998;**66**(1):96-102

[33] Fehr T, Sykes M. Tolerance induction in clinical transplantation. Transplant Immunology. 2004;**13**(2):117-130

[34] Lechler RI, Garden OA, Turka LA. The complementary roles of deletion and regulation in transplantation tolerance. Nature Reviews. Immunology. 2003;**3**(2):147-158

[35] Scandling JD, Busque S, Dejbakhsh-Jones S, Benike C, Millan MT, Shizuru JA, et al. Tolerance and chimerism after renal and hematopoietic-cell transplantation. The New England Journal of Medicine. 2008;**358**(4):362-368

[36] Kawai T, Sachs DH, Sprangers B, Spitzer TR, Saidman SL, Zorn E, et al. Long-term results in recipients of combined HLA-mismatched kidney and bone marrow transplantation without maintenance immunosuppression. American Journal of Transplantation. 2014;**14**(7):1599-1611

[37] Hardinger KL, Brennan DC, Klein CL. Selection of induction therapy in kidney transplantation. Transplant International: Official Journal of the European Society for Organ Transplantation. 2013;**26**(7):662-672

[38] Nashan B, Moore R, Amlot P, Schmidt AG, Abeywickrama K, Soulillou JP. Randomised trial of basiliximab versus placebo for control of acute cellular rejection in renal allograft recipients. CHIB 201 International Study Group. Lancet. 1997;**350**(9086):1193-1198

[39] Charpentier B, Rostaing L, Berthoux F, Lang P, Civati G, Touraine JL, et al. A three-arm study comparing immediate tacrolimus therapy with antithymocyte globulin induction therapy followed by tacrolimus or cyclosporine A in adult renal transplant recipients. Transplantation. 2003;**75**(6):844-851

[40] Flechner SM. Reviewing the evidence for de novo immunosuppression with sirolimus. Transplantation Proceedings. 2008;**40**(10 Suppl):S25-S28

[41] Verghese PS, Dunn TB, Chinnakotla S, Gillingham KJ, Matas AJ, Mauer MS. Calcineurin inhibitors in HLA-identical living related donor kidney transplantation. Nephrology, Dialysis, Transplantation. 2014;**29**(1):209-218

[42] Masson P, Henderson L, Chapman JR, Craig JC, Webster AC. Belatacept for kidney transplant recipients. The Cochrane Database of Systematic Reviews. 2014;(11):CD010699

[43] Prashar R, Venkat KK. Immunosuppression minimization and avoidance protocols: When less is not more. Advances in Chronic Kidney Disease. 2016;**23**(5):295-300

[44] Miller LW. Cardiovascular toxicities of immunosuppressive agents. American Journal of Transplantation. 2002;**2**(9):807-818

[45] Scantlebury V, Shapiro R, Fung J, Tzakis A, McCauley J, Jordan M, et al. New onset of diabetes in FK 506 vs cyclosporine-treated kidney transplant recipients. Transplantation Proceedings. 1991;**23**(6):3169-3170

[46] Ponticelli C. Calcineurin-inhibitors in renal transplantation. Too precious to be abandoned. Nephrology, Dialysis, Transplantation. 2000;**15**(9):1307-1309

[47] Halloran PF, Chang J, Famulski K, Hidalgo LG, Salazar ID, Merino Lopez M, et al. Disappearance of T cell-mediated rejection despite continued antibody-mediated rejection in late kidney transplant recipients. Journal of the American Society of Nephrology. 2015;**26**(7):1711-1720

[48] Halloran PF. T cell-mediated rejection of kidney transplants: A personal viewpoint. American Journal of Transplantation. 2010;**10**(5):1126-1134

[49] Einecke G, Broderick G, Sis B, Halloran PF. Early loss of renal transcripts in kidney allografts: Relationship to the development of histologic lesions and alloimmune effector mechanisms. American Journal of Transplantation. 2007;**7**(5):1121-1130

[50] Halloran PF, Famulski KS, Reeve J. Molecular assessment of disease states in kidney transplant biopsy samples. Nature Reviews. Nephrology. 2016;**12**(9):534-548

[51] Venner JM, Famulski KS, Badr D, Hidalgo LG, Chang J, Halloran PF. Molecular landscape of T cell-mediated rejection in human kidney transplants: Prominence of CTLA4 and PD ligands. American Journal of Transplantation. 2014;**14**(11):2565-2576

[52] Sharma VK, Bologa RM, Li B, GP X, Lagman M, Hiscock W, et al. Molecular executors of cell death--differential intrarenal expression of Fas ligand, Fas, granzyme B, and perforin during acute and/or chronic rejection of human renal allografts. Transplantation. 1996;**62**(12):1860-1866

[53] Walch JM, Zeng Q, Li Q, Oberbarnscheidt MH, Hoffman RA, Williams AL, et al. Cognate antigen directs CD8+ T cell migration to vascularized transplants. Journal of Clinical Investigation. 2013;**123**(6):2663-2671

[54] Adams AB, Williams MA, Jones TR, Shirasugi N, Durham MM, Kaech SM, et al. Heterologous immunity provides a potent barrier to transplantation tolerance. Journal of Clinical Investigation. 2003;**111**(12):1887-1895

[55] Chalasani G, Dai Z, Konieczny BT, Baddoura FK, Lakkis FG. Recall and propagation of allospecific memory T cells independent of secondary lymphoid organs. Proceedings of the National Academy of Sciences of the United States of America. 2002;**99**(9):6175-6180

[56] Glimcher LH, Townsend MJ, Sullivan BM, Lord GM. Recent developments in the transcriptional regulation of cytolytic effector cells. Nature Reviews. Immunology. 2004;**4**(11):900-911

[57] Lipson EJ, Bagnasco SM, Moore J, Jang S, Patel MJ, Zachary AA, et al. Tumor regression and allograft rejection after administration of anti-PD-1. The New England Journal of Medicine. 2016;**374**(9):896-898

[58] Brändle D, Joergensen J, Zenke G, Bürki K, Hof RP. Contribution of donor-specific antibodies to acute allograft rejection: Evidence from B cell-deficient mice. Transplantation. 1998;**65**(11):1489-1493

[59] Epstein MM, Di Rosa F, Jankovic D, Sher A, Matzinger P. Successful T cell priming in B cell-deficient mice. Journal of Experimental Medicine. 1995;**182**(4):915-922

[60] Sarwal M, Chua MS, Kambham N, Hsieh SC, Satterwhite T, Masek M, et al. Molecular heterogeneity in acute renal allograft rejection identified by DNA microarray profiling. The New England Journal of Medicine. 2003;**349**(2):125-138

[61] Hippen BE, DeMattos A, Cook WJ, Kew CE, Gaston RS. Association of CD20+ infiltrates with poorer clinical outcomes in acute cellular rejection of renal allografts. American Journal of Transplantation. 2005;**5**(9):2248-2252

[62] Tsai EW, Rianthavorn P, Gjertson DW, Wallace WD, Reed EF, Ettenger RB. CD20+ lymphocytes in renal allografts are associated with poor graft survival in pediatric patients. Transplantation. 2006;**82**(12):1769-1773

[63] Zarkhin V, Kambham N, Li L, Kwok S, Hsieh SC, Salvatierra O, et al. Characterization of intra-graft B cells during renal allograft rejection. Kidney International. 2008;**74**(5):664-673

[64] Bagnasco SM, Tsai W, Rahman MH, Kraus ES, Barisoni L, Vega R, et al. CD20-positive infiltrates in renal allograft biopsies with acute cellular rejection are not associated with worse graft survival. American Journal of Transplantation. 2007;**7**(8):1968-1973

[65] Kirk AD, Hale DA, Mannon RB, Kleiner DE, Hoffmann SC, Kampen RL, et al. Results from a human renal allograft tolerance trial evaluating the humanized CD52-specific monoclonal antibody alemtuzumab (CAMPATH-1H). Transplantation. 2003;**76**(1):120-129

[66] Cao Q, Harris DC, Wang Y. Macrophages in kidney injury, inflammation, and fibrosis. Physiology (Bethesda, Md.). 2015;**30**(3):183-194

[67] Lee S, Huen S, Nishio H, Nishio S, Lee HK, Choi BS, et al. Distinct macrophage phenotypes contribute to kidney injury and repair. Journal of the American Society of Nephrology. 2011;**22**(2):317-326

[68] Halloran PF, Afrouzian M, Ramassar V, Urmson J, Zhu LF, Helms LM, et al. Interferon-gamma acts directly on rejecting renal allografts to prevent graft necrosis. The American Journal of Pathology. 2001;**158**(1):215-226

[69] Halloran PF, Miller LW, Urmson J, Ramassar V, Zhu LF, Kneteman NM, et al. IFN-gamma alters the pathology of graft rejection: Protection from early necrosis. Journal of Immunology. 2001;**166**(12):7072-7081

[70] Afrouzian M, Ramassar V, Urmson J, Zhu LF, Halloran PF. Transcription factor IRF-1 in kidney transplants mediates resistance to graft necrosis during rejection. Journal of the American Society of Nephrology. 2002;**13**(5):1199-1209

[71] Terasaki PI. A personal perspective: 100-year history of the humoral theory of transplantation. Transplantation. 2012;**93**(8):751-756

[72] Kissmeyer-Nielsen F, Olsen S, Petersen VP, Fjeldborg O. Hyperacute rejection of kidney allografts, associated with pre-existing humoral antibodies against donor cells. Lancet. 1966;**2**(7465):662-665

[73] Patel R, Terasaki PI. Significance of the positive crossmatch test in kidney transplantation. The New England Journal of Medicine. 1969;**280**(14):735-739

[74] Loupy A, Viglietti D, Mengel M. Complement inhibition in HLA-incompatible kidney transplants: Persisting antibody-mediated injury despite marked decrease of clinical ABMR. The New England Journal of Medicine. 2015;**15**(5):1139-1140

[75] Everly MJ. Incidence and hazards of alloantibodies in renal transplantation. Clinical Transplants. 2013;313-317

[76] Butler CL, Valenzuela NM, Thomas KA, Reed EF. Not all antibodies are created equal: Factors that influence antibody mediated rejection. Journal of Immunology Research. 2017;**2017**:7903471

[77] Wang H, Arp J, Liu W, Faas SJ, Jiang J, Gies DR, et al. Inhibition of terminal complement components in presensitized transplant recipients prevents antibody-mediated rejection leading to long-term graft survival and accommodation. Journal of Immunology. 2007;**179**(7):4451-4463

[78] Valenzuela NM, McNamara JT, Reed EF. Antibody-mediated graft injury: Complement-dependent and complement-independent mechanisms. Current Opinion in Organ Transplantation. 2014;**19**(1):33-40

[79] Akiyoshi T, Hirohashi T, Alessandrini A, Chase CM, Farkash EA, Neal Smith R, et al. Role of complement and NK cells in antibody mediated rejection. Human Immunology. 2012;**73**(12):1226-1232

[80] Csencsits K, Burrell BE, Lu G, Eichwald EJ, Stahl GL, Bishop DK. The classical complement pathway in transplantation: Unanticipated protective effects of C1q and role in inductive antibody therapy. American Journal of Transplantation. 2008;**8**(8):1622-1630

[81] Jane-Wit D, Manes TD, Yi T, Qin L, Clark P, Kirkiles-Smith NC, et al. Alloantibody and complement promote T cell-mediated cardiac allograft vasculopathy through noncanonical nuclear factor-κB signaling in endothelial cells. Circulation. 2013;**128**(23):2504-2516

[82] Venner JM, Hidalgo LG, Famulski KS, Chang J, Halloran PF. The molecular landscape of antibody-mediated kidney transplant rejection: Evidence for NK involvement through CD16a Fc receptors. American Journal of Transplantation. 2015;**15**(5):1336-1348

[83] Valenzuela NM, Hickey MJ, Reed EF. Antibody subclass repertoire and graft outcome following solid organ transplantation. Frontiers in Immunology. 2016;7:433

Chapter 9

The Way from Renal Calcifications and Urinary Crystals to Kidney Stones: An Important Aspect in the Pathogenesis of Calcium Nephrolithiasis

Johannes M. Baumann

Additional information is available at the end of the chapter

http://dx.doi.org/10.5772/intechopen.70598

Abstract

The formation of calcium (Ca) stones occurs in an initial phase by fixed growth on kidney calcifications consisting either of intratubular crystal accumulations protruding in renal calices (Randall's plugs) or of interstitial hydroxyapatite deposits (Randall's plaques) broken through the covering epithelial layers. Crystal aggregation (AGN) seems to be responsible for stone growth during crystalluria. This chapter reports on new aspects of the AGN of calcium oxalate being the most frequent stone compound and tries to explain why despite the widespread occurrence of kidney calcifications and crystalluria not everybody forms stones. Urinary crystals normally are protected from AGN by coats of urinary macromolecules (UMs) which by their identical electronegative charge create zones of electrostatic repulsion. At high urinary concentration or ionic strength respectively, these zones are compressed and can be bridged by self-aggregated UMs. Self-AGN occurs in concentrated urine by the adsorption of UMs on free surfaces like Randall's plugs or plaques. High oxalate excretion and high urine concentration favoring intratubular crystal accumulation, breaking of epithelial layers on Randall's plaques and self-AGN of UMs are most deleterious factors in Ca stone formation and have to be avoided by stone metaphylaxis.

Keywords: calcium nephrolithiasis, crystalluria, Randall's plaques and plugs, urinary macromolecules, calcium oxalate aggregation

1. Introduction

The pathogenesis of kidney stones that often are accompanied by very painful colic and can lead to renal failure and even to the loss of a kidney is far from being clear. In Western populations, nephrolithiasis has reached a prevalence up to 10% [1]. Kidney stones are composed of crystal aggregates within an organic matrix. Long times stone formation mainly was ascribed to a pathological excretion of substances being involved in crystal formation. Fourier transform infrared spectroscopy being now commonplace for stone analysis shows that calcium oxalate (CaOx) is the most frequent stone compound. For calcium nephrolithiasis, the most frequent stone disease and the topic of this chapter, the important substances are calcium, oxalic and citric acid the latter being a calcium chelator [2]. However, not all stone formers show a pathological excretion of these compounds, and some anomalies also are found in urine of people without stone formation. Later on, stone research was focused on urinary macromolecules (UMs, mainly proteins and some glycosaminoglycans) being an integral part of the stone matrix and some of them promoting or inhibiting the crystallization of stone minerals [3]. In the meantime, more than 70 of such substances were isolated [4, 5], and 11 of them containing anionic residues like carboxyglutamic acid, phosphate and sialic acid are thought to be relevant for stone formation [6]. But anomalies with respect to excretion or composition of these UMs were exclusively found in some small groups of patients [7].

Modern urological endoscopy which allows the inspection of the whole renal cavity showed that calcium oxalate and phosphate stones comprising about 80% of all concretions [8] generally start by a fixed growth on papillary calcifications, which were already described as potential source of nephrolithiasis in 1937 by Randall [9]. Recently much work was done to elucidate the pathogenesis of these calcifications being present either as interstitial deposits of calcium phosphate (Randall's plaques) or as intratubular accumulation of calcium oxalate crystals (Randall's plugs) [10–12]. These calcifications when protruding into renal calyces can induce stone formation either by heterogeneous nucleation of new crystals or more probably by the aggregation (AGN) of crystals during crystalluria. The initial fixation on kidney calcifications allows stones to grow to a critical size where they cannot be washed out anymore by the urine flow and where they become symptomatic. However, the finding of kidney calcifications and crystalluria is much more frequent than stone disease [3], and Randall's plaques can persist during some decades without or with only minimal stone formation [13]. Therefore, the question raises whether special crystallization conditions in urine might be responsible for stone formation by the apposition of new crystals on Randall's plaques and plugs. This question stimulated us to an intensive study of the formation and especially the AGN of calcium oxalate crystals being with 60% the most frequent stone compound [8]. Experiments were directly performed in urine where like in other biological mediums, crystals as well as Randall's plaques and plugs always are coated by proteins [14]. Instead of the study of individual compounds thought to be involved in stone formation, the overall effect of UMs was compared to that one of urine and urinary ultrafiltrate. UMs were isolated either by a hemofiltration procedure or by temporary adsorption on Ca phosphate to which urinary proteins have a high affinity.

2. Measurement of calcium oxalate (CaOx) crystallization in urine

An approved test system which uses an increase of the rate of particle sedimentation as measure for crystal AGN was modified [15]. Contrary to current crystal production in standardized and protein-free solutions and with a long period of crystal ripening, CaOx was directly produced in urine by an oxalate titration [16]. Crystallization was followed monitoring optical density (OD) by a spectrophotometer. Typical crystallization curves are shown in **Figure 1A** and **C**. During a titration period of 15 min with the addition of 0.1 mM/min of sodium oxalate, a rapid increase of OD indicating crystal formation is observed. From the time lag of this increase, the critical oxalate addition to induce crystallization can be calculated and used as a measure for the metastability of urine with respect to CaOx crystallization. At the end of titration, maximal OD reflecting particle concentration in solutions [15] is determined, and magnetic stirring is stopped. Following the further course during at least 30 min, two different types of curves are observed. One type (**Figure 1A**) is characterized by a continuous slow OD decrease, which by scanning electron microscopy (SEM) of the sediment (**Figure 1B**) mainly can be attributed to the sedimentation of single crystals of CaOx monohydrate. From this low −mdOD/dt, the sedimentation rate of single crystals and an average particle size can be calculated [17]. The other type of curve is represented in **Figure 1C**. After an initial phase of slow OD decrease varying from 7 to 35 min and called suspensions stability, a rapid decline of OD is observed which by SEM of the sediment (**Figure 1D**) can be attributed to crystal AGN. Since OD mainly reflects particle concentration, the rapid OD decrease can be explained by an increased particle clearing in the observation field of the spectrophotometer. This high clearing bases on the one hand on an accelerated sedimentation of crystal aggregates (the sedimentation rate increases with particle diameter in square) and on the other hand on the diminution of particle concentration by the integration of a lot of single crystals into few large aggregates. Interestingly, the rapid

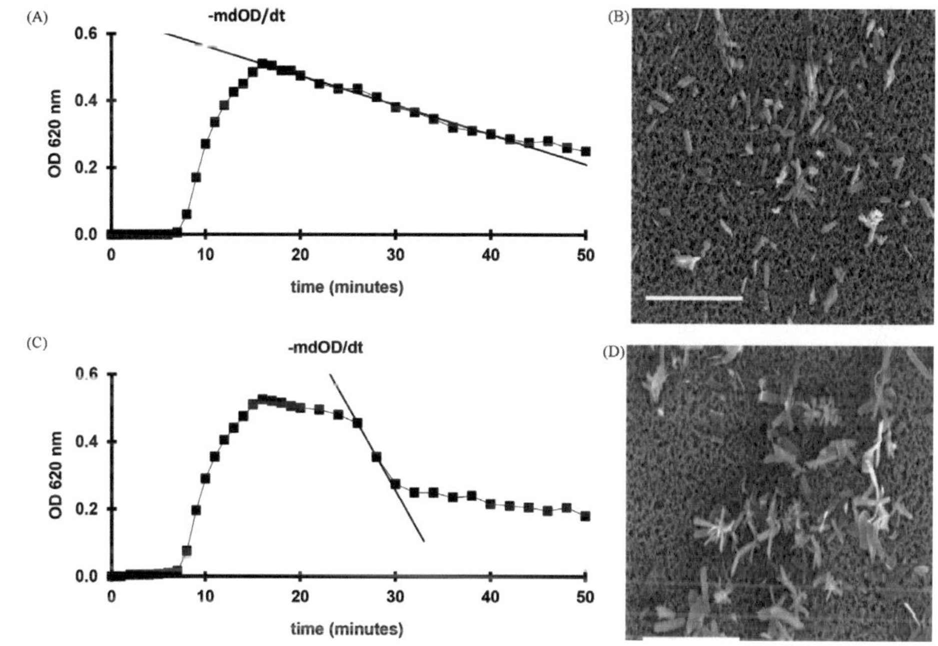

Figure 1. Crystallization curves (CC) of urine and scanning electron microscopy (SEM) of sediments: (A) urine with inhibition of CaOx AGN in CC (low maximal rate of OD decrease, −mdOD/dt) and (B) mainly with single crystals of CaOx monohydrate and only a few small aggregates in SEM, (C) urine with intensive AGN (high −mdOD/dt) in CC, and (D) large aggregates predominating in SEM. Bars on SEM indicating 20 μm.

OD decrease reflecting AGN stops after on average 30% of OD has disappeared by AGN [16]. Therefore, AGN in crystal suspensions seems to be limited to a critical OD or particle concentration. The maximal OD decrease observed in our experiments is expressed as maximal OD change per minute (−mdOD/dt).

UM solutions and urinary ultrafiltrate (UF) were obtained using a hemofilter the excluding limit of the dialysis membrane being 5 kDa [18]. To gain UF urine was placed on one side of the membrane and the filtrate collected on the other side. UMs were isolated by dialyzing urine against bi distilled water. This procedure showed a volume recovery of 96% and thus allowed the isolation of UMs in their almost original concentration. UM solutions also were prepared by Ca phosphate precipitation in urine, which was induced by the addition of sodium hydrogen phosphate at pH 7.0 [19]. After centrifugation and discharge of the supernatant, the precipitate was dissolved in distilled water buffered to pH 5.0 and with a volume corresponding to the urine volume used for precipitation. To obtain comparable results experiments in urine, ultrafiltrate and UM solutions were performed at identical pH, Na, and Ca concentration.

3. Crystallization conditions of CaOx in urine and within the kidney

CaOx crystallization in urine is a complex process. It occurs when the product of ion activities of Ca and oxalic acid ($Ca_a \times Ox_a$) exceeds a critical value called formation product (FP). In filtered urine, this FP was found to be very high. It exceeded about 14 times the product of ion activities ($Ca_e \times Ox_e$) observed in urine after equilibration with CaOx crystals in excess, the ratio $Ca_a \times Ox_a/Ca_e \times Ox_e$ being a measure for the state of saturation [2]. Ion activities and thus crystallization tendency of calcium and oxalic acid are reduced by the formation of highly soluble complexes of Ca with citric acid and of Ox with magnesium. These complexes reduce the concentrations of Ca and Ox being disposable for crystallization. The influence of stone forming substances, chelators, and pH on the state of urinary saturation with respect to CaOx can be calculated by special computer programs [20] or experimentally be tested [21]. Equilibration experiments performed with CaOx crystals in 76 urines from recurrent calcium stone formers demonstrated that supersaturation with respect to CaOx was only significantly ($p < 0.001$) correlated with urinary Ox concentration. The same experiments performed with brushite on the other hand showed that Ca phosphate saturation mainly is governed by Ca concentration and pH. Also clinical observations demonstrated that hyperoxaluria generally is much more important for the genesis of CaOx stones than hypercalciuria [22]. In 60 urines, an average addition of 0.64 mM Ox without a significant difference between stone patients and controls was necessary to induce CaOx crystallization [16]. Such high urinary Ox concentrations are apart from rare cases of primary hyperoxaluria exclusively observed after excessive Ox ingestion [23]. Nevertheless, crystalluria is a frequent finding. Crystals are found in 9–48% urines of stone patients and in 2–26% of healthy controls [24]. The discrepancy between clinical and experimental observations can be explained by heterogeneous crystal nucleation where preformed surfaces of Ca phosphate crystals, damaged renal tubular cells, and cellular debris in urine [3] allow the formation of CaOx far below the high FP necessary for spontaneous nucleation. Cellular debris comprises about 50% of urinary deposits [25].

For stone formation, crystals have to be retained in the kidney. This seems for single crystals hardly to be possible. In the nephron, Ox normally reaches a sufficient concentration for CaOx crystallization at the end of collecting ducts (CD), but at extremely high Ox concentrations, crystallization already can occur in the descending loop of Henle (DLH) [26]. Both situations are schematically indicated in **Figure 2**. Even at the high Ox concentrations necessary to induce crystal formation in DLH crystallization is a relative slow process compared to urinary transit time (UT) through the nephron. Following CaOx crystallization in urine by repeated measurement of the ionic Ca decay by a ion selective electrode shows that even after an extreme Ox addition of 1 mM crystallization reaches during an average transit time through the nephron of 3 min only about half of its final value (**Figure 3**). The figure demonstrates that the study of crystals in urine which previously has remained several times in the bladder hardly can be representative for the situation in the kidney. For the end of the nephron when crystals have passed inner tubular diameters of minimal 15–60 μm, maximal crystal diameters of 4 μm were calculated [27]. The discrepancy of crystals size and tubular dimensions is even more pronounced when crystallization starts at the end of collecting ducts where crystals only can grow during a few seconds until they reach the renal papilla (**Figure 2**). Therefore, for the formation of obstructing plugs, crystals have to aggregate as demonstrated

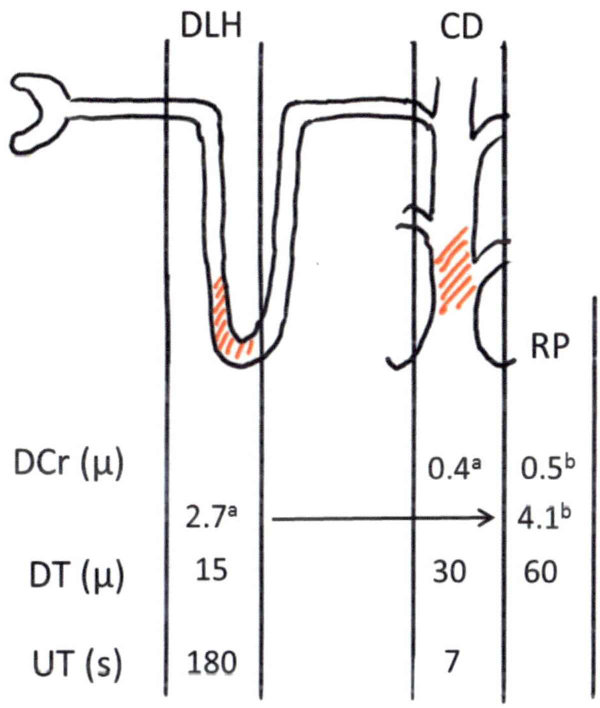

Figure 2. Localization of CaOx crystallization in the nephron (hatched areas): descending loop of Henle (DLH), collecting duct (CD), renal papilla (RP), maximal crystal diameter (DCr) expected at nucleation site ([a]), at RP ([b]), minimal inner tubular diameter (DT), urinary transit time (UT) to RP.

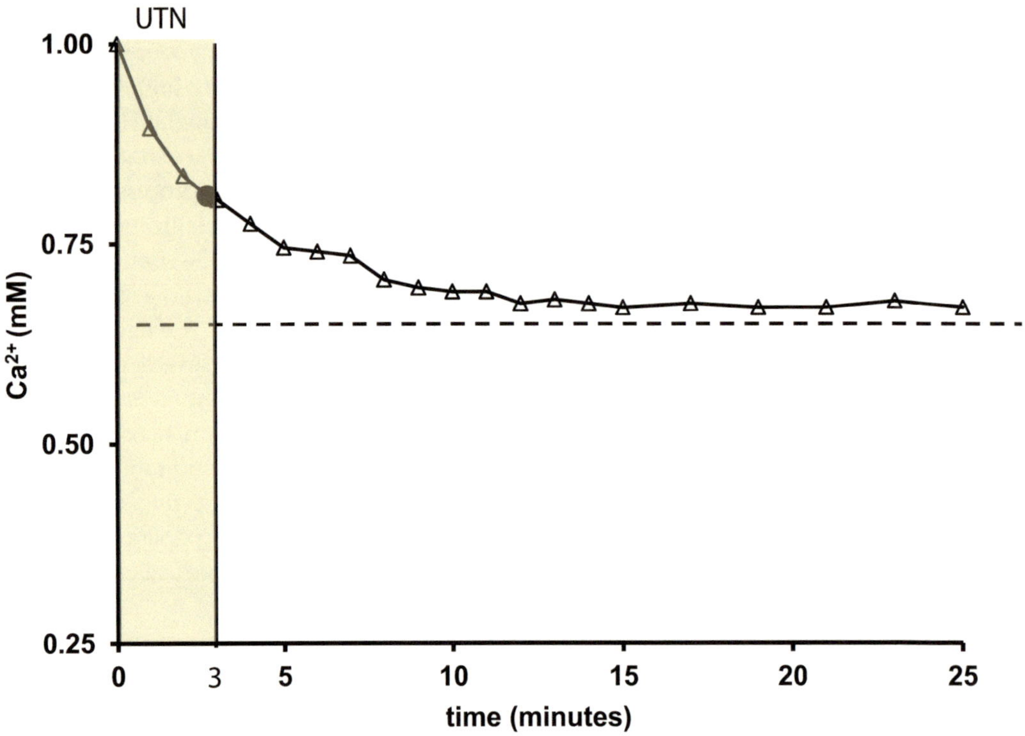

Figure 3. Ionic Ca (Ca^{2+}) decay after addition of 1 mM Ox to urine: half time (•) and endpoint of crystallization (dashed line), average urinary transit time through the nephron (UTN).

by the finding of large crystal aggregates on micro photographs of Randall's plugs [10]. AGN also seems to be responsible for the acquisition of CaOx on Randall's plaques and generally for the growth of calcium stones [28].

4. Crystal aggregation (AGN) in urine and within the kidney

Already in 1969, crystal AGN was found to be an important element in stone formation. In a study of six patients with short-term stone recurrence and six healthy controls, patients showed contrary to the controls 3 h after Ox ingestion large CaOx aggregates with diameters up to 200 μm in their urine [29]. However, in our crystallization test, AGN could also be produced by high Ox addition in 11 urines of 30 healthy people but less frequent than in urine of unselected stone patients (20/30, $p < 0.05$) [16]. Interestingly, this AGN started with a delay of 15–35 min being not only beyond the average urinary transit time (UT) of 3 min in the nephron but also beyond an average UT in the renal pelvis of 12 min [30]. Crystal AGN seems thus to depend on urinary Ox or crystal concentration respectively and on an induction time also called suspensions stability.

For AGN, particles have to collide. Under physiological conditions (without stirring or shaking), this collision occurs by particle sedimentation or Brownian motion (diffusion). At maximal crystal concentrations of 24,000 crystals/ml being observed during crystalluria [27], only 2.5×10^{-5} collisions per minute can be expected by diffusion within the short UT through the nephron [17]. Sedimentation on the other hand can accumulate under these conditions on a tubular wall being in horizontal position 1.3 crystals/min and on kidney calcifications or stone surfaces 624 crystals/cm^2 and minute. These accumulation rates are positively correlated with particle diameter in square and particle concentration whereas collision rates increase by particle concentration in square [17]. To get some insight in AGN processes within an appropriate observation time, studies have to be performed in highly concentrated crystal suspensions where AGN mainly occurs on the basis of diffusion. For the measurement of CaOx AGN in urine, Ox additions of 1.5 mM were necessary. Even under these extreme conditions, urine showed a high inhibitory activity with respect to CaOx AGN. AGN only was observed in 31 of 60 urines and always with some delay [16].

Inhibition of AGN can be ascribed to an electrical surface potential which allows identically charged particles only to near to critical distance where diffusion or sedimentation is compensated by electrostatic repulsion [31]. Also lower surface potentials act as intermediate barrier, which slows down AGN by the fact that numerous attempts are necessary to overcome electrostatic repulsion. This may explain the delay of AGN which was always observed in urine. In urine, crystals are coated by urinary macromolecules (UMs) which provide by their anionic residues an electronegative surface potential in the order of −15 mV [18]. Scanning electron microscopic pictures of CaOx crystals being incubated in albumin or globulin solutions showed protein coats on the crystals with diameters of 10–20 nm [14]. UM coats can be composed as mentioned in the Introduction by more than 70 different proteins [5]. Confronted with such multiple substances often with an unknown influence on crystallization processes, we decided to center our studies on whole urine, on UM solutions which were directly isolated from urine and on albumin being a frequent compound of urinary crystals and stones [3].

Although the adsorption of proteins like prothrombin fragment 1 and albumin was ascribed to a face-specific interaction between Ca in the lattice of CaOx crystals and selected anionic groups in the proteins [32], the coating of surfaces by UMs can also be a rather unspecific process. As **Figure 4** shows, not only crystals but also latex beads can be easily coated by UMs. This coating bases on a hydrophobic effect between proteins and latex. By Zetasizer analysis, latex beads showed after the incubation in UM solutions, an increase of particle diameters by 40 μm corresponding to an UM coat of 20 μm. A pH change in the UM solution from 6.0 to 5.0 diminished the negative surface potentials of the coated beads from −34 to −24 mV and produced a massive increase of particle diameters or AGN, respectively. This pH effect which bases on a reduced ionization of the anionic protein residues by an increased H^+ concentration demonstrates that surface potentials are essential for the inhibition of AGN. Further experiments which were performed with latex beads in almost electrolyte and especially Ca-free albumin solutions showed that the AGN of UM-coated particles too can base on a hydrophobic effect [19].

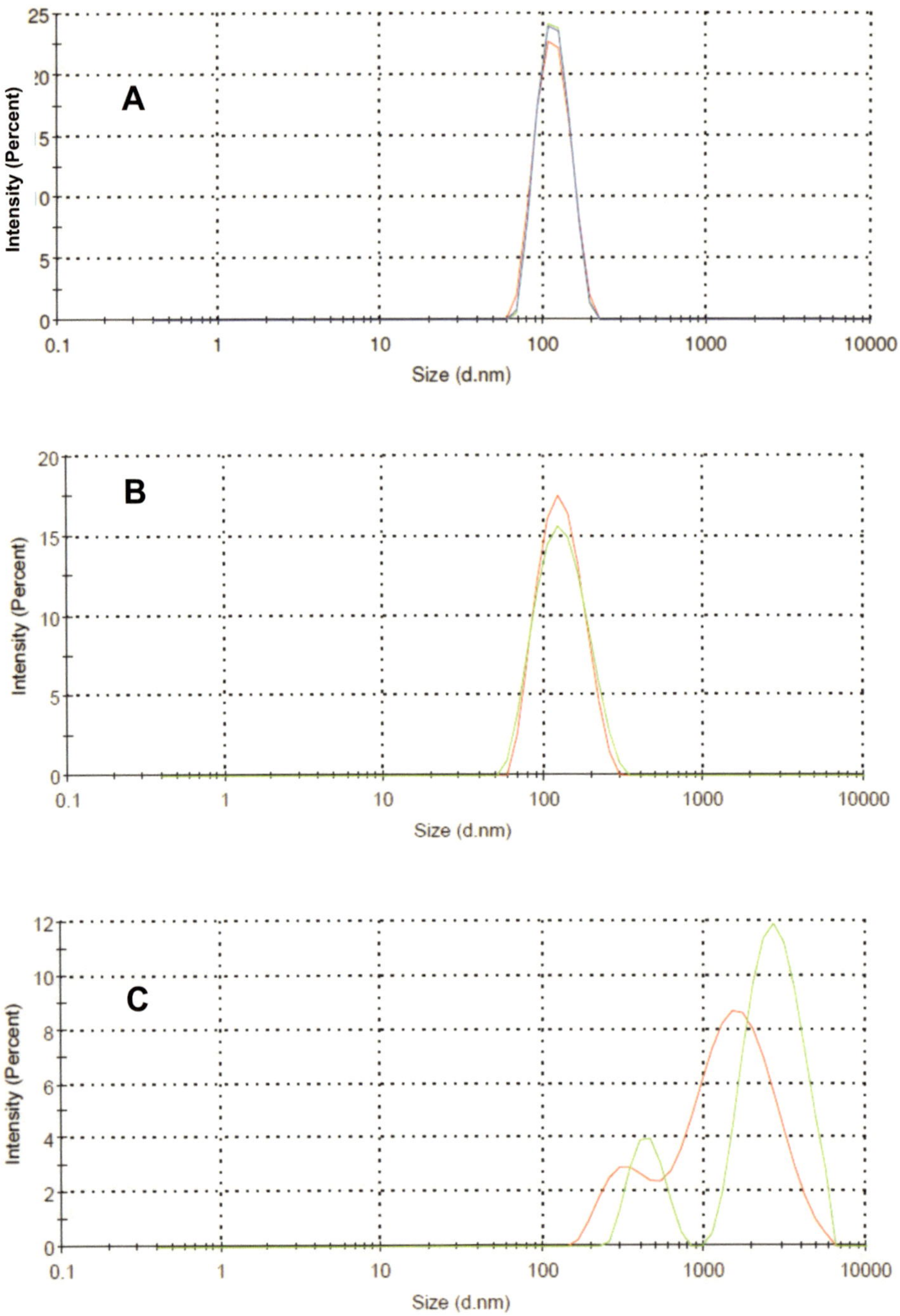

Figure 4. Affinity of urinary macromolecules (UMs) to latex beads (LBs) measured by particle size distribution (PSD) within a 2-min interval: (A) PSD of LBs before incubation in UM solution, (B) after incubation, (C) pH change from 6.0 to 5.0 in suspension of latex in UM solution showing from the left to the right curve a progressive increase of particle size due to AGN of the coated latex beads.

Pathological UMs with reduced anionic groups are found to be responsible for crystal AGN in urine [33–35] and were observed in urine of some stone patients [36–38]. However, also dialysis in a hemofilter abolishes the inhibitory activity of UMs [16]. All UM solutions obtained by dialysis from 29 urines with previously low maximal sedimentation rates showed a massive increase of −mdOD/dt indicating AGN (**Figure 5**). In order to find low molecular weight substances which might be responsible for the inhibition of AGN, crystallization tests were repeated in urinary ultrafiltrate (UF) with an identical result as obtained in the UM solution. Also a loss of important substances by the adsorption on the large surface of the hemofilter could be excluded by repeating crystallization tests in UM solutions where UMs were isolated only by temporary adsorption on Ca phosphate and consecutive dilution as described above. Further experiments performed with albumin brought an explanation for this peculiar loss of AGN inhibition after temporary contact with large surfaces. Albumin at high concentration has a tendency to self-AGN [39], which is demonstrated in **Figure 6A**. By the measurement of particle size distribution (PSD) immediately after the preparation of an albumin solution (AS) in a high urinary concentration of 20 mg/l, a main peak at 10 nm being typical for albumin and a lower second peak around 1000 nm were found. Two minutes later, the main peak was somewhat diminished and peaks around 350 and 4100 nm became visible indicating progressive self-AGN of albumin. However, in the CaOx crystallization test performed in AS, only a minimal acceleration of sedimentation was observed (**Figure 7A**). The diluted Ca phosphate precipitate of AS on the other hand showed in PSD that all extracted albumin was

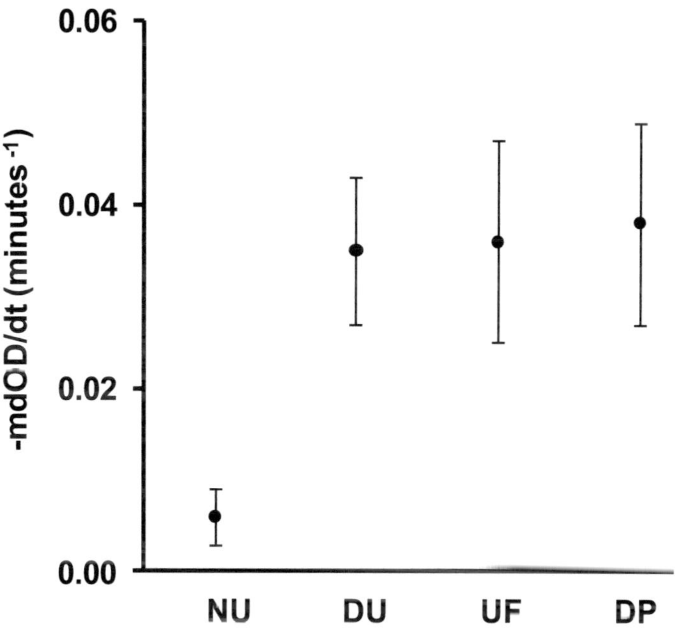

Figure 5. Effect of UM isolation on inhibition of CaOx AGN (low −mdOD/dt): native urine (NU), dialyzed urine (DU), ultrafiltrate (UF), and dissolved Ca phosphate precipitates of urine (DP) ($n = 29$, $x \pm SD$, NU vs. DU, UF and DP $p < 0.001$).

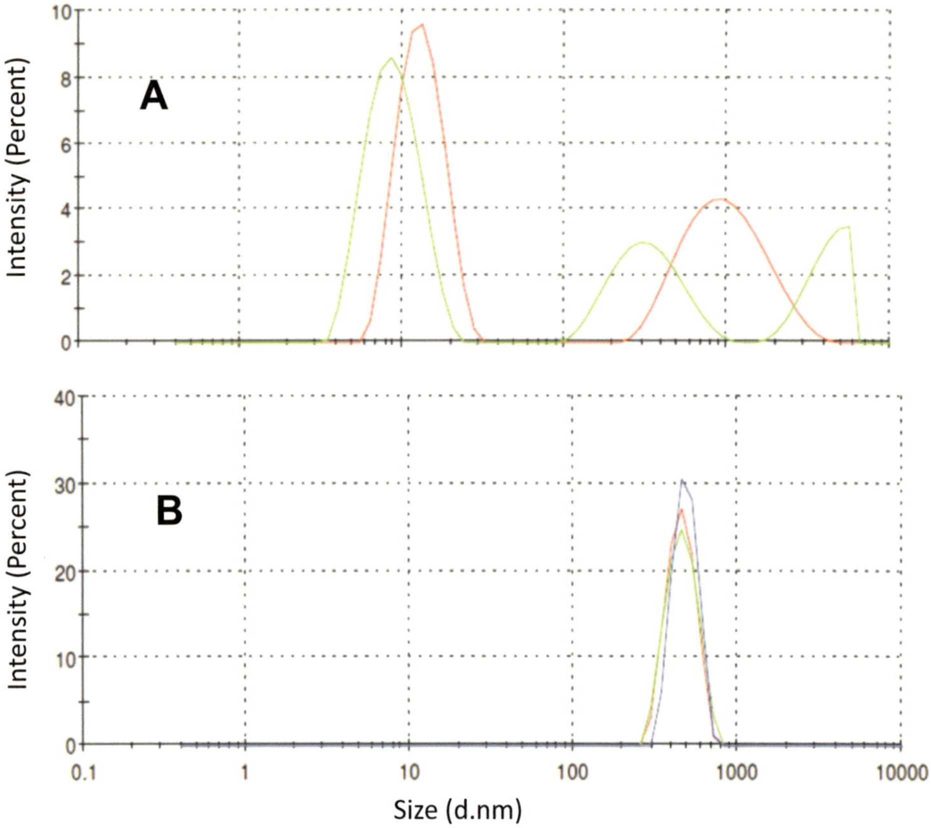

Figure 6. Particle size distribution (PSD) of albumin: (A) PSD in albumin solution in high urinary concentration (AS, 20mg/l) and (B) PSD in dissolved Ca phosphate precipitate of AS (DPA).

aggregated into a high single peak at 480 nm (**Figure 6B**) and in the crystallization test, a rapid OD decrease being characteristic for intensive crystal AGN was found (**Figure 7B**). These observations demonstrate that crystal AGN also occurs in the presence of normal but self-aggregated UMs. UM aggregates with increasing size like aggregated albumin obviously can bridge critical distances of electrostatic repulsion and connect crystals probably by hydrophobic binding to their UM coats. Scanning electron microscopy of Ca Ox crystals being incubated in gamma globulin solutions showed at crystal convergence of some aggregates large amounts of amorphous material suggesting a crystal binding by aggregated proteins [14].

The formation of Randall's plugs seems to be a product of crystal AGN. Randall's plugs are observed as origin of kidney stones at states of massive chronic supersaturation of urine either with respect to CaOx as found in primary hyperoxaluria or with respect to Ca phosphate in primary hyperparathyroidism [40]. Under these conditions, crystallization as mentioned

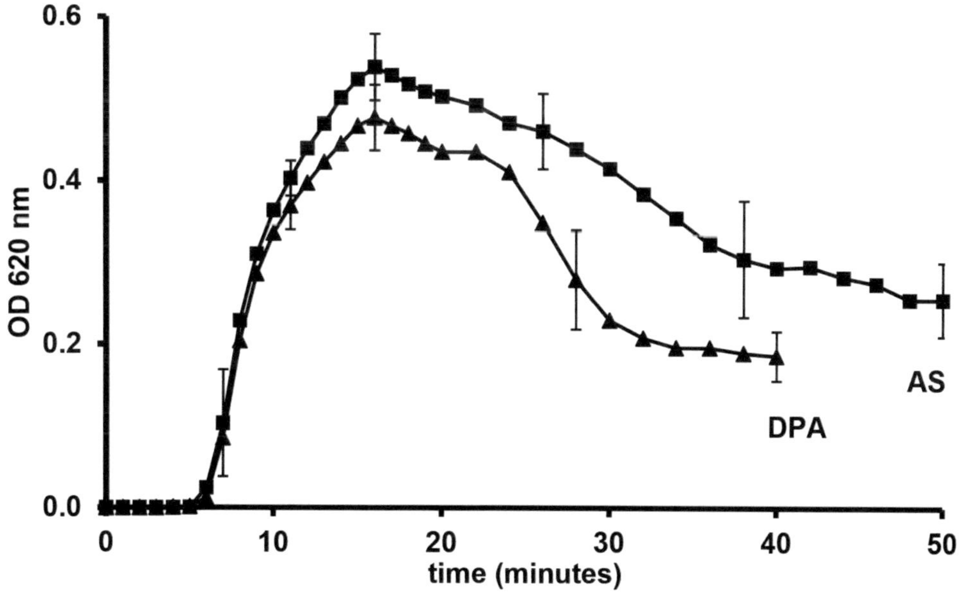

Figure 7. Crystallization curve of AS and DPA: AS shows with a relative low −mdOD/dt inhibition of CaOx AGN, and a high −mdDO/dt in DPA indicates massive AGN ($n = 5$, $x \pm$ SD, $p < 0.01$).

above already can start in DLH. During their way through the nephron, crystals can drop by sedimentation on tubular walls where they stick and together with following crystals can form large crystal accumulations. Such accumulations probably are an ideal platform for the adsorption and self-AGN of UMs. Massive crystalluria and even hyperoxaluria are known to damage tubular cells and thus to favor the sticking of crystals on tubular walls [41]. Damaged tubular cells produce pathological proteins which also favor this sticking and the AGN of the crystals [3]. Furthermore, basement membrane denuded by its epithelial layer can induce heterogeneous nucleation of CaOx [42]. These mechanisms can provoke massive crystal aggregates which protruding from ducts of Bellini into renal calices can raise stone formation in the kidney as observed by urological endoscopy [40].

5. CaOx AGN in the presence of hydroxyapatite (HAP), a possible model for stone formation on Randall's plaques (RPLs)

Idiopathic Ca nephrolithiasis where by definition no metabolic or endocrinologic disorders like primary hyperoxaluria or hyperparathyroidism are found is the most frequent stone disease and generally starts by stone growth on RPLs [10–12, 40]. RPLs are subepithelial deposits of Ca phosphate in the renal papilla which by disruption of the covering epithelial layer can come in contact with urine and give raise to stone growth. The Ca phosphate deposits, mainly HAP, are a consequence of the transformation of epithelial cells into an osteoplastic phenotype with an increased production of bone-specific proteins like osteopontin (OP) favoring tissue mineralization [12]. Histological analysis with immunohistochemistry or infrared spectroscopy of RPLs with an adherent stone showed that the RPLs consisted of an OP matrix with HAP deposits, whereas the adherent stone in addition to OP and HAP contained Tamm-Horsfall glycoprotein (THG) and CaOx crystals [40]. Stone formation on RPLs thus seems to occur at the interface of HAP and CaOx crystals being embedded in proteins like OP and THG which like albumin have a tendency to self-AGN [3]. The osteoplastic transformation of epithelial cells which mainly occurs in the loop of Henle was ascribed to vascular or metabolic disorders since in epidemiological studies, stone disease was found to be associated with hypertension, myocardial infarction, diabetes, or metabolic syndrome [12]. However, RPLs seem to be very frequent and not always associated with stone disease. High-resolution radiography of 50 consecutive sets of cadaveric kidneys showed in 57% radiographic evidence consistent with RPLs [43]. In an older study, in all kidneys of 100 randomly selected autopsies, some papillary calcifications were found but only in seven cases of kidney stones [44]. Urological endoscopy revealed RPLs even in 43% of cases not being related to stone disease [45]. The mechanisms involved in the progression of a RPL to a kidney stone are far from being clear. One of these processes is breaking of epithelial layers, which brings the calcifications of RPLs in contact with pelvic urine [12]. A further unknown factor is the formation of CaOx crystals on the denuded and protein-coated HAP of RPLs. Therefore, we tried to mimic this formation by the study of CaOx crystallization in the presence UM-coated HAP (cHAP). Contrary to previous studies performed immediately after thawing of frozen urine, 15 freshly voided urines of five healthy men were examined.

To prepare cHAP, commercially available HAP crystals (0.05 mg/ml) were incubated at 37° during at least 30 min in one portion each of 15 urines from healthy persons [46]. After centrifugation and discharge of the supernatant, the crystals were suspended in a second portion of the same urine. Ca and pH were adapted to the standard values of 2 mM and 6.0, respectively, used in the tests. CaOx crystallization tests as described above were performed in urine with and without the cHAP suspension. By this procedure, a high −mdOD/dt indicating AGN was observed in 8 of 15 urines performed with cHAP, whereas in the test performed without cHAP, only one of the 15 urines showed a high −mdOD/dt. Interestingly, urines with and without cHAP-induced AGN significantly ($p < 0.01$) could be distinguished by their sodium concentration (**Figure 8**) being an indicator for urinary ionic strength [47]. A high ionic strength seems to favor AGN, whereas urine dilution abolished the cHAP-induced AGN. All urines with an initially high −mdOd/dt showed after dilution and adaption of Ca and pH to the initial values only a slow OD decrease being typical for the sedimentation of single crystals without AGN. Urinary dilution down to 33% did not disturb urinary inhibitory activity with respect to not cHAP-related CaOx AGN, which is in agreement with the finding that urine even diluted to 20% is still an excellent inhibitor of the AGN of CaOx crystals [48]. The promotion of AGN by a high ionic strength can be explained by its influence on the extension on electrostatic surface potentials (ESPs). In electrolyte-containing solutions, ESP exponentially decreases with increasing distance from negatively charged particles by a cation accumulation (in our experiment of sodium) [31]. In concentrated urine with a high

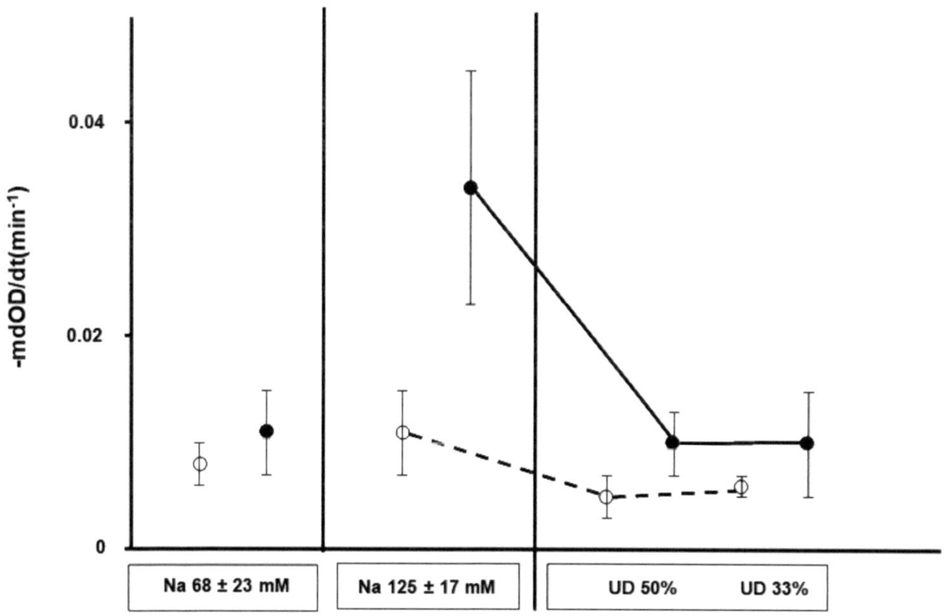

Figure 8. CaOx AGN (increase of −mdOD/dt) induced by UM-coated hydroxyapatite (cHAP) in urine: crystallization test without (o) and with the addition of 0.05 mg/ml cHAP (•) at low and at high sodium concentrations (Na) and after urinary dilution (UD) (n = 8, x ± SD).

ionic strength, ESP is compressed to a few nanometers where crystals can approach to distances where self-aggregated UMs can take over their bridging effect.

To get more information about CaOx AGN being induced by cHAP, supplementary experiments were performed in solutions of albumin in a high urinary concentration (AS, 20 mg/l). The comparison of experiments performed in AS and in concentrated urine showed almost identical results (**Figure 9**). A high inhibitory activity with respect to CaOx AGN of AS and urine was abolished by the cHAP addition and also in the dissolved Ca phosphate precipitates (DPs) of urine and AS. Under the special conditions of our experiments, albumin seems to be an ideal substance to mimic UM effects. Adsorption on surfaces favors self-AGN of UMs as demonstrated with respect to albumin and thus can turn inhibitors to promoters of AGN [46]. Ca phosphates are excellent substrates for UM adsorption [5]. HAP of RPLs being denuded from their epithelial cells is therefore an ideal platform to initiate stone formation by the adsorption and self-AGN of UMs. Since the effect of UMs or albumin on CaOx AGN was identical when adsorbed on HAP or when being in solution after temporary adsorption, HAP of RPLs is more likely to act as a mediator of crystal AGN than as a heterogeneous nucleator for CaOx formation as suggested by others [12]. Indeed, scanning electron microscopy of urinary sediments after HAP-induced CaOx AGN showed in agreement with findings on RPLs large CaOx aggregates which were in the surroundings but not in direct contact with the HAP crystals [49].

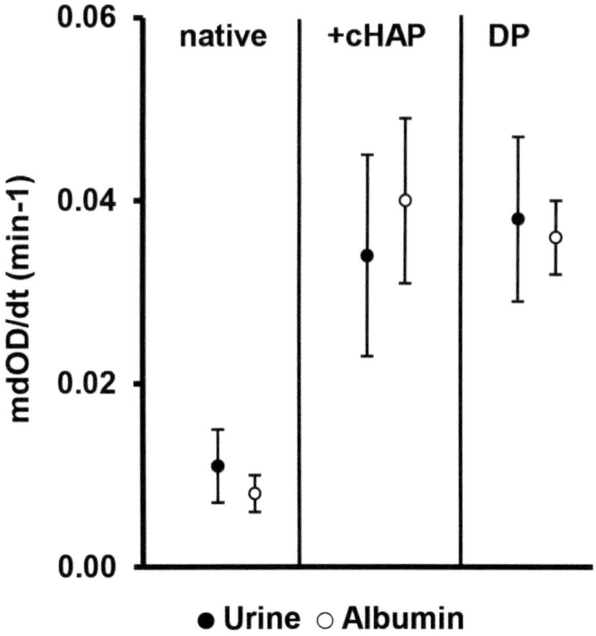

Figure 9. Almost identical results obtained in crystallization test (CT) performed with concentrated urine (•) and albumin solution (AS, 20 mg/l (o): CT performed in native urine or AS (native), in urine or AS with UM or albumin coated HAP (+cHAP) and in dissolved Ca phosphate precipitates of urine or AS (DP) ($n = 8$, $x \pm$ SD).

6. Summary and conclusions

The formation of Ca stones in the kidney during crystalluria seems to base on crystal AGN either on Randall's plugs or on plaques. Urine has, as demonstrated by our study, a high inhibitor capacity with respect to CaOx AGN. Coating of crystals by electronegative charged UMs creates zones of electrostatic repulsion between the crystals which under normal conditions and within the short urinary transit time in the kidney hardly can be overwhelmed by diffusion or sedimentation being responsible for particle collision and thus AGN. Zones of electrostatic repulsion are reduced in the presence of pathological UMs with a lack of anionic residues or in concentrated urine with a high ionic strength. UMs with a lack of negatively charged anionic groups create an insufficient surface potential on UM-coated crystals. At high ionic strength, the extent of surface potentials is compressed by an increased accumulation of cations. Under these conditions, zones of electrostatic repulsion probably can be bridged by normal but self-aggregated UMs. Self-AGN occurs by the adsorption of UMs on surfaces especially of HAP with its high affinity to UMs. The AGN of UM-coated particles like urinary crystals or latex beads probably mainly bases on a hydrophobic effect between the large hydrophobic protein segments. This effect can occur either directly between pathological UM coats or is mediated by self-aggregated but normal UMs.

Stone formation on Randall's plugs mainly occurs at high urinary supersaturation with respect to Ca salts as observed in primary hyperoxaluria or in hyperparathyroidism both with high recurrence rates of stone formation. At such states of chronic urinary supersaturation, crystallization already can start in the descending loop of Henle and crystals during their way through the nephron can stick to tubular walls and by sedimentation can accumulate further crystals. Tubular cells damaged by massive crystalluria favor crystal sticking and produce pathological UMs, which enhance crystal AGN. Crystal accumulates are ideal platforms for the adsorption of UMs and their self-AGN and thus for crystal AGN. By such mechanisms, large crystal plugs can be formed which when protruding out from ducts of Bellini into the renal calices may give raise to stone formation. Whereas in hyperparathyroidism nephrolithiasis can be cured by parathyroidectomy, the treatment of primary hyperoxaluria is extremely difficult but not the topic of this chapter. However, in stone metaphylaxis, a high fluid intake is essential which apart from urinary supersaturation also reduces ionic strength and urinary transit time through the collecting ducts and the renal pelvis.

The formation of Randall's plaques (RPLs) being the origin of most idiopathic Ca stones seems to be a complex process of biomineralization. RPLs are frequent but not always connected with stone disease. Even in the case of nephrolithiasis, stone formation on a RPL can take decades, whereas other RPLs in the same kidney can remain stone free [13]. Idiopathic Ca nephrolithiasis often is characterized by long stone free intervals [50]. In these cases, stone formation seems more to be the result of a coincidence of noisy factors than a real disease. A most dangerous constellation is an excessive ingestion of Ox rich food (e.g., chocolate) in combination with a poor fluid intake. After excessive Ox intake, a threefold increase of urinary Ox was observed [23]. High urinary Ox and consecutive crystal concentrations can, as mentioned above, induce the secretion of pathological UMs and destroy epithelial layers of RPLs. The consequence is that HAP deposits come in contact with crystals in a concentrated urine where self-AGN and AGN are enhanced by a high ionic strength and a high UM concentration. Therefore, for idiopathic Ca stone patients, dietary Ox restriction and a high fluid intake are mandatory. However, only the last measure is evidence based [51]; since in studies of stone metaphylaxis, the compliance of patients especially of those with long stone-free intervals often is rather poor.

Author details

Johannes M. Baumann

Address all correspondence to: johannes.denise.baumann@bluewin.ch

Stone Research Center Biel, Biel, Switzerland

References

[1] Romero V, Akpinar H, Assimos DG. Kidney stones: A global picture of prevalence, incidence and associated risk factors. Reviews in Urology. 2010;**12**(2-3):e86-e96

[2] Baumann JM, Affolter B. From crystalluria to kidney stones, some physicochemical aspects of calcium nephrolithiasis. World Journal of Nephrology. 2014;**3**(4):256-267

[3] Khan SR, Kok DJ. Modulators of urinary stone formation. Frontiers in Bioscience. 2004;**9**:1450-1482

[4] Thurgood LA, Wang T, Chataway TK, Ryall RL. Comparison of the specific incorporation of intracrystalline proteins into urinary calcium oxalate monohydrate and dehydrate crystals. Journal of Proteome Research. 2010;**9**(9):4745-4757

[5] Thurgood LA, Ryall RL. Proteomic analysis of proteins selectively associated with hydroxyapatite, brushite, and uric acid crystals precipitated from human urine. Journal of Proteome Research. 2010;**9**(10):5402-5412

[6] Robertson WG. Do "inhibitors of crystallization" play any role in the prevention of kidney stones? A critique. Urolithiasis. 2017;**45**:53-56

[7] Jaggi M, Nakagawa Y, Zipperle L, Hess B. Tamm-Horsfall protein in recurrent calcium kidney stone formers with positive family history: Abnormalities in urinary excretion, molecular structure and function. Urological Research. 2007;**35**:55-62

[8] Mandel NS, Mandel IC, Kolbach-Mandel AM. Accurate stone analysis: The impact on disease diagnosis and treatment. Urolithiasis. 2017;**45**:3-9

[9] Randall A. The origin and growth of renal calculi. Annals of Surgery. 1937;**105**:1009-1027

[10] Daudon M, Bazin D, Letavernier E. Randall's plaques as the origin of calcium oxalate kidney stones. Urolithiasis. 2015;**43**(Suppl 1):5-11

[11] Evan AP, Worcester EM, Coe FL, Williams J Jr, Lingemann JE. Mechanisms of human kidney stone formation. Urolithiasis. 2015;**43**(Suppl 1):19-32.

[12] Khan RS, Canales BK. Unified theory on the pathogenesis of Randall's plaques and plugs. Urolithiasis. 2015;**43**(Suppl 1):109-123

[13] Kok DJ, Boellaard W, Ridwan Y, Levchenko VA. Timeless of the "free-particle" and "fixed-particle" models of stone-formation: Theoretical and experimental investigations. Urolithiasis. 2017;**45**(1):33-41

[14] Khan SR, Finlayson B, Hackett RL. Stone matrix as proteins adsorbed on crystal surfaces: A microscopic study. Scanning Electron Microscope. 1983;**1**:379-385

[15] Hess B, Nakagawa Y, Coe FL. Inhibition of calcium oxalate monohydrate crystal aggregation by urine proteins. The American Journal of Physiology. 1989;**257**:F99-F106

[16] Baumann JM, Affolter B, Casella R. Aggregation of freshly precipitated calcium oxalate crystals in urine of calcium stone patients and controls. Urological Research. 2011;**6**:421-427

[17] Baumann JM, Affolter B, Meyer R. Crystal sedimentation and stone formation. Urological Research. 2010;**38**:21-27

[18] Baumann JM, Affolter B, Caprez U, Clivaz C, Glück Z, Weber R. Stabilization of calcium oxalate suspension by urinary macromolecules, probably an efficient protection from stone formation. Urologia Internationalis. 2007;**79**:267-272

[19] Baumann JM, Affolter B, von Arx U, Noël M. Alteration of urinary macromolecules by adsorption on surfaces, probably an important factor in urolithiasis. Urolithiasis. 2013;**41**(6):467-474.

[20] Brown CM, Ackermann DK, Purich DL. EQUIL93: A tool for experimental and clinical urolithiasis. Urological Research. 1994;**22**:119-126

[21] Ackermann D, Baumann JM. Chemical factors governing the state of saturation towards brushite and whewellite in urine of calcium stone formers. Urological Research. 1987;**15**:63-65

[22] Robertson WG, Peacock M. The cause of idiopathic calcium stone disease: Hypercalciuria or hyperoxaluria? Nephron. 1980;**26**(3):105-110

[23] Balcke P, Zazgornik J, Sunder-Plassmann G, Kiss A, Hauser AC, Gremmel F, Derfler K, Stockenhuber F, Schmidt P. Transient hyperoxaluria after ingestion of chocolate as a high risk factor for calcium oxalate calculi. Nephron. 1989;**51**:32-34

[24] Fogazzi GB. Crystalluria: A neglected aspect of urinary sediment analysis. Nephrology Dialysis Transplantation. 1996;**11**:379-387

[25] Marickar YM, Salim A. Photomicrography of urinary deposits in stone clinic. Urological Research. 2009;**37**:359-368

[26] Robertson WG. Kidney models of calcium oxalate stone formation. Nephron Physiology. 2004;**98**:21-30

[27] Kok DJ, Khan SR. Calcium oxalate nephrolithiasis, a free or fixed particle disease. Kidney International. 1994;**46**:847-854

[28] Saw NK, Rao PN, Kavanagh JPA. Nidus, crystalluria and aggregation: Key ingredients for stone enlargement. Urological Research. 2008;**36**:11-15

[29] Robertson WG, Peacock M, Nordin BE. Calcium crystalluria in recurrent renal-stone formers. Lancet. 1969;**2**:21-24

[30] Finlayson B, Reid F. The expectation of free and fixed particles in urinary stone disease. Investigative Urology. 1978;**15**:442-448

[31] Müller RH. Zetapotential und Partikelladung in der Laborpraxis. Stuttgart: Wissenschaftliche Verlagsgesellschaft; 1996

[32] Cook AF, Grover PK, Ryall RL. Face-specific binding of prothrombin fragment 1 and human serum albumin to inorganic and urinary calcium oxalate monohydrate crystals. BJU International. 2009;**103**:826-835

[33] Webber D, Rodgers AL, Sturrock ED. Glycosylation of prothrombin fragment 1 governs calcium oxalate crystal nucleation and aggregation, but not crystal growth. Urological Research. 2007;**35**:277-285

[34] Wang L, Guan X, Tang R, Hoyer JR, Wierzbicki A, De Yoreo JJ, Nancollas GH. Phosphorylation of osteopontin is required for inhibition of calcium oxalate crystallization. Journal of Physical Chemistry B. 2008;**112**:9151-9157

[35] Viswanathan P, Rimer JD, Kolbach AM, Ward MD, Kleinman JG, Wesson JA. Calcium oxalate monohydrate aggregation induced by aggregation of desialylated Tamm-Horsfall protein. Urological Research. 2011;**39**:269-282

[36] Coe FL, Nakagawa Y, Asplin J, Parks JH. Role of nephrocalcin in inhibition of calcium oxalate crystallization and nephrolithiasis. Mineral and Electrolyte Metabolism. 1994;**20**(6):378-384

[37] Webber D, Radcliffe CM, Royle L, Tobiasen G, Merry AH, Rodgers AL, Sturrock ED, Wormald MR, Harvey DJ, Dwek RA, Rudd PM. Sialylation of urinary prothrombin fragment 1 is implicated as a contributory factor in the risk of calcium oxalate kidney stone formation. FEBS Journal. 2006;**273**:3024-3037

[38] Kolbach AM, Afzal O, Halligan B, Sorokina E, Kleinman JG, Wesson JA. Relative deficiency of acidic isoforms of osteopontin from stone former urine. Urological Research. 2012;**40**:447-454

[39] Cerini C, Geider S, Dussol B, Hennequin C, Daudon M, Veesler S, Nitsche S, Boistelle R, Berthézène P, Dupuy P, Vazi A, Berland Y, Dagorn JC, Verdier JM. Nucleation of calcium oxalate crystals by albumin: Involvement in the prevention of stone formation. Kidney International. 1999;**55**:1776-1786

[40] Coe FL, Evan AP, Worcester EM, Lingeman JE. Three pathways for human kidney stone formation. Urological Research. 2010;**38**:147-160

[41] Kahn SR. Calcium oxalate crystal interaction with renal tubular epithelium, mechanism of crystal adhesion and its impact on stone development. Urological Research. 1995;**23**:71-79

[42] Khan SR, Masiamini SA, Atmani F, Glenton PA, Opalko FJ, Thamilselvan S, Hammett-Stabler C. Membranes and their constituents as promoters of calcium oxalate crystal formation in human urine. Calcified Tissue International. 2000;**66**(2):90-96

[43] Stoller ML, Low RK, Shami GS, McCormick VD, Kerschmann RL. High resolution radiography of cadaveric kidneys: Unraveling the mystery of Randall's plaque formation. Journal of Urology. 1996;**156**(4):1263-1266

[44] Haggitt RC, Pitcock JA. Renal medullary calcifications: A light and electron microscopic study. Journal of Urology. 1971;**106**:342-347

[45] Low RK, Stoller ML. Endoscopic mapping of renal papillae for Randall's plaques in patients with urinary stone disease. Journal of Urology. 1997;**158**(6):2062-2064

[46] Baumann JM, Affolter B. The paradoxical role of urinary macromolecules in the aggregation of calcium oxalate: A further plea to increase diuresis in stone metaphylaxis. Urolithiasis. 2016;**44**(4):311-317

[47] Guerra A, Allegri F, Meschi T, Adorni G, Prati B, Nouvenne A, Novarini A, Maggiore U, Fiaccadori E, Borghi L. Effects of urine dilution on quantity, size and aggregation of calcium oxalate crystals induced in vitro by an oxalate load. Clinical Chemistry and Laboratory Medicine. 2005;**43**:585-589

[48] Kok DJ, Papapoulos SE, Bijvoet OL. Crystal agglomeration is a major element in calcium oxalate urinary stone formation. Kidney International. 1990;**37**:51-56

[49] Baumann JM, Affolter B, Caprez U, Henze U, Lauper D, Maier F. Hydroxyapatite induction and secondary aggregation of calcium oxalate, two important processes in calcium stone formation. Urological Research. 2001;**29**:417-422

[50] Strohmaier WL. Course of calcium stone disease without treatment. What can we expect? European Urology. 2000;**37**:339-344

[51] Fink HA, Akornor JW, Garimella PS, MacDonald R, Cutting A, Rutks IR, Monga M, Wilt TJ. Diet, fluid, or supplements for secondary prevention of nephrolithiasis: A systematic review and meta-analysis of randomized trials. European Urology. 2009;**56**:72-80

Section 5

Genitourinary Pathophysiology

An Overview on Prostate Pathophysiology: New Insights into Prostate Cancer Clinical Diagnosis

Gustavo Ferreira Simoes, Paula Sakuramoto,
Caroline Brito dos Santos,
Nilva Karla Cervigne Furlan and
Taize Machado Augusto

Additional information is available at the end of the chapter

http://dx.doi.org/10.5772/intechopen.74269

Abstract

The prostate is an accessory gland of the male reproductive tract, and its presence is universal in mammals. It is committed to the prostatic fluid production and storage, which is released with other semen components during ejaculation. Such fluid contributes to increasing motility and fertility of the spermatozoa, and the neutralization of the vagina, thus playing an important role in fertilization. Few pathological complications, often progressively aggravated with age, can affect this gland (i.e. benign and malignant proliferative changes; all to be described next in this chapter). Nowadays, the neoplastic expansion is the main motivator and contributor for studies on enlightening of growth regulation mechanisms and physiology of the prostate.

Keywords: physiology, pathology, benign prostatic hyperplasia, prostate cancer, biomarkers

1. Prostate anatomy

The human prostate is a pelvic gland located under the urinary bladder and in front of the rectum, and it is composed by glandular and non-glandular structures surrounded by one same capsule [1–3]. It consists mainly of muscular-fibrous tissue, which it is subdivided into about 50 tubule-alveolar glands [4], at the lateral and posterior segment of the urethra, which drain to 20–30 small prostatic ductules opening in the prostate, or close to the posterior wall of the prostatic urethra [5–8]. The prostatic secretion, which accounts for approximately 20% of the seminal fluid, confers a characteristic odor of this flowing, and participates in the activation of spermatozoa [8]. The ducts of the prostatic glands open into a sulcus located on each side of the urethral ridge, called the prostatic sinus. The prostate is traversed throughout the prostatic portion of the urethra, from the base to the apex, with a slightly curved course in the anterior-posterior direction, and closer to its anterior face [5–8].

The prostate is anatomically described as an inverted pyramid whose apex is the lowest portion, and which is located about 1.5 cm behind the lower border of the pubic symphysis and is directly related to the upper face of the urogenital diaphragm. The base of the prostate gland is in a horizontal plane that passes through the middle part of the pubic symphysis, and it is directly related to the cervix of the bladder and the inner ostium of the urethra. Inferior-lateral surfaces are convex and are separated from the superior fascia of the pelvic diaphragm by a venous plexus, and are related to the pubococcygeal muscles [6–9]. The posterior surface is flattened and triangular, and it is related to the bladder of the rectum. The anterior surface is narrow and separated from the pubic symphysis by retropubic fat tissue. The upper part is related to the seminal glands and to the lower extremities of the vas deferens, and near its base presents small depressions for the entrance of the ejaculatory ducts [6].

Despite not being clearly distinguished anatomically, the following prostate lobes are traditionally defined: right, left and a middle lobe [5–8]. In pathology, the prostate is described in different zones (peripheral zone, central zone, transition zone and anterior fibro-muscular zone) [9]. The right and left lobes are not isolated from each other, being connected, prior to the urethra, by the isthmus of the prostate, constituted by fibromuscular tissue. Their muscular fibers represent the superior continuation of the external sphincter muscle of the urethra to the cervix of the bladder, and it is devoid of glandular tissue. The middle lobe, of variable size, is the part of the prostate that protrudes internally from the upper part of the posterior face of the organ, between the ejaculatory duct and the urethra [5–8]. However, structurally, the middle lobe is indeed inseparable from the right and left lobes. In each prostate lobe we can identify four lobules: (I) Posterior-Inferior, located posterior to the urethra, and inferior to the ejaculatory ducts. It constitutes the face of the prostate, palpable to digital rectal examination; (II) Lateral-Inferior, directly lateral to the urethra, forming the major part of the right or left lobe; (III) Superomedial, deeply to the inferoposterior lobe, surrounding the ipsilateral ejaculatory duct; (IV) Anteromedial, deeply to the inferolateral lobe, directly lateral to the proximal portion of the prostatic urethra.

The superior fascia of the pelvic diaphragm reflects in the superior direction from the visceral fascia of the pelvis to envelop the prostate, and then continues superiorly over the bladder. The portion covering the prostate is dense and fibrous, being called the fascia of the prostate. It is located externally to the prostate capsule and is separated from it, laterally and anteriorly, by the loose connective tissue harboring the prostatic venous plexus. The fascia of the prostate fuses anteriorly with the tendinous arch of the pelvic fascia, which at the level of the pube is called the medial puboprostatic ligament [5–7]. Smooth muscle fibers fulfill this ligament, and it is called the puboprostatic muscle. The lateral puboprostatic ligament extends from the fascia of the prostate to the tendon arch of the pelvic fascia. Inferior to the puboprostatic ligaments, the prostate associates with the medial borders of the pubococcygeus muscle, and from this point the muscle fibers extend in the superior direction to fuse with the fascia of the prostate, forming the prostate lifting muscle. Later, the fascia of the prostate is separated from the tunica of the rectum by the rectovesical septum [6, 10].

The prostatic arteries are usually direct branches of the inferior bladder artery from one of the branches of the internal iliac artery. In some cases, it may be a branch of the internal pudendal artery, or the medial rectal artery [5–7, 10]. The veins draining the prostate girdle, to form the prostatic venous plexus, located in the fascia of the prostate. The prostatic venous plexus continuous superiorly with the bladder venous plexus, and communicates posteriorly with the internal vertebral venous plexus. The lymphatic vessels of the prostate drain into the internal iliac lymph nodes [5–7, 10]. Finally, the prostate is innervated by sympathetic fibers from the lower hypogastric plexus. These fibers innervate smooth muscle fibers and blood vessels [5–7, 10].

2. Prostate gland hormonal regulation

There are considerable variations related to the prostate anatomy, biochemistry and pathology of several mammal species. In humans, the sexual accessory tissues (or glands) produce high concentration of several biologically active substances, such as fructose, citric acid, spermine, prostaglandins, zinc, proteins including immunoglobulins, and specific enzymes (i.e. esterases and phosphatases) [11].

The growth, differentiation and maintenance of the activity of the prostate gland [12] are mainly controlled by androgens, which is the basis of the anti-androgenic therapies for the treatment of primary prostate cancer. The development and physiology of the prostate is also directly modulated by somatothrophic hormones (such as insulin, prolactin and growth hormone), retinoic acid and estrogen [13, 14], as well as a biomolecular scenario of complex interactions between the epithelium and stroma [15], which sum up to a complicated and poorly understood regulatory mechanism.

Receptors type androgen receptor (AR) and estrogen receptor (ER) are responsible for mediating the physiological effects of androgens and estrogens, respectively [16, 17]. Briefly, the receptor located in the cytoplasm binds to testosterone or dihydrotestosterone, dissociates a heat shock protein (HSP), dimerizes, and it is translocated to the nucleus, where, together with a variety of co-activators and co-repressors, activates or inactivates different sets of genes [18]. The classic AR has 110 kDa and several features in common with members of the nuclear receptor family, such as estrogen receptors, progesterone, thyroid hormones, and peroxisome proliferator-activated receptors (PPARs) [19].

Testosterone and dihydrotestosterone (DHT) act through AR. The AR primarily functions as a transcription factor. It is an extremely important molecule, responsible for the primary male sex differentiation (formation of gonads and external genitalia), and for the pubertal acquisition of the male secondary characteristics (events associated with puberty and adolescence) [20]. It is also liable for most cases of complete androgen insensitivity (resulting in infertile XY karyotype female) [21], and it is deeply associated with the origin of prostate tumors and, particularly, with the recurrence of androgen independent cancer [22–24].

The most striking androgen dependence of the prostate gland is observed by hormonal or surgical castration. In a rat model, removal of the testes results in prostate involution to approximately 10% of its original size after 21 days. Epithelial cells death and stroma reorganization are responsible by such event [25]. Similar to AR, estrogen receptors (ERs) belong to the family of nuclear receptors. The two subtypes, ERα and ERβ, have different physiological roles. They share homology with each other, but are the products of different genes [26]. Both ERα and ERβ are expressed in the prostate. In adults, ERα and ERβ are preferentially found in the stroma and in the epithelium, respectively [27]. Similarly to the AR, ER expression might be suppressed by methylation of its promoters, and this epigenetic alteration was suggested to be involved in both benign prostatic hyperplasia and prostate cancer development [28, 33].

The action of estrogens on prostatic ductal morphogenesis and cell differentiation is complex [14]. However, a brief exposure of rodents to estrogens during neonatal development causes irreversible and dose-dependent effects on morphology, cellular organization and function of the gland [29, 30]. Reduced prostate size at adulthood was associated with decreased responsiveness at puberty due to reduced AR content [31]. The reduced AR levels were justified by increased proteasomal degradation of AR protein at postnatal day 10 [32].

Estrogen exposure to occasional doses during the gestation period causes increased concentrations of androgen receptor in mice, ductal budding and prostate weight later in the adulthood [34]; whereas the neonatal exposure to high doses compromises the growth epithelial differentiation, and accounts for changes in the secretory function, as well as for incidence of prostatic intraepithelial neoplasia (PIN) and prostatitis [14, 29]. The effect of high doses of estrogens on the neonatal prostate is due not only to the changes in the androgen concentrations, via permanent actions on the hypothalamic-gonadal pituitary gland, but also due to direct effects on the prostate gland, since the administration of testosterone is not able to reverse those effects [35]; this phenomena is known as estrogenic *imprinting*.

High doses of estrogen administered in adult animals function as castration, resulting in the inhibition of the hypothalamic-pituitary-gonadal axis, by suppression of the gonadotrophin releasing hormone, and consequent blockage of the hormone testosterone by the testes [36, 37]. Nonetheless, such effects can be reversed (contrary to those observed in neonates), by replacing testosterone or dihydrotestosterone hormones.

It is well established that some of the circulating androgens are converted into estrogens in various peripheral tissues by the enzyme aromatase [38]. The aromatase was also identified in the human prostate, suggesting that this gland is able to perform the aromatization reaction and it is a feasible local source of estrogen production [39]. Estrogens acts in target cells all over the body and in addition to sexual organs they influence growth, health and cell activity. Despite early work of estrogens used as therapy for androgen-resistant prostate cancer, it can be critical in predisposing prostate cancer.

Estrogens also participate in several pathological changes in the prostate; among the very well described pathologies is the induction of chronic inflammation [40, 41], squamous metaplasia reported in several species of mammals [42–44], and human prostate cancer [45].

There are several pathological complications, including benign and malign proliferative alterations, often aging escalate-associated, that affect prostate gland. So, studies focusing on the growth regulation and physiology of the prostate are very precious to understand the origin and progression of these pathologies.

3. Benign prostate hyperplasia (BPH)

Benign prostate hyperplasia (BPH) is a common urological issue that causes prostate enlargement in men after 40-years-old. It is a noncancerous augmentation of the prostate gland size, with stromal and glandular epithelial hyperplasia in the transition zone. It is estimated that 50% of 50 year old, and 75% of 80 year old men could have some lower urinary tract symptom (LUTS). In such condition the urethra can be partially or totally blocked, resulting in urinary retention, weak urination stream, incomplete bladder emptying and hesitancy; and so carrying secondary problems as urinary tract infections, bladder stones and chronic kidney disease, culminating in kidney failure. The LUTS is reflection of the hormonal changes rising with age, and resulting in abnormal stromal and epithelial cell proliferation (hyperplasia) in the transition zone of the prostate. The molecular etiology of these events remains unclear, but few studies attempt to correlate it to sex steroids hormones [46], also known as gonadocorticoids and gonadal steroids, that interact with vertebrate androgen and estrogen receptors. It is important to mention that the BPH is generally not a precursor lesion to a prostate cancer (PCa) condition.

Some animal models studies, including dogs and chimpanzees, have been performed in order to understand the prostate conditions. Chimpanzees sporadically suffer from age-associated BPH, and are the closest match to human prostate gland. Throughout the time, dogs are like human counterpart because they develop BPH containing distinct nodules of hyperplasia with diffuse areas of compression of the rectum producing constipation, a symptom opposed to the urinary retention in men [47, 48]. In order to supply these deficiencies, some transgenic animal models using other normal mammal species were developed. Prostate-specific 15-LOX-2 transgenic mouse and PPAR∂ knockdown mice naturally develop increased prostate size with age, in addition to epithelial-hyperplasia, and prostatic intraepithelial neoplasia progression [49, 50].

4. Prostate cancer

Nearly 14 million new cases of cancer occurred worldwide during 2012 [51], generating around 8.2 million deaths. More than a half of cancer deaths arose in countries of medium or low human development index (HDI). The four most common types, in this order were lung, female breast, bowel and PCa. Among malignant neoplasms that affect men, PCa is the most common, after non-melanoma skin tumors, especially in the male population from the sixth decade of life. This is a recognized public health problem, since according to data from the Mortality Information System (MIS), 13,773 deaths were caused by PCa in Brazil in 2013 [52].

Considering the statistics worldwide, PCa prevalence is only beaten by lung cancer in men. Unlike some types of tumors, the incidence of PCa has increased over the years. There are two main factors for this association: the improvement of diagnostic methods and the extended life expectancy of men over the years; since PCa has slow growth and its incidence is age-associated, it is very comprehensible the increased detection of this malignant neoplasia lately in the years. The origin of PCa and the several processes giving direction to PCa carcinogenesis are still unclear, but often are assumed that several components may influence it, among which stands out: diet, genetic, hormonal, and environmental factors; all currently being widely investigated in the literature.

The treatment of PCa can be very controversial because there are many variables, such as the patient's age, prostatic specific antigen (PSA) concentrations and the stage of the tumor. Patients in inoperable conditions, due to age, are treated with hormone therapy or radiation. The most common hormone therapy for PCa is the androgen deprivation, since the prostate gland is a highly androgen dependent gland, and because the majority of prostate tumors originate from androgen-dependent glandular epithelial cells of the prostate [53]. The therapies in use for PCa will be best addressed later in this chapter.

5. Clinical diagnosis and biomarkers for PCa

The diagnosis and follow-up of PCa patients are often difficult because of the absence of specific markers that could change accordingly to the status of disease, the best therapy, and the existence of future complications caused by the chosen treatment.

For several decades many researchers joined efforts to study biomarkers of prognosis and treatment for PCa. Almost 50-years, PSA measurement represented the best marker for PCa. The primary idea was to substitute the digital rectal examination by PSA screening; nevertheless this was not possible despite the low specificity and false positive rate, as it is also observed in BPH [54]. No significant progress in the use of PSA as a precise biomarker of PCa was achieved during the past years.

Beyond this scenario, advances in genetic testing for PCa risk and new molecular diagnostic assays have been designed to improve diagnostic accuracy and treatment decision beyond prostate-specific antigen (PSA) testing. PSA is a protein of the kallikrein family synthesized in the prostatic epithelium and secreted in the seminal fluid. From its discovery in 1970 to the present day, it is a diagnostic tool used as a tumor marker for early diagnosis, treatment and monitoring of patients with neoplasia in conjunction with the rectal examination. However, many studies have questioned the use of this biomarker for a diagnosis, due to the exponential increase in the diagnosis of PCa and, consequently, the increase of unnecessary hormonal, radiotherapeutic, chemotherapeutic and surgical treatments such as radical prostatectomy [55, 56]. PSA evaluation is performed by its measurement in serum using immunoassay (34 kDa). Normal values vary according to the method used. In most tests, values of up to 2.5 ng/mL are allowed as normal. If this value is higher, it is indicated to request the dosage of fractionated PSA, which relates total PSA to free PSA (fPSA). The result is expected to be equal to or greater than 20%; if it is lower, there is a probability that it is a PCa [57]. However, this test does not have 100% of specificity or sensitivity, insofar as there is PCa whose PSA is not altered, and there are other transient factors that can raise serum PSA levels, such as prostatitis

[58], benign prostatic hyperplasia [59], prostatic biopsies [60] and trauma, due to prostatic cell lysis releasing PSA into the bloodstream [61].

Despite results enhancing detection at earlier stage and decreasing the number of metastatic patients, the use of prostate-specific antigen (PSA) to detect PCa has low specificity, unnecessary biopsies and frequently mistaken diagnoses. Also, PCa has various features so prognosis following diagnosis is greatly variable. Hence, there is a requirement for new prognostic biomarkers, particularly to differentiate between inactive and aggressive forms of the disease, to improve clinical management of PCa patients. Research continues into finding additional markers that may allow this goal to be attained.

In order to improve the specificity of PSA as a tumor biomarker, tests called PHI (Prostatic Health Index), that predicts the risk of having PCa and 4 K score™ (predicts the risk of having high-risk of PCa) were launched on the American and European markets [62]. 4 K score™ blood test combines 4 prostatic biomarkers (total PSA, fPSA, intact PSA, and human kallekrein 2(hK2)) with the age of the patient, the digital rectal exam (DRE) findings (presence of a nodule or not), and the result of previous biopsies [63]. The higher the score, the greater the probability of finding tumor cells in a biopsy (Gleason ≥ 7). This test combination is interesting because it does not allow unnecessary biopsies to be performed, whereas post-operative, as well as any surgery, has risks and can lead to future complications for the patient, affecting his quality of life.

Another non-invasive test available is the ExoDxTM Prostate (IntelliScore) Test18, which, through urinalysis, assesses the risk of developing invasive PCa, and thereby target the best treatment by molecular analysis of three specific genes in exosome and microvesic RNAs released by tumor cells, called extracellular vesicles (further discussed in this chapter) [64]. These related genes (*ERG*, *PCA3* and *SPDEF*) are most commonly related to tumor progression and, consequently, its aggressiveness and invasion [65].

It is important to note that these tests are not accessible to the entire population, either because of the high cost of the technology, or because some countries have still not approved it. Thus, the main diagnostic method used nowadays for the screening and detection of the PCa remains PSA testing and rectal examination (DRE). If the results of these exams are altered, a biopsy is necessary to confirm the diagnosis, and determine the aggressiveness and prognosis of the cancer. This is done by histological analysis of the biopsied tissue, following classification according to the Gleason Scale. This system consists of the sum of 2 values that represent the degree of the tumor, and that determine the dominant cellular pattern and the most frequent cellular pattern, respectively. Tumor grades range from 1 to 5, the former representing more differentiated and prostate restricted tumors, while the latter represents totally undifferentiated tumors that have normally infiltrated the glandular stoma. The score, therefore, ranges from 2 (1 + 1) to 10 (5 + 5), and values below 4 on the Gleason Scale represent a well differentiated PCa; between 5 and 7, an intermediate PCa; and between 8 and 10, advanced PCa [66]. The determination of the degree and stage of cancer allows classification into high, intermediate and low risk categories.

The clinical picture of castrated-resistant prostate cancer (CRPC) is quite heterogeneous, ranging from the asymptomatic increase in the PSA indices to the distant metastasis (commonly bone metastasis), with an important impairment of the patient's quality of life [66]. This is a reflection of the complexity and diversity of biomolecular alterations already found in biopsies. Tumor progression is related to a number of genetic changes that can affect AR, signaling cascades, apoptosis mechanisms and cell regulation, or, as in many cases, a combination of all of them [67].

Biomolecular techniques, such as fluorescent *in situ* hybridization (FISH) and Microarray, for example, have identified a variety of key factors genes, oncogenes and tumor suppressor genes, related to the development and progression of PCa [68, 69]. The use of molecular techniques also allowed the identification of some genes related to the suppressive function of metastasis, opening a new perspective for researching the phenomenon of tumor invasion to other tissues and, with that, to identify and elucidate new indicators of prognosis, or even PCa target therapies. As example, some studies have focused attention on the CDH1 gene and its protein expression, located on chromosome 16q22, which encodes the E-cadherin, a glycoprotein responsible for cell-cell adhesion, an important cellular function that prevents EMT in tumor progression [70].

The Metastatic prostate adenocarcinoma (metPA) is diagnosed by immunohistochemistry. Nowadays very promising biomarkers have been used to determine prostatic origin of metPA, such as prostate specific membrane antigen (PSMA) and NKX3.1 [71]. PSMA is a type II membrane protein not secreted and is expressed in all forms of prostate tissue, but it is expressed at high levels on malignant prostate cells with limited extraprostatic expression [72]. Many approaches to target PSMA include DNA-based vaccines, as well as passive administration of monoclonal antibodies (PSMA-mAb), including 7E11.C5.3, that has already been approved by USA FDA (Food and Drug Administration); the medication is commercially available as ProstaScint® [72, 73].

Compared to PSA, PSMA is upregulated with androgen deprivation, and its expression was correlated with cancer aggressiveness and poor prognosis, while PSA decreases with androgen deprivation [72]. PSMA was also evaluated in PCa using PET molecular imaging system. After all, PSMA is not specific only to prostate gland; it is expressed in other normal tissues (such as salivary glands, duodenal mucosa, renal tubular cells, and neuroendocrine cells in the colon), and in malignant cells (renal cell carcinomas, colon carcinomas, and endothelial cells that surround or are into the tumors) [74].

Although multiple independent studies sought to demonstrate evidence that genetic variations may be independent predictors of PCa risk in addition to family history and serum PSA levels, the challenge in the years to come will be to introduce these new gene-based diagnostic and prognostic tests in algorithms integrating the other known risk factors including age, ethnicity, family history and PSA level to better tailor diagnostic and therapeutic strategies for PCa.

5.1. The extracellular vesicles (exosomes) and PCa: beyond classical biomarkers

Several studies have related to novel PCa biomarkers that can precisely detect, and treat, types of aggressive cancer by headlining circulating tumor cells (CTCs) and circulating extracellular vesicles (EVs) **(Figure 1)**. Notably, EVs are released by almost all the cells, and brings lots of molecular information. The study based on EVs provides lots of information about its content,

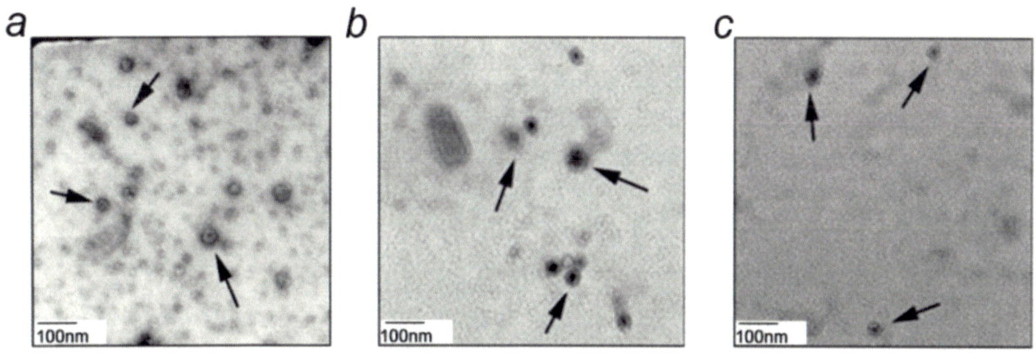

Figure 1. Representative TEM images of exosomes derived from (a) C42 PCa cell line, (b) LNCaP xenograft serum and (c) patient plasma by ultracentrifugation method. Exosomes were negatively stained with 2% uracyl acetate after removal of moisture. Arrows indicate cup-shaped structures which are identified as exosomes (30–100 nm in diameter). From: Kharmate et al. [86]. Online available at: http://journals.plos.org/plosone/article?id=10.1371/journal.pone.0154967.

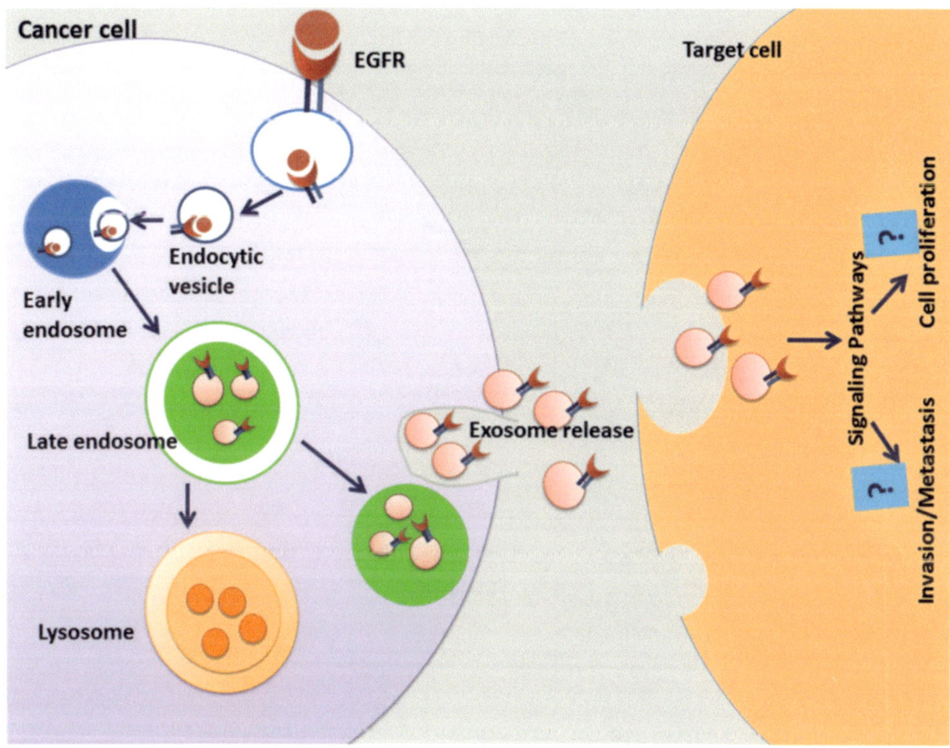

Figure 2. *Schematic representation of possible role of EGFR-exosomes in cancer progression.* Ligand binding induces rapid activation and internalization of EGFR and endocytosis. Whether EGFR escapes lysosomal degradation and is released extracellularly via exosomes is unknown. The transfer of EGFR via exosomes may significantly alter the tumor microenvironment and could be relevant to progression of an aggressive PCa. From: Kharmate et al. [86]. Online available at: http://journals.plos.org/plosone/article?id=10.1371/journal.pone.0154967.

such as: lipids, proteins, nucleic acids and metabolites [75, 76]. All of each can be isolated in small volumes from body fluids, just by using some steps of ultracentrifugation, as a non-invasive method to monitor disease progression, and are proposed to function as tumor-specific molecular signatures. They are small structures (50–150 nm) that carry genetic and/or nongenetic materials from tumor cells. Recent study analyzed the presence of CD9 and CD63 (a housekeeping exosome marker) positive EVs, demonstrating that patients with metastatic cancer and detectable CTCs have higher CD9 detectable in plasma [77]. The CD9 positive EVs were found higher in plasma of PCa patients compared to HPB patients, and were related to paracrine signaling that contributes to PCa progression [77]. *In silico* reanalysis of genes involved in vesicular trafficking demonstrated that the expression of required well-known endosomal sorting complexes, such as *RAB27A, RAB27B* and *VPS36,* are downregulated in patients with advanced PCa [78].

Other studies suggest possible micro-RNAs roles in PCa [79] due to their recruitment to EVs present in various human body fluids; they are miR-2909 and miR-615-3p, which was detected in urinary-exosomal of PCa patients [80, 81]. Also EVs was useful to monitor the response to radiation therapy, in the search for a personalized treatment according to different profiling levels [82].

Biomarkers	Biomarkers Measurement	Sample	Recommendation
Prostate Health Index (PHI)	PSA, fPSA, [−2]proPSA	serum	Approved by the Food and Drug Administration (FDA) * Related to PCa aggressiveness
4K*score*	PSA, fPSA, iPSA, hK2	serum	The test provides information about the probability of having a high-risk PCa * Related to PCa aggressiveness
PCA3 *score*	*m*RNA *PCA3* in relation to *m*RNA *PSA*	urine obtained after prostate massage	Approved by the Food and Drug Administration (FDA) * Inconclusive results about its relationship with PCa aggressiveness
*mi*RNAs and other exosomal biomarkers	No standardized methodology	blood and urine	Directly related to development and progression of cancer No standardized methodology Preliminary results

Table 1. Biomarkers in PCa detection and prognosis.

Additionally to androgens (as described in Section 3), prostate physiology is, in part, regulated by the epidermal growth factor (EGF), whose action is mediated by its receptor (EGFR). EGFR is one of the mediators of cell proliferation, and its overexpression has been associated with aggressiveness and invasion of PCa. It has been described and identified as an important anti-PCa target, and some inhibitors of EGFR were tested with limited effectiveness in prostate cancer patients; they are Gefitinib, Lapatinib, and Erlotinib [83–85]. Recently, EGFR was also observed in EVs (**Figure 2**) of PCa patients [86].

Previous studies have demonstrated that PSA can be detectable in plasma and urine derived EV's [87]. Logozzi et al. [88] demonstrated that an acid microenvironment (such as the tumor microenvironment), functions as a key factor for the exosomal releasing, and determines the quality and quantity of released vesicles, including the ones containing PSA, an enzyme that needs an acidic microenvironment for full activation, in PCa.

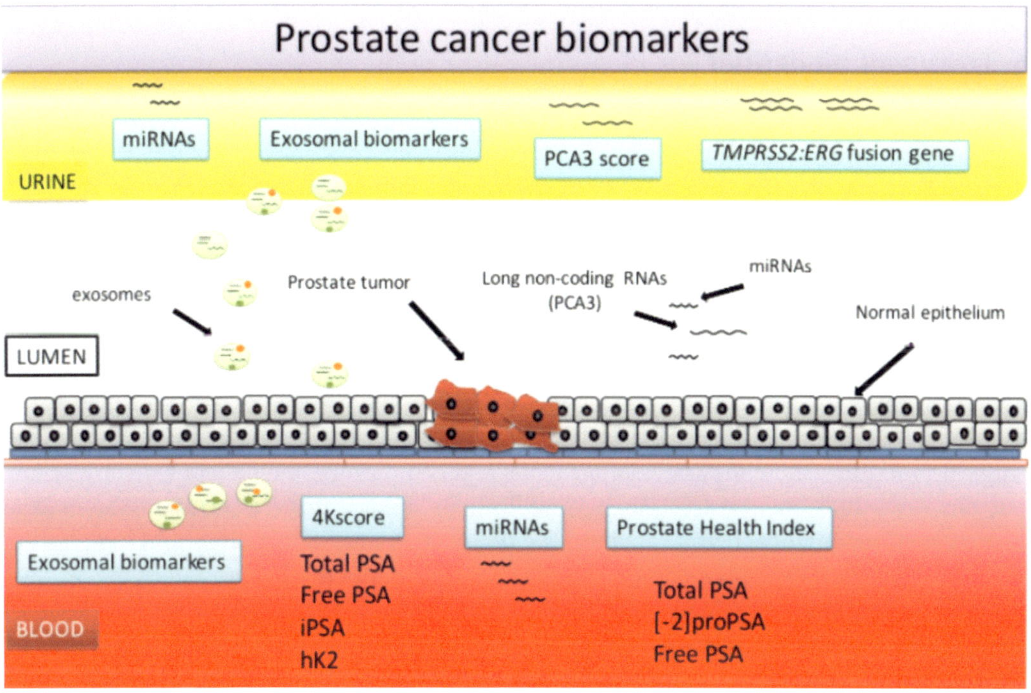

Figure 3. The prostate specific antigen (PSA) remains the most used biomarker in the management of early prostate cancer (PCa), in spite of the problems related to false positive results and overdiagnosis. New biomarkers have been proposed in recent years with the aim of increasing specificity and distinguishing aggressive from non-aggressive PCa. The emerging role of the prostate health index and the 4Kscore: both are blood-based tests related to the aggressiveness of the tumor, which provide the risk of suffering PCa and avoiding negative biopsies. Furthermore, the use of urine has emerged as a non-invasive way to identify new biomarkers in recent years, including the *PCA3* and *TMPRSS2: ERG* fusion gene. Available results showed PCA3 score usefulness to decide the repetition of biopsy in patients with a previous negative result, although its relationship with the aggressiveness of the tumor is controversial. More recently, aberrant the microRNA expression in PCa has been reported by different authors. The utility of circulating and urinary microRNAs in the detection and prognosis of PCa has also been explored. Although several of these new biomarkers have been recommended by different guidelines, large prospective and comparative studies are necessary to establish their value in PCa detection and prognosis. From: Filella and Foj [69]. Online available at: http://www.mdpi.com/1422-0067/17/11/1784

To summarize, in recent years, many new promising PCa biomarkers have been identified **(Table 1) (Figure 3)**, and found to be associated with tumor aggressiveness. Multiplied studies showed the utility of the PHI, the 4Kscore™ and the PCA3 score to reduce the number of unnecessary prostate biopsies in PSA tested men. Actually, these biomarkers have been recommended for different guidelines. Still, large prospective studies, avoiding bias due to selection of patients according to PSA serum levels, are necessary to compare the value of these biomarkers. Also, new efforts are necessary to standardize the methodology for the measurement of exosomal and non-exosomal miRNAs, in order to analyze accurately their usefulness in the management of patients with early PCa. Finally, the combined role of these biomarkers together with magnetic resonance imaging data should be elucidated [89].

Adapted from: Filella and Foj [69]. (*Recommended by the National Comprehensive Cancer Network).

6. Treatment modalities for PCa

PCa treatment is variable, and it is chosen according to the staging of the cancer and, mainly, according to the patient's own preference. Since this type of cancer has slow growth, the presence of low-risk groups, where tumor is diagnosed still *in situ*, is indicative of an active surveillance treatment in which the patient only accompanies the tumor through regular PSA testing, and digital touch every 3–6 months [90]. During this follow-up period, if the existence of a tumor progression is observed, radiotherapy or surgery is indicated by total removal of the prostate gland (radical prostatectomy).

Radical prostatectomy may be the first choice of the patient who opts for complete removal of the gland, by caution of future metastasis. It is an effective procedure, however, just like any surgical procedure, there may be complications and compromise the patient's quality of life. For this procedure, the most common complications are the urinary incontinence, erectile dysfunction, and inguinal hernia; anyhow, the prognosis tends to be positive and long-lasting [91]. Nonetheless, some tumors may recur over time even after radical prostatectomy. In such cases, it is important to evaluate whether the recurrence was local or occurred at a distance (lymph nodes or other organs, such as liver, bone, or lung).

Hormone therapy is usually used in patients with lymph node involvement or distant metastasis. It consists of reducing androgen concentrations to the level of castration. This can be done by surgical method through bilateral orchiectomy, or through drugs that act on the androgen receptor (AR) pathways; the latter being more commonly used nowadays. At first, hormone deprivation therapy has great effects on the control of advanced PCa. However, it is known that part of the cases evolves to the state of CRPC. The mechanisms responsible for progression of tumor growth, despite hormonal blockade, have not been fully elucidated yet. Current studies have shown that molecular changes in the androgen receptor (AR) are related to such progression. Among these changes, it is relevant to mention the overexpression of AR, mutations in the

http://dx.doi.org/10.5772/intechopen.74269

AR gene that allow its activation by other endogenous steroids, increased production of growth factors activating AR even in the absence of androgen, changes in co-regulatory proteins and upregulation of enzymes related to androgen synthesis [92].

There are two drug lines for hormone therapy; the first line accounts for the central blockers that constitute the agonists of gonadotrophin-releasing hormone (GnRH agonists), and the peripheral androgen receptor blockers. Usually they are used in a comminuted way, since the central blockers, for example, Leuprolide (Lupron) and Gosserelin Acetate (Zoladex), acts through the interruption of the pituitary feedback mechanism, inhibiting LH realizing by the pituitary gland, and leading to a decreased testoterone production [63]. However, because these drugs initially boosted testosterone production, the combination with peripheral androgen receptor blockers, such as Bicalutamide (Casodex), Flutamide (Flutamide) and Androcur (Androcur), shall be indicated due to their binding capacity to the ARs in a way that inhibits androgenic stimulation, deactivating their genetic expression [93].

The second line of therapy is most commonly used when PCa is resistant to the first-line hormonal therapies stage. Abiraterone Acetate (Zytiga) is a drug that primarily acts on the adrenal gland through the inhibition of the 17α-hydroxylase/C17, 20-lyase (CYP17) enzyme, essential for androgen biosynthesis in tissues [94, 95]. Enzalutamide (Xtandi) is another drug of this therapeutic line that works by inhibiting androgen receptors, their signaling pathways, and is able to act on anti-androgen-resistant tumor cells.

It is important to emphasize that hormonal therapy is a palliative treatment, in that it acts to contain the progression of advanced PCa, and not its elimination. In this context, given the scarcity of effective treatments for these types of tumors, it is promising to still search for new biomarkers capable of not only diagnosing PCa early, but also being able to evaluate its aggressiveness and prognosis.

Author details

Gustavo Ferreira Simoes[1,2], Paula Sakuramoto[3], Caroline Brito dos Santos[3], Nilva Karla Cervigne Furlan[4] and Taize Machado Augusto[4]*

*Address all correspondence to: taizea@gmail.com

1 Research Associate at Department of Structural and Functional Biology, Biology Institute, UNICAMP, Campinas-SP, Brazil

2 Faculty of Medicine of Santa Casa de Sao Paulo, Department of Morphology, FCMSCSP, Sao Paulo-SP, Brazil

3 Undergraduated Medical Student at Faculty of Medicine of Jundiai, Jundiai-SP, Brazil

4 Department of Morphology and Basic Pathology, Faculty of Medicine of Jundiai, Jundiai-SP, Brazil

References

[1] Price D. Comparative aspects of development and structure in the prostate. National Cancer Institute Monograph. 1963;**12**:1-27

[2] Pfau A, Caine M. In: Spring-Mills E, Hafez ESSE, editors. Male Accessory Sex Glands. Elsevier-North-Holland, New York; 1980. p. 357

[3] McNeal JE, Villers AA, Redwine EA, Freiha FS, Stamey TA. Histologic differentiation, cancer volume, and pelvic lymph node metastasis in adenocarcinoma of the prostate. Cancer. 1990 Sep 15;**66**(6):1225-1233

[4] Ham A, Cormark DH. Histologia. Guanabara–Koogan. 9ª ed. Rio de Janeiro; 1991

[5] Dangelo JG, Fattini CA. Anatomia Sistemica e Segmentar. 3° ed. São Paulo-SP: Editora Atheneu; 2011. ISBN: 8573798483

[6] Gardner E, Gray DJ, O'rahilly R. Anatomia. 4° ed. Rio de Janeiro-RJ: Editora Guanabara Koogan; 1988. ISBN: 9788527717519

[7] Gray H. Anatomia. 29° ed. Rio de Janeiro-RJ: Editora Guanabara Koogan; 1988. ISBN: 9788527712781

[8] Moore KL, Dalley AF, Agur AMR. Anatomia Orientada para a Clínica. 7° ed. Rio de Janeiro-RJ: Editora Guanabara Koogan; 2014. ISBN: 9788527725170

[9] McNeal JE. Regional morphology and pathology of the prostate. American Journal of Clinical Pathology. 1968 Mar;**49**(3):347-357

[10] SNELL RS. Anatomia Clínica para Estudantes de Medicina. 5° ed. Rio de Janeiro-RJ: Editora Guanabara Koogan; 2000. ISBN: 9788527705257

[11] García-Flórez M, Oliveira CA, Carvalho HF. Early effects of estrogen on the rat ventral prostate. Brazilian Journal of Medical and Biological Research. 2005;**38**(4):487-497

[12] Cunha GR, Donjacour AA, Cooke PS, Mee S, Bigsby RM, Higgins SJ, Sugimura Y. The endocrinology and developmental biology of the prostate. Endocrine Reviews. 1987;**8**:338-362

[13] Webber MM. Polypeptide hormones and the prostate. Progress in Clinical and Biological Research. 1981;**75B**:63-88

[14] Prins GS, Birch L, Habermann H, Chang WY, Christopher T, Oliver P, Bieberich C. Influence of neonatal estrogens on rat prostate development. Reproduction, Fertility, and Development. 2001;**13**:241-252

[15] Lee C, Sensibar JA, Dudek SM, Hiipakka RA, Liao S. Prostatic ductal system in rats: Regional variation in morphological and functional activities. Biology of Reproduction. 1990;**43**:1079-1086

[16] Gelmann E. Molecular biology of the androgen receptor. Journal of Clinical Oncology. 2002;**20**:3001-3015

[17] Sasaki M, Kaneuchi M, Fujimoto S, Tanaka Y, Dahiya R. Hypermethylation can selectively silence multiple promoters of steroid receptors in cancers. Molecular and Cellular Endocrinology. 2003;**202**:201-207

[18] Heinlein CA, Chang C. The roles of androgen receptors and androgen-binding proteins in nongenomic androgen actions. Molecular Endocrinology. 2002;**16**(10):2181-2187

[19] Jacobs MN, Dickins M, Lewis DF. Homology modelling of the nuclear receptors: human oestrogen receptorbeta (hERbeta), the human pregnane–X–receptor (PXR), the Ah receptor (AhR) and the constitutive androstane receptor (CAR) ligand binding domains from the human oestrogen receptor alpha (hERalpha) crystal structure, and the human peroxisome proliferator activated receptor alpha (PPARalpha) ligand binding domain from the human PPARgamma crystal structure. The Journal of Steroid Biochemistry and Molecular Biology. 2003;**84**:117-132

[20] Sisk CL, Foster DL. The neural basis of puberty and adolescence. Nature Neuroscience. 2004;**7**(10):1040-1047

[21] Dohle GR, Smit M, Weber RF. Androgens and male fertility. World Journal of Urology. 2003;**21**(5):341-345

[22] Feldman BJ, Feldman D. The development of androgen –independent prostate cancer. Nature Reviews. Cancer. 2001;**1**(1):34-45

[23] Lee DK, Chang C. Endocrine mechanisms of disease: Expression and degradation of androgen receptor: mechanism and clinical implication. The Journal of Clinical Endocrinology and Metabolism. 2003;**88**(9):4043-4054

[24] Heinlein CA. ChangC. Androgen receptor in prostate cancer. Endocrine Reviews. 2004; **25**(2):276-308

[25] Augusto TM, Felisbino SL, Carvalho HF. Prostatic remodeling after castration involves heparanase activation. Cell and Tissue Research. 2008;**332**(2):307-315

[26] Yang YJ, Zhang YL, Li X, Dan HL, Lai ZS, Wang JD, Wang QY, Cui HH, Sun Y, Wang YD. Contribution of eIF–4E inhibition to the expression and activity of heparanase in human colon adenocarcinoma cell line: LS–174T. World Journal of Gastroenterology. 2003;**9**:1707-1712

[27] Weihua Z, Lathe R, Warner M, Gustafsson JA. An endocrine pathway in the prostate, -diol and CYP7B1, regulates the prostate growth. β, 17β- androstane-3α, AR, 5βER. Proceedings of the National Academy of Sciences of the United States of America. 2002;**99**: 13589-13594

[28] Li SC, Chen GF, Chan PS, Choi HL, Ho SM, Chan FL. Altered expression of extracellular matrix and proteinases in Noble rat prostate gland after long–term treatment with sex steroids. Prostate. 2001;**49**:58-71

[29] Prins GS, Birch L, Greene GL. Androgen receptor localization in different cell types of the adult rat prostate. Endocrinology. 1992;**129**:3187-3199

[30] Augusto TM, Bruni-Cardoso A, Damas-Souza DM, Zambuzzi WF, Kühne F, Lourenço LB, Ferreira CV, Carvalho HF. Oestrogen imprinting causes nuclear changes in epithelial cells and overall inhibition of gene transcription and protein synthesis in rat ventral prostate. International Journal of Andrology. 2010;**33**(5):675-685

[31] Putz O, Schwartz CB, Kim S, GA LB, Cooper RL, Prins GS. Neonatal low and high-dose exposure to estradiol benzoate in the male rat: I. Effects on the prostate gland. Biology of Reproduction. 2001;**65**(5):1496-1505

[32] Woodham C, Birch L, Prins GS. Neonatal estrogen down-regulates prostatic androgen receptor through a proteosome-mediated protein degradation pathway. Endocrinology. 2003;**144**(11):4841-4850

[33] Li LC, Chui R, Nakajima K, Oh BR, Au HC, Dahiya R. Frequent methylation of estrogen receptor in prostate cancer: correlation with tumor progression. Cancer Research. 2000;**3**: 702-706

[34] Nonneman DJ, Ganjam VK, Welshons WV, Vom Saal FS. Intrauterine position effects on steroid metabolism and steroid receptors of reproductive organs in male mice. Biology of Reproduction. 1992;**47**:723-729

[35] Huang L, Pu Y, Alam S, Birch L, Prins GS. Estrogenic regulation of signaling pathways and homeobox genes during rat prostate development. Journal of Andrology. 2004;**25**: 330-337

[36] Neubauer B, Blume C, Cricco R, Greiner J, Mawhinney M. Comparative effects and mechanisms of castration, estrogen anti–androgen, and anti–estrogen–induced regression of accessory sex organ epithelium and muscle. Investigative Urology. 1981;(4):229-234

[37] Thompson SA, Rowley DR, Heidger PM Jr. Effects of estrogen upon the fine structure of epithelium and stroma in the rat ventral prostate gland. Investigative Urology. 1979;(1):83-89

[38] Simpson E, Rubin G, Clyne C. Local estrogens biosynthesis in males and females. Endocrine-Related Cancer. 1999;**6**:131-137

[39] Tsugaya M, Harada N, Tozawa K. Aromatase mRNA levels in benign prostatic hyperplasia and prostate cancer. International Journal of Urology. 1996;**3**:292-296

[40] Bianco JJ, McPherson SJ, Wang H, Prins GS, Risbridger GP. Transient neonatal estrogen exposure to estrogen-deficient mice (aromatase knockout) reduces prostate weight and induces inflammation in late life. The American Journal of Pathology. 2006;**168**:1869-1878

[41] Prins GS, Huang L, Birch L, Pu Y. The role of estrogens in normal and abnormal development of the prostate gland. Annals of the New York Academy of Sciences. 2006;**1089**:1-13

[42] Doré M, Chevalier S, Sirois J. Estrogen–dependent induction of cyclooxygenase–2 in the canine prostate in vivo. Veterinary Pathology. 2005;(1):100-103

[43] Risbridger GP, Wang H, Frydenberg M, Cunha G. The metaplastic effects of estrogen on mouse prostate epithelium: proliferation of cells with basal cell phenotype. Endocrinology. 2001;(6):2443-2450

[44] Nevalainen MT, Harkonen PL, Valve EM, Ping W, Nurmi M, Martikainen PM. Hormone regulation of human prostate in organ culture. Cancer Research. 1993;(21):5199-5207

[45] Barrett-Connor E, Garland C, McPhillips JB, Khaw KT, Wingard DL. A prospective, population-based study of androstenedione, estrogens, and prostatic cancer. Cancer Research. 1990;**50**(1):169-173

[46] Asiedu B, Anang Y, Nyarko A, Doku DA, Amoah BY, Santa S, Ngala RA, Asare GA. The role of sex steroid hormones in benign prostatic hyperplasia. The Aging Male. 2017;**20**:17-22

[47] DeKlerk DP, Coffey DS, Ewing LL, et al. Comparison of spontaneous and experimentally induced canine prostatic hyperplasia. The Journal of Clinical Investigation. 1979;**64**:842-849

[48] Berry SJ, Strandberg JD, Saunders WJ, Coffey DS. Development of canine benign prostatic hyperplasia with age. Prostate. 1986;**9**:363-373

[49] Suraneni MV, Schneider-Broussard R, Moore JR, Davis TC, Maldonado CJ, Li H, Newman RA, Kusewitt D, Hu J, Yang P, Tang DG. Transgenic expression of 15-lipoxygenase 2 (15-LOX2) in mouse prostate leads to hyperplasia and cell senescence. Oncogene. 2010;**29**:4261-4275

[50] Jiang M, Fernandez S, Jerome WG, He Y, Yu X, Cai H, Boone B, Yi Y, Magnuson MA, Roy-Burman P, Matusik RJ, Shappell SB, Hayward SW. Disruption of PPARgamma signaling results in mouse prostatic intraepithelial neoplasia involving active autophagy. Cell Death and Differentiation. 2010;**17**:469-481

[51] Cancer Research UK. Prostate Cancer Incidence Statistics. 2017. Available from: http://www.cancerresearchuk.org/health-professional/cancer-statistics/statistics-by-cancer-type/prostate-cancer/incidence

[52] Brazilian National Institute of Cancer (INCA). Rio de Janeiro, Brazil. Available: http://www.inca.gov.br.

[53] Cunha GR, Donjacour AA, Cooke PS, Mee S, Bigsby RM, Higgins SJ, Sugimura Y. The endocrinology and developmental biology of the prostate. Endocrine Reviews. 1987;**8**(3):338-362

[54] Hoffman RM. Clinical practice. Screening for prostate cancer. The New England Journal of Medicine. 2011;**365**:2013-2019

[55] Qaseem A, Barry MJ, Denberg TD, et al. Screening for prostate cancer: a guidance statement from the Clinical Guidelines Committee of the American College of Physicians. Annals of Internal Medicine. 2013;**158**:761

[56] Reis RB, Cassini MF. Prostatic Specific Antigen (PSA). Nardozza Júnior A, Zerati Filho M, Reis RB. In: Urologia Fundamental. Sao Paulo, Brazil, Planmark; 2010. pp. 189-194

[57] Brazilian Society of Urology. Available from: http://sbu-sp.org.br/old/publico-geral/materia_doencas.php?id=17

[58] Kawakami J, Siemens DR, Nickel JC. Prostatitis and prostate cancer: implications for prostate cancer screening. Urology. 2004;**64**:1075

[59] Mao Q, Zheng X, Jia X, et al. Relationships between total/free prostate-specific antigen and prostate volume in Chinese men with biopsy-proven benign prostatic hyperplasia. International Urology and Nephrology. 2009;**41**:761

[60] Tchetgen MB, Oesterling JE. The effect of prostatitis, urinary retention, ejaculation, and ambulation on the serum prostate-specific antigen concentration. The Urologic Clinics of North America. 1997;**24**:283

[61] Jung K, Meyer A, Lein M, et al. Ratio of free-to-total prostate specific antigen in serum cannot distinguish patients with prostate cancer from those with chronic inflammation of the prostate. The Journal of Urology. 1998;**159**:1595

[62] Vickers AJ, Scardino PT, Lilja H, Linder V, Steinmiller D; Opko Diagnostics, LLC, ou Artic Partners Ab. Methods and apparatuses for predicting risk of prostate cancer and prostate gland volume. United States patente US9672329 B2. 2017 Jun 6

[63] Vickers AJ, Cronin AM, Aus G, et al. A panel of kallikrein markers can reduce unnecessary biopsy for prostate cancer: data from the European Randomized Study of Prostate Cancer Screening in Goteborg, Sweden. BMC Medicine. 2008;**6**:19

[64] ExomeDx. Exome Diagnostics announces launch of ExoDx® Prostate (IntelliScore), a completely non-invasive liquid biopsy test to help rule out high-grade prostate câncer [Internet]. [Plublished 2016 Sep 7]. Available from: http://www.exosomedx.com/news-events/press-releases/exosome-diagnostics-announces-launch-exodxr-prostateintelliscore-completely.

[65] McKiernan J, Donovan MJ, O'Neill V, Bentink S, Noerholm M, Belzer S, Skog J, Kattan MW, Partin A, Andriole G, Brown G, Wei JT, Thompson IM, Carroll P. A novel urine exosome gene expression assay to predict high-grade prostate cancer at initial biopsy. JAMA Oncology. 2016;**2**(7):882-889

[66] Kumar V, Abbas AK, Fausto N. Robbins & Coltran: Patologia - Bases patologicas das doenças. 8ª ed. Rio de janeiro: Elsevier; 2010

[67] Zoladex: Goserelin acetate. AstraZeneca. Available from: https://www.zoladex.com/

[68] Inoue T, Segawa T, Kamba T, Yoshimura K, et al. Prevalence of skeletal complications and their impact on survival of hormone refractory prostate cancer patients in Japan. Urology. 2009;**73**:1104-1109

[69] Fradet Y. Biomarkers in prostate cancer diagnosis and prognosis:beyond prostate-specific antigen. Current Opinion in Urology. 2009;**19**(3):243-246

[70] Filella X, Foj L. Prostate Cancer Detection and Prognosis: From Prostate Specific Antigen (PSA) to Exosomal Biomarkers. International Journal of Molecular Sciences. 2016;**17**(11):1784

[71] Qiu L-X, Li T-T, Zhang J-B, Zhong W-Z, Bai J-L, Liu B-R, Zheng M-H, Qian X-P. The E-cadherin (CDH1) −160 C/A polymorphism and prostate cancer risk: a meta-analysis. European Journal of Human Genetics. 2009;**17**:244-249

[72] Jia L, Jiang Y, Michael CW. Performance of different prostate specific antibodies in the cytological diagnosis of metastaticprostate adenocarcinoma. Diagnostic Cytopathology. 2017. DOI: 10.1002/dc.23809 [Epub ahead of print]

[73] Chang SS. Overview of Prostate-Specific Membrane Antigen. Revista de Urología. 2004;**6** (Suppl 10):S13-S18

[74] Muthumani K, Marnin L, Kudchodkar SB, Perales-Puchalt A, Choi H, Agarwal S, Scott VL, Reuschel EL, Zaidi FI, Duperret EK, Wise MC, Kraynyak KA, Ugen KE, Sardesai NY, Joseph Kim J, Weiner DB. Novel prostate cancer immunotherapy with a DNA-encoded anti-prostate-specific membrane antigen monoclonal antibody. Cancer Immunology, Immunotherapy. 2017. DOI: 10.1007/s00262-017-2042-7 [Epub ahead of print]

[75] Hossein Jadvar P. PSMA PET in Prostate Cancer. Journal of Nuclear Medicine. 2015;**56**: 1131-1132

[76] Lo Cicero A, Stahl PD, Raposo G. Extracellular vesicles shuffling intercellular messages: for good or for bad. Current Opinion in Cell Biology. 2015;**35**:69-77

[77] Chevillet JR, Kang K, Ruf IK, Briggs HA, Vojtech LN, Hughes SM, Cheng HH, Arroyo JD, Meredith EK, Gallichotte EN. Quantitative and stoichiometric analysis or the microRNA content of exosomes. Proceedings of the National Academy of Sciences of the United States of America. 2014;**111**:14888-14893

[78] Soekmadji C, Riches JD, Russell PJ, et al. Modulation of paracrine signaling by CD9 positive small extracellular vesicles mediates cellular growth of androgen deprived prostate cancer. Oncotarget. 2017;**8**(32):52237-52255

[79] Worst TS, Meyer Y, Gottschalt M, Weis CA, von Hardenberg J, Frank C, Steidler A, Michel MS, Erben P. RAB27A, RAB27B and VPS36 are downregulated in advanced prostate cancer and show functional relevance in prostate cancer cells. International Journal of Oncology. 2017;**50**:920-932

[80] Endzeliņš E, Melne V, Kalnina Z, Lietuvietis V, Riekstina U, Llorente A, Line A. Diagnostic, prognostic and predictive value of cell-free miRNAs in prostate cancer: a systematic review. Molecular Cancer. 2016;**15**(1):41

[81] Valentino A, Reclusa P, Sirera R, Giallombardo M, Camps C, Pauwels P, Crispi S, Rolfo C. Exosomal microRNAs in liquid biopsies: future biomarkers for prostate cancer. Clinical & Translational Oncology. 2017;**19**:651-657

[82] Wani S, Kaul D, Mavuduru RS, Kakkar N, Bhatia A. Urinary-exosomal miR-2909: A novel pathognomonic trait of prostate cancer severity. Journal of Biotechnology. 2017;**259**:135-139

[83] Malla B, Zaugg K, Vassella E, Aebersold DM, Dal Pra A. Exosomes and exosomal microRNAs in prostate cancer radiation therapy. International Journal of Radiation Oncology, Biology, Physics. 2017;**98**(5):982-995

[84] Ciardiello F, Caputo R, Bianco R, Damiano V, Pomatico G, De Placido S, et al. Antitumor effect and potentiation of cytotoxic drugs activity in human cancer cells by ZD-1839 (Iressa), an epidermal growth factor receptor-selective tyrosine kinase inhibitor. Clinical Cancer Research: An Official Journal of the American Association for Cancer Research. 2000;**6**(5):2053-2063

[85] Sirotnak FM, She Y, Lee F, Chen J, Scher HI. Studies with CWR22 xenografts in nude mice suggest that ZD1839 may have a role in the treatment of both androgen-dependent and androgen-independent human prostate cancer. Clinical Cancer Research: An Official Journal of the American Association for Cancer Research. 2002;**8**(12):3870-3876

[86] Sridhar SS, Hotte SJ, Chin JL, Hudes GR, Gregg R, Trachtenberg J, et al. A multicenter phase II clinical trial of lapatinib (GW572016) in hormonally untreated advanced prostate cancer. American Journal of Clinical Oncology. 2010;**33**(6):609-613

[87] Kharmate G, Hosseini-Beheshti E, Caradec J, Chin MY, Tomlinson Guns ES. Epidermal growth factor receptor in prostate cancer derived exosomes. PLoS One. 2016;**11**(5):e0154967

[88] Mitchell PJ, Welton J, Staffurth J, Court J, Mason MD, Tabi Z, Clayton A. Can urinary exosomes act as treatment response markers in prostate cancer? Journal of Translational Medicine. 2009;**7**:4

[89] Logozzi M, Angelini DF, Iessi E, Mizzoni D, Di Raimo R, Federici C, Lugini L, Borsellino G, Gentilucci A, Pierella F, Marzio V, Sciarra A, Battistini L, Fais S. Increased PSA expression on prostate cancer exosomes in in vitro condition and in cancer patients. Cancer Letters. 2017;**403**:318-329

[90] Porpiglia F, De Luca S, Bertolo R, Passera R, Mele F, Manfredi M, Amparori D, Morra I, Fiori C. Robot-Assisted extended pelvic lymph nodes dissection for prostate cancer: Personal Surgicaal technique outcomes. International Braz J Urol. 2015;**41**(6):1209-12019

[91] Hamdy FC, Donovan JL, Lane JA, et al. 10-Year Outcomes after Monitoring, Surgery, or Radiotherapy for Localized Prostate Cancer. The New England Journal of Medicine. 2016; **375**:1415

[92] National Cancer Institute. Prostate Cancer Treatment (PDQ®) – Patient Version [Internet]. [Update 2016 Jul 7]. Available from: https://www.cancer.gov/types/prostate/patient/prostate-treatment-pdq#section/_142.

[93] Chen Y, Clegg NJ, Scher HI. Anti-androgens and androgen-depleting therapies in prostate cancer: new agents for an established target. The Lancet Oncology. 2010;**10**:981-991

[94] UpToDate [Internet]. Dawson NA (MD): Patient education: Treatment for advanced prostate cancer (Beyound the Basics). [Update 2017 Aug].

[95] Zytiga: Abiratenone acetate. Janssen-Cilag Oncology. Available From: https://www.zytiga.com/

Polycystic Ovary Syndrome, Pathophysiology, and Reproductive Health Implications

Bassim Alsadi

Additional information is available at the end of the chapter

http://dx.doi.org/10.5772/intechopen.70848

Abstract

Polycystic ovary syndrome (PCOS) is one of the most common endocrine disorders in women of reproductive age. The clinical picture characterized by both endocrine disorders (hyperandrogenism, menstrual cycle disorders, obesity) and metabolic alteration with implications for women's health and reproductive and metabolic consequences. Leventhal described for the first time a syndrome characterized by polycystic ovaries associated with menstrual cycle disorders, hirsutism, and obesity. The pathophysiology and other metabolic disorders that make the PCOS more complex than originally described are the most common cause of infertility linked to chronic anovulation. In fact, this is a multifactorial disorder that involves the hypothalamus, pituitary, ovary, adrenal, and peripheral adipose tissues, which are simultaneously involved in the pathogenesis of the syndrome.

Keywords: infertility, polycystic ovary (PCO), polycystic ovarian syndrome (PCOS), menstrual irregularities, acne, hirsutism, anovulation, obesity, hyperandrogenism, insulin resistance and hyperinsulinemia, metformin

1. Introduction

Polycystic ovary syndrome (PCOS) is a common endocrine disorder among women of reproductiveage. It was described for the first time by Stein and Leventhal in 1935 [1].

The PCOS Consensus Workshop Group has proposed a review of diagnostic criteria, defining PCOS as the presence of at least two of the following criteria together [2]:

- Oligo-anovulation
- Hyperandrogenism with clinical or biochemical signs
- Polycystic ovary appearance on ultrasound examination

In order to establish the diagnosis of PCOS, it is important to exclude other disorders with a similar clinical presentation, such as congenital adrenal hyperplasia, Cushing's syndrome, and androgen-secreting tumors.

2. Clinical presentation and clinical components in polycystic ovary syndrome (PCOS)

2.1. Menstrual irregularities in women with polycystic ovary syndrome (PCOS)

This often occurs during the adolescent period at the menarche with menstrual irregularities mainly oligomenorrhea or less frequently amenorrhea. Over 70% of women with PCOS spontaneously reach menstrual regularity in the fourth decade of their life with metabolic dysfunction mainly in perimenopausal age [3]. The chronic state of anovulation present in these patients will produce amenorrhea and oligomenorrhea. An elevated pulse frequency for the luteinizing hormone (LH) has been documented [4]. The increased pulse frequency of the hypothalamic gonadotropin-releasing hormone (GnRH) promotes the transcription of the LH beta-subunit compared to the follicle-stimulating hormone (FSH) beta-subunit [5]. It is unclear whether this increase in pulse frequency is due to an inherent anomaly of the GnRH pulse generator or caused by low progesterone levels due to the chronic state of anovulation as progesterone slows down the GnRH pulse generator [6].

Most women with this syndrome exhibit oligomenorrhea with irregular vaginal bleeding episodes. The cause of such bleeding is not always referred to ovulation but may be caused by a sudden drop in plasma estrogen levels [7].

Increased ovarian androgen biosynthesis in the polycystic ovary syndrome results from abnormalities at all levels of the hypothalamic-pituitary-ovarian axis [8]. The etiopathogenesis of PCOs is multifactorial; all these factors act by creating a vicious circle that eventually leads to the syndrome. It is not yet clear at present what pathogenic event that triggers the chain reaction that leads to hyperandrogenism. The clinical manifestation of PCOs is the result of a series of alterations of physiological mechanisms, so there is not always a full expression of this syndrome. PCOs usually occur in puberty with menstrual disorders, hirsutism, and obesity. Alongside endocrine disorders, there are also metabolic disorders which, however, become more and more evident with the progress of time until they become predominant after menopause.

3. Obesity

Obesity is present in 30–60% of patients with PCOS with body mass index (BMI) greater than 30 kg/m^2 and is often associated with a state of hyperinsulinism. However, even in this case, the cutoff choice can be discussed and modified on the basis of geographical and socioeconomic considerations. The presence of obesity in women with PCOS results in worsening in the metabolic and reproductive outcomes [9].

Obese women with PCOS compared to women with normal weight with PCOS have increased prevalence of glucose intolerance and type 2 diabetes mellitus [10], higher prevalence of hirsutism [11], greater risk of metabolic syndrome, and therefore cardiovascular disease [12, 13]. Obesity increases the prevalence of obstructive sleep apnea in patients with PCOS [14].

A lipolysis dysregulation in PCOS patients has been documented [15], as an increased lipolysis of visceral fat resulting in an increase in free fatty acids released directly into the portal circulation. The free fatty acid levels in the hepatic portal circulation are the major modulators of hepatic gluconeogenesis [16]. This increased visceral fat lipolysis may be one of the mechanisms for increased risk of glucose intolerance [17].

In obese women with PCOS, physical activity and low-calorie diet intake lead to an improvement in ovarian function and reduction of the risk of type 2 diabetes mellitus [18]. Exercise and weight control are highly recommended because of their direct effect not only on the metabolic framework but also on ovarian function and restoration of fertility [19]. Success in treating obesity requires a multidisciplinary approach involving the dietician, the psychologist, and the physician.

4. Hirsutism

The perception of hirsutism as a problem depends on cultural and ethnic factors. The commonly used Ferriman-Gallwey score for clinical evaluation and score above 8 is considered diagnostic [20]. The fact remains that it is an extremely subjective assessment.

The incidence of hirsutism in Caucasian women is 60–70%, while in Japanese women is 30% [21].

In PCOS patients, hyperinsulinism also contributes to increased adrenal androgen secretion in part by increasing adrenal sensitivity to adrenocorticotropic hormone (ACTH) action [22].

4.1. Acne

It is a polymorphic dermatitis sustained by a chronic inflammatory process of the hair follicle. In the genesis of acne, four pathological events are distinguished: follicular channel hyperkeratosis, sebaceous hypersecretion, bacterial proliferation, and inflammation.

Chronic hyperandrogenism causes an increase in sebaceous secretion, thus forming a cystic collection resulting in bacterial overlap and thereby stimulating the inflammatory process. It has been estimated roughly that one-third of PCOS patients have acne [23, 24].

4.2. Infertility

The main cause of infertility in PCOS women is chronic anovulation. However, subfertility may be related to the increase of plasma LH levels in the follicular phase of the cycle, causing a resumption of the second meiotic division of the oocyte and the release of premature ovocytes [25]. High levels of luteinizing hormone (LH) found in polycystic ovary syndrome seem to be related to increased frequency of spontaneous abortions. Other factors that connect PCOS and spontaneous abortion are not yet well known; however, various factors involved in steroidogenesis, folliculogenesis, oocyte maturation, and reduced endometrial receptivity contribute to this vicious cycle between PCOS and abortion [26].

4.3. Insulin resistance and hyperandrogenism in PCOS

There are numerous evidence that polycystic ovary syndrome (PCOS) is a disorder characterized by insulin resistance and hyperinsulinemia.

Insulin resistance is a condition for which a normal insulin concentration produces attenuated biological effects in cases where pancreatic function is intact, leading to compensatory hyperinsulinemia. The presence of insulin resistance does not imply systematic glucose intolerance, and blood glucose may be normal.

Prospective and retrospective observational studies show that at least 40% of women with PCOS exhibit glucose intolerance and that in the 10–20% will develop type 2 diabetes mellitus later in their life between the age of 55 and 65 years [27, 28].

Prior to the development of glucose intolerance, the defect of insulin secretion may remain latent and only occur in conditions that increase insulin resistance, such as the onset of gestational diabetes or a glucose intolerance in the case of corticosteroid treatment.

The molecular mechanism responsible for insulin resistance in PCOS appears to be unique and specific for this syndrome and different from the one present in obesity. Altered phosphorylation of the insulin receptor has been described, resulting in a lack of signal transduction [29].

The ovarian tissue in women with PCOS remains sensitive to the action of insulin, although there is a systemic resistance to insulin.

Ovarian stimulation seems to involve a signal transduction system other than glucose transport, in particular a different second messenger, probably inositol phosphoglycan [30, 31].

Insulin and insulin-like growth factor 1 (IGF-1) are important regulators of ovarian function and directly and indirectly affect ovarian steroidogenesis and androgenic status. Insulin acts directly on the ovarian cells of the theca by activating cytochrome P450 c17alpha hydroxylase and 17,20-lyase activity (key enzyme in the synthesis of androgens) and also synergistically promotes the synthesis of androgen induced by the LH.

Insulin acts indirectly by suppressing the circulating levels of sex hormone-binding globulin (SHBG), resulting in increased free testosterone, and the fraction of the bioavailable hormone for tissues.

Finally, insulin may suppress liver synthesis of IGF-1-binding protein (IGFBP-1), thereby increasing the bioavailability of IGF-1, another important regulator of androgenic ovarian synthesis. It also appears that insulin may act at the hypothalamus level by modifying the pulsed secretion of LH, thus also affecting ovarian steroidogenesis (**Figure 1**) [32, 33].

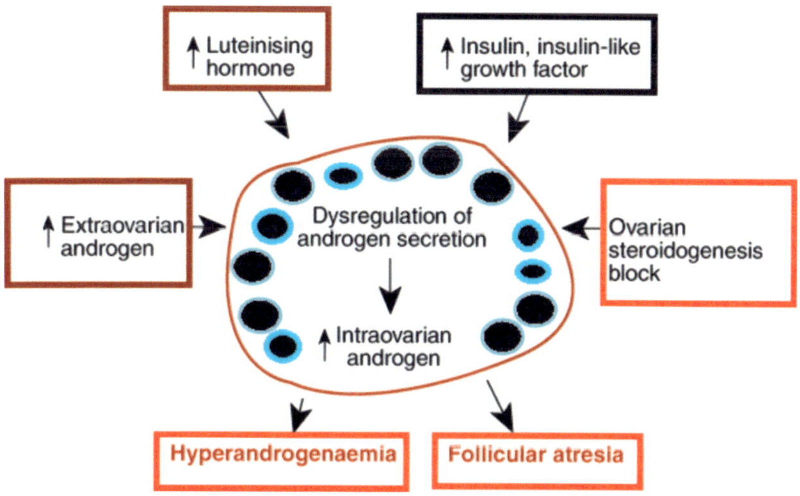

Figure 1. Factors involved in altering follicular steroidogenesis.

There is currently no insulin resistance screening test, whereas a criterion for defining metabolic syndrome has been established that includes components associated with insulin resistance syndrome including visceral obesity, hypertension, fasting hyperglycemia, and dyslipidemia [34]. Other groups add the oral glucose tolerance test (OGTT) to evaluate the fasting blood glucose and at a distance of 2 hours after an oral dose of 75 g of glucose [34].

These characteristics make women with PCOS at increased risk of metabolic syndrome, defined in the past as X syndrome or insulin resistance syndrome [35]. Metabolic abnormalities in women with PCOS therefore require a change in the clinical approach to this syndrome, recognizing that this condition is chronic and with possible long-term consequences. The metabolic disorders linked to insulin resistance usually become predominant with age advancement (**Figure 2**).

The most common metabolic disorders are those that are traditionally linked to insulin resistance and usually become predominant with age advancement.

4.4. Role and issues of ultrasound in the diagnosis of PCOS

Initially, Adams's ultrasound criteria have been used for ultrasound assessment of the ovaries in women with PCOS which required 10 or more follicles with a diameter of 2–10 mm around an hyperechogenic stroma [37, 38]. Although they are still the most widely used, Adams' criteria are not universally accepted for the diagnosis of polycystic ovary basically because there is a considerable overlap between the normal ultrasound aspect and that of polycystic ovaries regarding the number of follicles and the size of the ovaries, and therefore no reliable cutoff has been identified with satisfactory sensitivity and specificity.

Transvaginal ultrasound is the most commonly used for diagnosis of polycystic ovary (PCO). Ultrasound criteria were subsequently modified resulting in increased ovarian volume (>10 cm^3) and the presence of >12 follicles in diameter of 2–9 mm in at least one ovary for PCOS diagnosis [39].

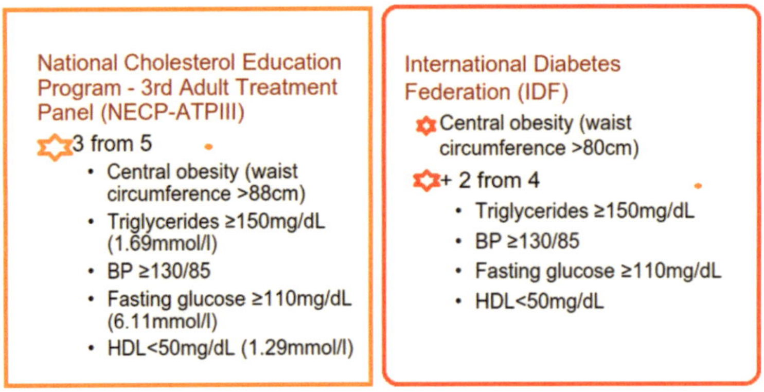

Figure 2. Criteria for metabolic syndrome [36].

Women who use oral contraceptives should be excluded from this criterion as they modify ovarian morphology in healthy women and probably even in women with polycystic ovary [2].

The prevalence of polycystic ovary depending on the age of women: 21.6% in women <35 years and 7.9% in women >35 years [40].

The ultrasound aspect of polycystic ovary can be an isolated finding in asymptomatic patients as well as patients with typical clinical and biochemical manifestations of PCOS may have morphologically normal ovaries.

The variability of the ultrasound description of ovarian morphology (number and location of follicles, hyperechogenic stroma) is a fact even though recent studies consider the increase in ovarian volume (>10 cm^3) as the most reliable criterion for ultrasound evaluation of PCOS [41].

The characteristic ultrasound feature is an increase in ovarian stroma vascularization at Doppler ultrasound [42, 43], which in turn may be related to changes in ovarian morphology. It is necessary to clarify the correlation between ovarian volume and stromal vascularization with ovarian steroidogenesis in patients with PCOS. It is believed that vascular endothelial growth factor (VEGF) plays an important role in increasing stromal flow in patients with PCOS (**Figure 3**) [44].

4.5. Combined oral contraceptive pills in PCOS patient

Combined oral contraceptives (COC) are the most widely used therapeutic option for treating menstrual irregularities. Oral contraceptives cause suppression of LH, resulting in a reduction in androgenic ovarian secretion. The estrogenic component of the combined oral contraceptive induces an increase in sex hormone-binding globulin (SHBG) hepatic synthesis. The various progestogen components of the COC have different effects on the circulating levels of the SHBG [45]. Combined oral contraceptives also significantly reduce the risk of endometrial cancer [45].

The COC pills containing ethinylestradiol and a progestogen with antiandrogenic activity (cyproterone acetate or drospirenone) are effective for the treatment of hirsutism in women

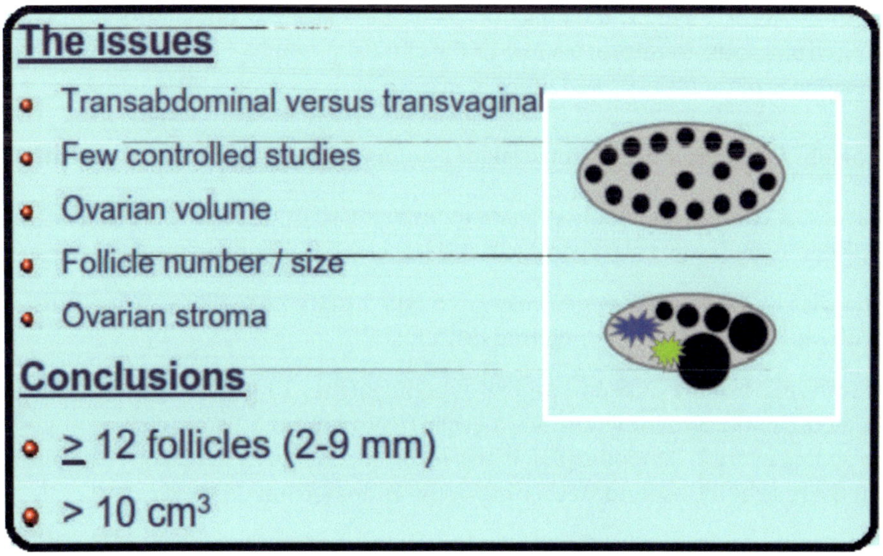

Figure 3. Ultrasound assessment of the polycystic ovary: international consensus definition [39].

with PCOS. The duration of this treatment for at least 6 months is related to the long physiological duration of the hair follicle, while the effect on acne is faster [46].

The best combined oral contraceptive for patients with PCOS is still not well identified. Recent studies have shown that COC therapy may at least partly cause a further worsening of insulin sensitivity in PCOS patients despite a significant reduction in circulating androgens [47, 48].

The effect of COC on insulin balance in women with PCOS remains uncertain. Although the use of combined oral contraceptives is not associated with increased risk of type 2 diabetes mellitus in the general population, studies in women with PCOS have shown mixed results, and this risk cannot be excluded [49].

4.6. Insulin-sensitizing drugs as new therapeutic approach in PCOS

In recent years, numerous studies have been conducted on the use of insulin-sensitizing drugs such as metformin in women with PCOS.

Considering the evidence that insulin resistance and hyperinsulinemia would play a pathogenic role in the development of polycystic ovary syndrome. Metformin improves insulin resistance by reducing glucose intestinal absorption and gluconeogenesis. It also increases the circulating levels of SHBG and FSH with improved ovarian steroidogenesis and normalization of follicular growth [50].

A systematic review evaluated the effectiveness of insulin-sensitizing drugs in women with PCOS. Metformin administration in women with PCOS is associated with a reduction in serum insulin levels and free and total testosterone levels [51]. In short-term therapies (3–6 months), it promotes spontaneous ovulation [51]. There is a decrease in blood pressure and LDL cholesterol, whereas the effect on body mass index is not significant [51]. Insulin-sensitizing drugs seem to improve some of the clinical parameters of PCOS, but there is not enough evidence of their safety and efficacy in long-term therapies [51].

4.7. Endometrial hyperplasia and the risk of endometrial cancer in PCOS patient

The presence of chronic anovulation leads to an increase of estrogen levels which, over the years, can lead to endometrial hyperplasia and increased risk for endometrial cancer [52].

In women with PCOS, there may be obesity and type 2 diabetes mellitus, two conditions associated with increased risk for endometrial cancer.

Women suffering from PCOS and severe oligomenorrhea (interval of more than 3 months between menstruations) or amenorrhea, a cyclic treatment for 12 days with a progestogen to induce bleeding every 1–3 months [53]. It also recommended a hysteroscopy and endometrial biopsy in the case of ultrasound thickening of the endometrium [53].

5. Conclusions

The natural history of the polycystic ovarian syndrome and the role of possible extra-ovarian factors such as obesity, insulin resistance, and environmental factors in the manifestations of the phenotype of PCOS are the subject of scientific debate.

The sonographic finding of polycystic ovary (PCO) appearance, even if isolated, needs more attention in its clinical evaluation.

Polycystic ovary (PCO) pathogenetic evolution toward a PCOS phenotype is not yet well codified. The pathogenesis of PCOS and its natural history are the determining factors for a real assessment of PCOS. However, longitudinal studies are needed to better clarify the pathophysiology of PCOS and its impact on reproductive health.

Author details

Bassim Alsadi

Address all correspondence to: balsadi@hotmail.com

North Tees and Hartlepool Hospitals NHS Foundation Trust, Stockton on Tees, UK

References

[1] Stein IF, leventhal NL. Amenorrhea associated with bilateral polycystic ovaries. American Journal of Obstetrics and Gynecology 1935;**29**:181-191

[2] Rotterdam ESHRE/ASRM Sponsored PCOS Consensus Workshop Group. Revised 2003 consensus on diagnostic criteria and long-term health risks related to polycystic ovary syndrome. Fertility and Sterility. 2004;**81**:19-24

[3] Elting MW, Korsen JM, et al. Women with polycystic ovary syndrome gain regular menstrual cycles when ageing. Human Reproduction 2000;**15**(1):24-28

[4] Waldstreicher J, Santoro NF, et al. Hyperfunction of the hypothalamic-pituitary axis in women with polycystic ovary disease: Indirect evidence for partial gonadotroph desensitization. The Journal of Clinical Endocrinology and Metabolism. 1988;**66**:165-172

[5] Haisenleder DJ, Dalkin AC, et al. Pulsatile gonadotropin-releasing hormone stimulus is required to increase transcription of the gonadotropin subunit genes: Evidence for differential regulation of transcription by pulse frequency in vivo. Endocrinology. 1991;**128**:509-517

[6] Eagleson CA, Gingrich MB, et al. Polycystic ovarian syndrome: Evidence that flutamide restores sensitivity of the gonadotropin-releasing hormone pulse generator to inhibition by estradiol and progesterone. The Journal of Clinical Endocrinology and Metabolism. 2000;**85**:4047-4052

[7] Legro RS. Polycystic ovary syndrome: The new millennium. Molecular and Cellular Endocrinology. 2001;**184**:87-93

[8] Ehrmann DA. Polycystic ovary syndrome. The New England Journal of Medicine. 2005; **352**:1223-1236

[9] Salehi M et al. Pathogenesis of polycystic ovary syndrome: What is the role of obesity? Metabolism. 2004;**53**:358-376

[10] Pasquali R, Fabbri R, et al. Effect of weight loss and antiandrogenic therapy on sex-hormone blood levels and insulin resistance in obese patients with polycystic ovaries. American Journal of Obstetrics and Gynecology. 1985;**154**:139-144

[11] Kiddy DS et al. Differences in clinical and endocrine features between obese and non-obese subjects with polycystic ovary syndrome: An analysis of 263 consecutive cases. Clinical Endocrinology. 1990;**32**:213-220

[12] Orio F Jr, Palomba S, et al. The cardiovascular risk of young women with polycystic ovary syndrome:An observational, analytical, prospective case-control study. The Journal of Clinical Endocrinology and Metabolism. 2004;**89**:3696-3701

[13] Ehrmann D, Schneider DJ, et al. Troglitazone improves defects in insulin action, insulin secretion, ovarian steroidogenesis, and fibrinolysis in women with polycystic ovary syndrome. The Journal of Clinical Endocrinology and Metabolism. 1997;**82**:2108-2116

[14] Vgontzas AN, Legro RS, et al. Polycystic ovary syndrome is associated with obstructive sleep apnea and daytime sleepiness: Role of insulin resistance. The Journal of Clinical Endocrinology and Metabolism. 2001;**86**:517-520

[15] EK I et al. A unique defect in the regulation of visceral fat cell lipolysis in the polycystic ovary syndrome as an early link to insulin resistance. Diabetes. 2002;**51**:284-292

[16] Montague CT et al. The perils of portliness: Causes and consequences of visceral adiposity. Diabetes. 2000;**49**:883-888

[17] Bergman RN. New concepts in extracellular signaling for insulin action: The single gateway hypothesis. Recent Progress in Hormone Research. 1997;**52**:359-385

[18] Saleh AM, Khalil HS. Review of nonsurgical and surgical treatment and the role of insulin sensitizing agents in the management of infertile women with polycystic ovary syndrome. Acta Obstetricia et Gynecologica Scandinavica. 2004;**83**:614-621

[19] Pettigrew R, Hamilton-Fairly D. Obesity and female reproductive function. British Medical Bulletin. 1997;**53**:341-358

[20] Ferriman D, Gallwey JD. Clinical assessment of body hair growth in women. The Journal of Clinical Endocrinology and Metabolism. 1961;**21**:1440-1447

[21] lobo R. Hirsutism in polycystic ovary syndrome: Current concepts. Clinical Obstetrics and Gynecology. 1991;**34**:817-826

[22] Lanzone A, Fulghesu AM, et al. Differential androgen response to adrenocorticotropic hormone stimulation in polycystic ovarian syndrome: Relationship with insulin secretion. Fertility and Sterility 1992;**58**:296-301

[23] Balen A, Conway G, et al. Polycystic ovary syndrome: The spectrum of the disorder in 1741 patients. Human Reproduction. 1995;**10**:2107-2111

[24] Eden JA. The polycystic ovarian syndrome presenting as resistant acne successfully treated with cyproterone acetate. Medical Journal of Australia. 1991;**155**:677-680

[25] Homburg R, Armar NA, et al. Influence of serum luteinising hormone concentration on ovulation, conception, and early pregnancy loss in polycystic ovary syndrome. BMJ. 1988;**297**:1024-1026

[26] Van der Spuy ZM, Dyer SJ. The pathogenesis of infertility and early pregnancy loss in polycystic ovary syndrome in Arulkumaran S (editor). Clinics in Obstetrics and Gynaecology. 2004;**18**(5):755-771

[27] Dunaif A. Current concepts in the polycystic ovary syndrome. Revista Médica. 2001; **52**:401-419

[28] Dunaif A, Segal KR, et al. Profound peripheral insulin resistance, independent of obesity, in polycystic ovary syndrome. Diabetes. 1989;**38**:1165-1174

[29] Dunaif A. Insulin resistance and polycystic ovary syndrome: Mechanisms and implications for pathogenesis. Endocrine Reviews. 1997;**18**:774-800

[30] Romero G, Garmy JC, Veldhuis JD. The involvement of inositol phosphoglycan mediators in the modulation of steroidogenesis by insulin and insulin – Like growth factor-1. Endocrinology. 1993;**132**:1561-1568

[31] Poretsky L et al. Phosphatidyl-inositol-3 kinase-independent insulin action pathway (s) in the human ovary. Journal of Clinical Endocrinology and Metabolism. 2001;**86**:3115-3119

[32] Nestler JE, Jakubovicz DJ. Lean women with polycystic ovary syndrome respond to insulin reduction with decrease in ovarian p450c17 alpha activity and serum androgens. Clinics in Endocrinology and Metabolism. 1997;**82**:4075-4079

[33] Poretsky L et al. The insulin-related ovarian regulatory system in health and disease. Endocrine Reviews 1999;**20**:535-582

[34] Bloomgarden ZT. American Association of Clinical Endocrinologists (AACE) consensus conference on the insulin resistance syndrome. Diabetes Care. 2003;**26**:1297-1303

[35] Sam S, Dunaif A. Polycystic ovary syndrome: Syndrome XX? Trends in Endocrinology and Metabolism. 2003;**14**:365-370

[36] Skilton MR, Moulin P, et al. A comparison of the NCEP-ATPIII, IDF and AHA/NHLBI metabolic syndrome definitions with relation to early carotid atherosclerosis in subjects with hypercholesterolemia or at risk of CVD: Evidence for sex-specific differences. Atherosclerosis. 2007;**190**(2):416-422

[37] Adams J, Franks S, Polson DW, et al. Multifollicular ovaries: Clinical and endocrine features and response to pulsatile gonadotropin releasing hormone. Lancet. 1985;**2**:1375-1379

[38] Adams J, Polson DW, Franks S. Prevalence of polycystic ovaries in women with anovulation and idiopathic hirsutism. British Medical Journal. 1986;**293**:355-359

[39] Balen AH, Laven JSE, Tan SL, Dewailly D. Ultrasound assessment of the polycystic ovary: International consensus definition. Human Reproduction Update. 2003;**9**:505-514

[40] Koivunen R, Laatikainen T, Tomas C, et al. The prevalence of polycystic ovaries in healthy women. Acta Obstetricia et Gynecologica Scandinavica. 1999;**78**:137-141

[41] Dewailly D, Ardaens Y, Robert Y. Ultrasound for the evaluation of PCOS. In: Azziz R, Nestler J, Dewailly D, editors. Androgen Excess Disorder in Women. Philadelphia: Lippincott-Raven Publishers; 1997. pp. 269-278

[42] Aleem FA, Predanic M. Transvaginal color Doppler determination of the ovarian and uterine blood flow characteristics in polycystic ovary disease. Fertility and Sterility. 1996;**65**:510-516

[43] Carmina E, Longo A, Lobo RA. Does ovarian blood flow distinguish between ovulatory and anovulatory patient with polycystic ovary syndrome? The European Journal of Obstetrics and Gynecology. 2003;**189**:1283-1286

[44] Agrawal R, Sladkevicius P, Engmann L, et al. Serum vascular endothelial growth factor concentration and ovarian stromal blood flow are increased in women with polycystic ovaries. Human Reproduction. 1998;**13**:651-655

[45] Vessey MP, Painter R. Endometrial and ovarian cancer and oral contraceptives-findings in a large cohort study. British Journal of Cancer. 1995;**71**:1340-1342

[46] Homburg R. Polycystic ovary syndrome-from gynecological curiosity to multisystem endocrinopathy. Human Reproduction. 1996;**11**:29-39

[47] Dalghren E, Landin K, et al. Effect of two antiandrogen treatment on hirsutism and insulin sensitivity in women with polycystic ovary syndrome. Human Reproduction. 1998;**13**:2706-2711

[48] Morin-Papunen LC, Vauhkonen I, et al. Endocrine and effects of metformin versus ethinylestradiol-cyproterone acetate in obese women with polycystic ovary syndrome. A randomized study. The Journal of Clinical Endocrinology and Metabolism. 2000; **85**:3161-3168

[49] Diamanti-Kandarakis E. A modern medical quandary: Polycystic ovary syndrome, insulin resistance, and oral contraceptive pills. The Journal of Clinical Endocrinology and Metabolism. 2003;**88**:1927-1932

[50] Moghetti P, Castello R, et al. Metformin effects on clinical features, endocrine and metabolic profiles, and insulin sensitivity in polycystic ovary syndrome: A randomized, double-blind, placebo-controlled 6-month trial, followed by open, long term clinical evaluation. The Journal of Clinical Endocrinology and Metabolism. 2000;**85**:139-146

[51] Lord JM, Flight IHK, Norman RJ. Insulin-sensitising drugs (metformin, troglitazone, rosiglitazone, pioglitazone, D-chiro-inositol) for polycystic ovary syndrome (Cochrane Review). Cochrane Database of Systematic Reviews. 2003;(3):CD003053

[52] Dahlgren E, Friberg LG, et al. Endometrial carcinoma: ovarian dysfunction-a risk factor for young women. European Journal of Obstetrics & Gynecology and Reproductive Biology. 1991;**41**:143-150

[53] Royal College of Obstetricians and Gynaecologists. Long-term Consequences of Polycystic Ovary Syndrome. Guideline No 33. London: RCOG; 2003